Street Children and Homeless Youth

Lewis Aptekar • Daniel Stoecklin

Street Children and Homeless Youth

A Cross-Cultural Perspective

Springer

Lewis Aptekar
San Jose State University
One Washington Square
San Jose, CA, USA

Daniel Stoecklin
University Institute Kurt Bösch (IUKB)
Sion, Switzerland

ISBN 978-94-017-7901-2 ISBN 978-94-007-7356-1 (eBook)
DOI 10.1007/978-94-007-7356-1
Springer Dordrecht Heidelberg New York London

Printed on acid-free paper

Springer is part of Springer Science+Business Media (www.springer.com)

Contents

Chapter 1
Introduction: A New Vision of Street Children and Homeless and Runaway Youth

We approach this work in five parts. The first chapter orients our readers to street children who live in the developing world, and homeless youth who are from the developed world who, when we refer to both, we call children in street situations (CSS).

We use this expression because we want to show the problem is not just with the children, it is also with the situations they face. The child "in a street situation" is a social actor, actively adapting his/her behaviour to the social context, by making use of what we call instrumental resources (activities, time, space) as well as symbolic ones (norms and values, relations, image of self, motivation, gender).

In Chapter 2 we discuss the homes children in street situations leave and why and how they cope once on the street. We talk about their families of origin and the careers they develop from leaving home to being fully engaged in street life, and we discuss what happens to them when they get older. We look at their mental health and examine comparative studies to see how they fare in comparisons with other poor and abused youth. By way of example, we offer a full view of two types of street children found in Latin America, *gamines* and *chupagruesos.*

We discuss the problems associated with their published demographics, particularly the numbers of children in street situations. These figures can be dubious because of mixing different categories of children: "children of the street", "children on the street", "homeless children", "abandoned children", "children in conflict with the law", "children in especially difficult circumstances", "exploitive child labour" and other categories that might be in included or excluded from the counting of children in street situations. Also, the numbers can be exaggerated to increase the feeling of insecurity and justify "cleaning-up the streets"; or underestimated to preserve the image of a humane country.

We ask why only a very small percentage of poor children go to live on the street. We also ask why the majority of abused children do not go to the streets. While we cannot offer a clear answer to these questions, we put forth evidence that suggests poverty is a necessary, but not sufficient, condition for street children and abuse is a necessary, but not sufficient, condition for homeless youth. We show the

L. Aptekar and D. Stoecklin, *Street Children and Homeless Youth: A Cross-Cultural Perspective*, DOI 10.1007/978-94-007-7356-1_1,

importance of gender differences in the explanation for the origins of street children and homeless youth.

In Chapter 3 we talk about the social lives of children in street situations, both within their important peer groups and in their interactions with their societies. Within their groups, we stress the importance of peer relations and gender differences and we talk about sexual abuse and drug use with reference to group function. We define their groups as a particular urban sub-culture and show how they are unlike gangs.

We also use cultural and historical information to see how different epochs and cultures define and interact with children in street situations. We found that social reactions fluctuate between violence, indifference and assistance. Ambivalent reactions are common. On the one hand, the civil politic pities "street child" and "homeless youth" as being deprived of family and childhood. But on the other hand, they fear their alleged delinquency. But these children and youth are not only victims or objects of pity; they are also actors trying to surmount their difficulties by creating a world that helps them survive.

We look at the construction of public opinion and show that in far too many places reactions have become so violent that the children are victims of murder and mayhem. One example is the 1993 murder in Rio de Janeiro where children were killed in front of the La Candelaria Church by death squads hired to "clean up the streets". (It is not especially surprising that the people the children fear most are the police.) We put forward a child-centred approach, emphasising the quality of the interactions between these children and the people that surround them.

What are the reasons for their violent and repressive reactions to street children and homeless youth, who are labelled a huge public nuisance yet mostly commit petty crimes? Is this because it is far easier (and cheaper) than addressing the larger economic and social problems such as poverty and abuse, or because the problem is intrinsic to definitions of target-groups by power brokers, or because the image of uncontrolled children in the street produces too much fear or guilt?

In the fourth chapter we turn our attention to research. We look into the unique problems of doing research with this group, including problems of validity, and we make suggestions on which methods to avoid and which to use in collecting data.

We talk about how the problems of definition have led to difficulties in determining the target population. We discuss the problems of sampling and show how random sampling can be used.

We show that the research paradigm can include children's rights, including a look into Participatory Action Research (PAR). We lament the lack of longitudinal studies and go over some of the common ethical considerations.

In Chapter 5 we discuss programs and policies. We demonstrate that the child is not just a "target" of intervention, but a participant: a social actor, a subject of rights. In the contexts where this approach has been developed, the intervention strategies tend to include the children themselves in the definition of the programme, from objective identification to intervention modalities.

Implementation of the UN Convention on the Rights of the Child (UNCRC) and control mechanisms should progressively help overcome the institutional limits mostly bound to the classical top-down approach. We found that the UNCRC is a key international instrument that bestows important yet difficult to administer human rights for children.

We also examine a variety of programs that serve these children, pointing out why we think some are better than others. We discuss the differences between the needs–based and human rights programs. We also discuss different programmatic models and show how a human rights approach can be used by classifying different levels of interventions. We critique several examples, offering suggestions including how to implement preventive approaches.

Finally, in the concluding chapter we tie together our point of view and offer recommendations about programs, policies and research. We show that funding must be oriented not just towards direct aid to the children but to the more systematic problems of poverty and abuse, particularly for prevention. To do this, we devise a public mental health model for children in street situations that combines primary, secondary and tertiary care.

There are hardships of working with children in street situations. We offer solace and methods for preventing burnout. This includes making a judgment about differences in child rearing that respects culture and individuality, but does not take away children's human rights. We also suggest giving a role to children in street situations so they can participate in the programs that serve them and the research that is done on them.

The book comes from our diverse and long experiences. A bit more than 25 years ago, Aptekar (1988) was on the streets with street children in Cali, Colombia. Since then his work has taken him to 4 continents and some 30 countries. Along the way, he has conducted ethnographic research with several groups of urban youth who are, as UNICEF says, "children of particularly difficult circumstances". These include children with psychosocial reactions to disasters (Aptekar 1994; Aptekar and Boore 1990), children traumatized by war (Aptekar and Abebe 2004; Aptekar and Giel 2002) and disabled children living in low income countries (Aptekar 1988). While hopefully there is more to come, Aptekar offers to readers of this book what he has learned about street children and homeless youth, programs, policies and research from a perspective of time and culture.

Stoecklin's (2000a) research on street children in China looked into the "out-of-plan" children, so-called "black babies". He asked if they would eventually end up marginalised in the streets and if, on the other hand, children living in the street are likely to labeled with the "out-of-plan" status. This appeared to be true for the majority of small children, mostly girls, who were begging in the streets of Shanghai.

Bringing to bear his sociological training, he explains that when specific social problems (poverty, abuse) are defined by special groups (children in street situations), there is a good chance that the definition will be tainted with some self-interest by the definers. He found that causes associated with poverty and leading to street life include family break-up and domestic violence, but also poor knowledge of one's rights, and a lack of access to the public space (inadequate political representation). Having no voice, slum children are mostly only taken into account once they have become street children, a public and visible issue, depicted as a public nuisance. This is how these children in special need are labelled children "in conflict with the law" (Stoecklin 2007).

His research confirms some important dimensions of street life: the time spent on the street, the child's age, the child's use of space (city center or periphery), and the child's social networks, norms and values, activities, image of self, motivation, and opportunities according to gender. From here, Stoecklin (2000b) developed six different individual profiles of children in street situations. Finally, he introduces a new method favoring the respect of the child's right to be heard (art. 12 UNCRC), that may inspire work with children in street situations (Stoecklin 2013).

References

Aptekar, L. (1988). *Street children of Cali*. Durham: Duke University Press.

Aptekar, L. (1994). *Environmental disasters in global perspective*. New York: G. K. Hall/Macmillan.

Aptekar, L., & Abebe, B. (1997). Conflict in the neighborhood: Street children and the public space. *Childhood, 4*(4), 477–490.

Aptekar, L., & Abebe, B. (2004). In the mouth of the lion: working with the displaced in Addis Ababa. In A. Pankhurst & F. Piguet (Eds.), *Proceedings of the workshop held by the Ethiopian society of Sociologists, Social Workers and Anthropologists and the United Nations Emergency Unit for Ethiopia* (pp. 338–370). Addis Ababa: Addis Ababa University Press.

Aptekar, L., & Boore, J. (1990, Summer). The emotional effects of disaster on children. *International Journal of Mental Health, 19*(2), 77–90.

Aptekar, L., & Giel, R. (2002). Walks in Kaliti: life in a destitute shelter for the displaced. In Joop de Jong (Ed.), *Trauma, war, and violence: Public mental health in socio-cultural context* (pp. 337–366). New York: Kluwer Academic/Plenum Publishers.

Stoecklin, D. (2000a). *Enfants des rues en Chine*. Paris: Karthala.

Stoecklin, D. (2000b). *A baseline survey of the street children of Chittagong City in Bangladesh*. Dhaka: Aparajeyo-Bangladesh.

Stoecklin, D. (2007). Children in street situations: A rights-based approach. In I. Rizzini, U. M. Butler, & D. Stoecklin (Eds.), *Life on the streets. Children and adolescents on the streets: Inevitable trajectories?* (pp. 77–97). Sion: Institut International des Droits de l'enfant.

Stoecklin, D. (2013, November). Theories of action in the field of child participation. In search of explicit frameworks. *Childhood*. Issue 4, pp. 443–457.

Chapter 2
Children in Street Situations: Street Children and Homeless Youth

The Value of Cross-Cultural Comparisons

Regardless of wealth, political ideology, government decree or religious affiliation, there is no place in the globe that has succeeded in eliminating homelessness. This is extraordinary when you consider that homelessness, particularly among children, is distinguished as a grave ethical failure. Among international instruments to protect homeless children, provide them with adequate services and let them participate in the solutions to street life or homelessness, the United Nations Convention on the Rights of the Child (UNCRC) is of primary importance. It is the most widespread international instrument, as it has been ratified by literally all of the States in the world with the notable exceptions of the USA, Somalia and South Sudan.

Yet non-domiciled children and youth still live in full public view without permission, even in the wealthiest nations in Europe, North America and Scandinavia. They are at once terrifying to the civil politic and, deprived of any capacity to join society, while at the same time considered too potentially hazardous to leave unattended. There are countless stories about non-domiciled youth belonging to delinquent gangs are involved in organized crime, pawns of drug cartels and war lords, and abducted into sexual slavery.

The persistence efforts to curb homelessness over time and place, have been immense but with very little result. This indicates that there are several things about these efforts that we do not yet know. For example, why do only a fraction of abused children leave home, and why are only a small percentage of the poor on the streets? And why, in any given household, do only some siblings become homeless? We plan to provide as many answers as possible, which we will do in a unique way, by looking at studies of non-domiciled children in a variety of cultures.

Looking from the perspectives of cultural differences and similarities can lead to many areas of information. We can learn how the safety net which is almost always wider and stronger in the developed world than it is in the developing world, and more protective in strong policies (coherent) than strong governments (dictatorships)

L. Aptekar and D. Stoecklin, *Street Children and Homeless Youth: A Cross-Cultural Perspective*, DOI 10.1007/978-94-007-7356-1_2,

or laissez faire States (uncaring), has a bearing on those who finally make the choice to leave home as well as those who continue on the street.

The cross-cultural view can also explain the value a State gives to children's welfare. We know from cross-cultural comparisons that the issue is not only financial. Cuba for example, has little money but the State does not allow non-domiciled children and youth to be without care (Lutjens 2000). Culture can tell us if leaving home has the same meaning to potential homeless youths. For instance, an American youth who is being abused at home, knows that if he or she leaves, there is a state agency that provides housing and shelter, as well as food and medical care. In contrast, a child from the Democratic Republic of Congo knows that leaving could lead to starvation. The problem is not only scientific but political (de Benitez 2011), and often heartbreaking.[1]

The number of AIDS related orphans is not going up in developed countries where there are few parentless children so the community and the State can find homes for them. In communities where there are many AIDS related orphans, the traditional kinship system of fostering by relatives or care by the State can no longer support all of them. Being an AIDS orphan presents different outcomes depending on the financial and social context of one's culture.

In some countries, the State actively refuses to support children in street situations, even if they could find the resources. Take the example of displaced people of the civil war living in camps in Addis Ababa, Ethiopia (Aptekar 2010). Many of the children living in these camps are war orphans, but the State has actively avoided helping them because these children are looked upon by the State as prior or potential combatants. Most of these children have families, but become street children not because they have lost everything and everyone, but because of political reasons.[2]

We can learn by cultural comparison that in the developing world as many as 90% of street children are not stateless and are not parentless or homeless. They are working children, who begin work at an age when children from higher social classes are in school. At the end of the day, rather than showing their parents their school papers, they show them the money they earned. They are in essence supporting a family, but one that is too poor to send their children to public school (Fig. 2.1).

Most of these children work because there is not enough food at home. Among these children, some stop living at home and become street children. Some poor children come from abusive families, but more often they do not. Cross-cultural comparisons tell us it would be a mistake to assume that abuse is more likely in lower than in higher income families (Aptekar 1994, 2004).

---

[1] See Table 4.1 (page 122) for one list of estimated numbers of street children worldwide.

[2] Their parents worked for several generations in what was Ethiopia, but became Eritrea when the war ended. They were forced by the international humanitarian effort back into their country of citizenship (Ethiopia). The new Ethiopian government accused them of fighting for Eritrean independence. Thus, they found themselves living in camps in Ethiopia amongst the enemy whose citizenship they shared.

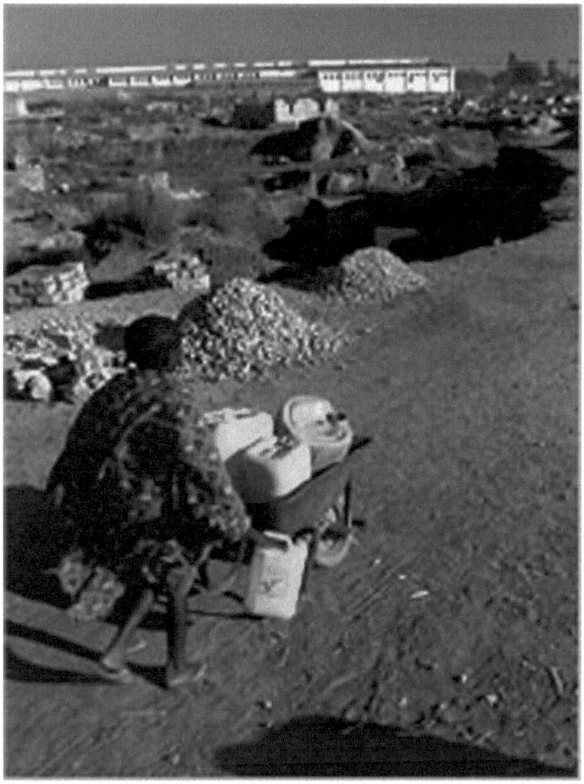

Fig. 2.1 Working child with wheel barrow

In the current epoch of global economic crisis, there is a wider separation between wealthy and poor leading to a reduction of social support networks for the poor. This had led to an increase in violence among gangs who occupy the vacuum left by the withdrawal of law enforcement and has resulted in a general trend of the State being more punitive toward its marginalized (Hagedorn 2006). Children who do not have a place to live are, across cultures, among the most marginalized. While gangs get stronger, children in street situations become further associated by the public and the press with violence. They receive more pejorative comments and more violent acts are committed against them.[3]

Finally, the cultural examination we bring to this work has taught that there are some children in street situations that seek the lure of street friendships and the freedom from a boring family life at home. In the cultural context, we must ask whether or not there are predisposing factors to homelessness.

[3]The strong identification of gang members with a cultural identity that replaces the loss of their former advantage, such as the "skin heads" of Great Britain, has led in some cases to more gangs becoming internationalized (the drug cartels, the sex trade).

Street Children

We use the term children in street situations to refer to homeless youth in the developed world **and** street children in the developing world. When we are talking about one and not the other we refer to their particular names.

Thus, when we are talking about street children we refer to children who live in the developing world and when we speak about homeless youth we assume they are living in the developed world. The term street child was first introduced by UNICEF following the UN International Year of the Child in 1979 (Veale et al. 2000). It was intended to deal with what UNICEF saw, mostly in Latin America at the time, but eventually throughout the developing world, as a newly emerging group of children working in the streets. Soon afterward, UNICEF (1986) and other international organizations claimed, without empirical evidence, that these "street children" were parentless and therefore in need of supervision and direction. Those working for international organizations also assumed street children came from the rural poor who had recently migrated to the capital, and could not cope with city life. To survive, they begged and stole and became drug "addicts".[4] The next assumption (again without empirical evidence) was that street children came from abused or neglectful homes and were therefore forced to survive on the streets.

After a time, UNICEF and other international organizations recognized that all of the children on the streets in the developing world who were working did not have the same family circumstances and hence developed new terms. Street children were "**of** the streets" meaning they did not go home at night. While working children who returned home at night to give what they earned to their families were called "children **on** the streets" (Fig. 2.2).

If you leave it up to the children to define street children, as Veale and Dona (2003) did in Rwanda, they would say that they are *mayibobo*, which refers to unaccompanied children working or living in the streets who do not have an adult to take care of them, no place to live, and who sleep where they want.

New situations are bringing children to the streets. Some are war orphans; others are stateless, because they are the children of illegal immigrants. Many of these children have simply disappeared from view, and therefore have lost access to their legal rights of protection. Having a child's identity officially acknowledged and registered is a fundamental human right, as stipulated by Article 7 of the Convention on the Rights of the Child. Registration enables a child to obtain a birth certificate, which is the most visible evidence of a government's legal recognition of the child as a member of society. A birth certificate is proof of the child's fundamental relationship with his or her parents and also determines nationality (UNICEF 2006).

Several additional factors appear central to increasing the risk of children becoming invisible: the lack or loss of formal identification; inadequate State protection

[4] Even today this is difficult to ascertain as non-empirical studies suggest that drug use among street children is between 20% and 90% (See Sherman and Plitt 2005).

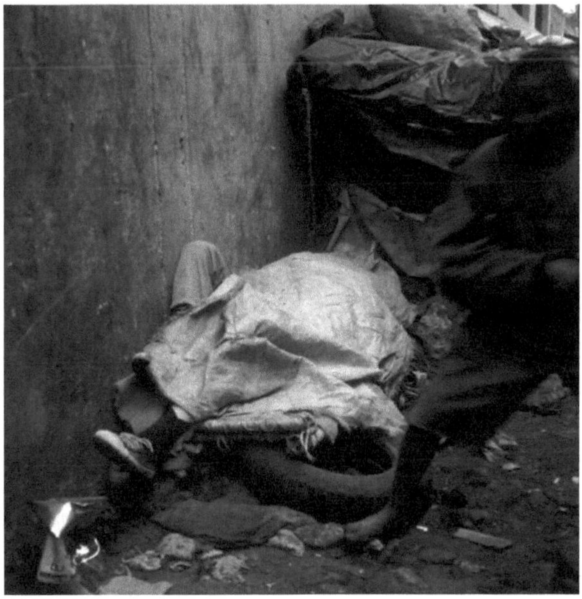

Fig. 2.2 Sleeping rough

for children without parental care; the exploitation of children through trafficking and forced labor; and premature entry of children into adult roles such as marriage, hazardous labor and combat. Children affected by these factors include those not registered at birth, refugees and displaced children, orphans, children in detention, children in early marriages, hazardous labor or combat, and trafficked and indentured children.

According to the latest UNICEF (2006) estimates, on average over 50% of births in the developing world (excluding China) each year go unregistered, a proportion that rises to 62% in sub-Saharan Africa. In South Asia, the share is higher still, at 70% of the total number of people displaced within their own countries by conflict or human rights violations, which amounts to roughly 25 million.

At the end of the millennium, there were an estimated 143 million orphans under the age of 18 in 93 developing countries. More than 16 million children were orphaned in 1 year alone. A major contributing factor to these alarming figures is the HIV/AIDS pandemic, without which the global number of orphans would be expected to decline.

Poverty is another factor underpinning early marriage. Marriage can be seen as a survival strategy for a girl – particularly if she marries an older and wealthier husband. In West Africa, for example, a UNICEF (2006) study showed a correlation between economic hardship and a rise in early marriage, even among some population groups that do not normally practice it.

A third of children between 5 and 17 years of age are engaged in child labor. Of these, nearly 70%, or 171 million children, were working in hazardous situations or conditions, such as in mines (Fig. 2.3), with chemicals and pesticides in agriculture

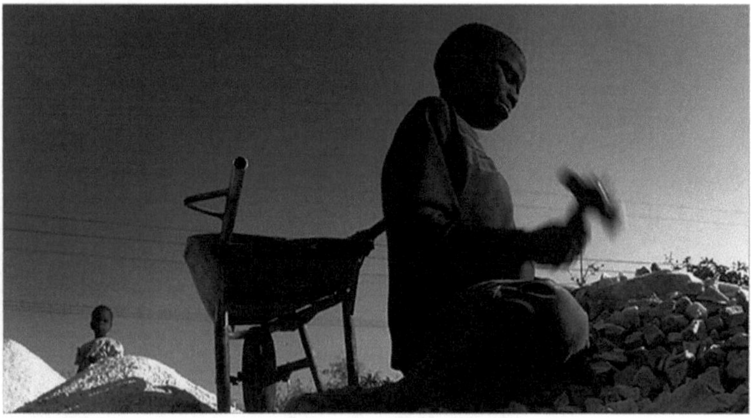

Fig. 2.3 Working child breaking up rocks with hammer

or with dangerous machinery. Some 73 million of them are less than 10 years old (UNICEF 2006).[5]

In Haiti, for example, 15-year-old domestic workers were found to be on average 4 cm shorter and 40 lb lighter than 15-year-olds not in domestic service in the same area (Giannini 2011). Rapid assessment research in El Salvador found that 66% of girls in domestic service reported having been physically (many of them sexually) or psychologically abused, and that the threat of sexual advances from employers was ever present (UNICEF 2006).

Because of AIDS related deaths, over 75 million children lost one parent, and 25 million have become "double" orphans (UNAIDS 2002). What percentage of them become street children?

In Turkey, the term street children refers to both those working and/or living in the streets (Ataov and Haider 2006). Children working on the street can be classified into two groups. The first group of children works on the street during the day, sometimes during the evening and night, but they go home to stay with their families. The second group of children, coming mainly from disintegrated families, work and live in the streets. The majority of children working in the streets in Turkey belong to the first group and are involved in selling small items, for example: napkins, chewing gum, water, nuts, ballpoint pens and others. The children in the second group, working and living in the streets, are involved in scavenging recyclable litter from containers in the streets and garbage dumps and then selling these things.

The origin of the street children phenomenon in Turkey is linked to wider issues. Internal migration and poverty alone cannot explain the street children phenomenon. Internal migration has an impact on the structure and function of families in many ways, but family problems are another contributing reason. Besides migration

[5] All numbers without clear empirical evidence should be suspect. They either come from NGOs or International Organizations who might use them to fight for a piece of the pie, or academics who might try to increase numbers to make their work seem more important.

and poverty, there are multiple causes behind the emergence of street children. Poor and dysfunctional families with problems such as alcoholism, physical or sexual child abuse or child neglect force children to leave home to live and/or to work in the streets.

Homeless Youth

There are two types of homeless youth; one is youth who are part of homeless families, which according to the U.S. Bureau of the Census (1999) are some 630,000 homeless between 6 and 16 years of age who live with their homeless families. The problem is considerable. Homeless families with children comprise 38% of the homeless population in the U.S. and homeless youth is the largest group of the homeless population (Menke 2000). Due to topic, time, and space limitations, we cannot deal with that group here. Instead we focus on those homeless youth who are living in the developed world without adults.

Homeless youth living without families are defined by the US Stewart and McKinney Homeless Assistance Act of 1987 as lacking a regular adequate nighttime residence, or as living in a shelter, institutional facility or a place not ordinarily used for sleeping such as on the floor in a friend's house (Smollar 1999; Stonge 2000). They have experienced at least one episode of a lack of housing for at least a week in the last month, and have no prospect of housing in the next month (Goering et al. 2002). There are between 1 and 1.5 million adolescents in the US who run away from home each year, which is about 2% of all American adolescents. In any given year, 3% of all families will have an adolescent who runs away and about an eighth of all Americans will run away at some point during their adolescent years (Shaffner 1999).[6]

The U.S. Department of Justice has four categories for non-domiciled youth. The greatest percent are (1) runaways (their choice, almost always has some push and pull factors). About 4% are forced out and are referred to as (2) throwaways, push-outs or castaways (National Runaway Switchboard 2001). There is even a smaller group of (3) lost, injured, or missing youth. There is also the (4) youth of illegal immigrants or who are illegal immigrants themselves, and who live on the streets because there is no housing for them.

In Canada, homeless youth are divided into "runners", who live on the street for a long period of time, and "in and outers", who use the streets intermittingly and only when necessary (Kufeldt and Nimmo 1987).[7]

Being homeless is against the law in most developed countries, as is running away from home in all states in the United States (US). In the U.S., running away is part of what is called a status offence, largely defined by the fact that the adolescents have

[6]The National Runaway Switchboard (2001) estimates a smaller number, about one million runaways each year.

[7]A study in Vancouver, Canada found that there were street gangs and "wannabe" groups, the latter much like the homeless youth of our discussion (Gordon 2004).

not yet reached the age of majority, which is somewhere between 16 and 21 years of age depending on the individual state statute. In addition to running away, status offenses include such acts as being out late at night, drinking alcohol, having sex, and being truant from school. Status offenders are picked up by state authorities and generally placed in a foster home or a state institution. Then they become foster youth, and not runaway youth, which means they will live under the direction of the government and will be taken out of the care of their families of origin (a response very unlikely in the developing world).

Homeless youth may be without shelter (sleeping on the streets, in parks, construction sites, rooftops, etc.) or in emergency shelters. They may also, as is the case of the "hidden homeless", be temporarily staying with another family, with friends, or with occasional acquaintances (Gaetz 2004a).

Comparisons Between Homeless Youth and Street Children

In the developing world, poverty is a necessary but not sufficient condition for a child to become a street child. Nearly 100% of street children come from poor families. In the developed world, poverty is neither a sufficient nor a necessary condition of homelessness.

While we say there are no street children in the developed world, it might be worthwhile to use our terms to explain what we do see on the streets in the developed world. In the developed world there are few poor runaways, at least according to Aptekar's observations of urban youth in downtown Portland, Oregon. The teenagers he saw were older and they come from the middle class rather than from the poverty found among street children in the developing world. The adolescent runaways in Portland hang out on the lawn of the main square in the city, dressing down in dirty clothes that are a far cry from the rags on street children in the developing world. They are not barefoot; in fact they are often shod in proper mountain gear. They seem to have plenty of cigarettes, and most have at least one electronic device. Street children in the developing world don't have the money to smoke many cigarettes, their hair is more likely to be shaved to avoid lice than be worn long and stylishly multicolored, and any electronic device would soon be fenced for something closer to the basics of existence.

Furthermore half the runaways in Portland are female, several times the 10–20% figure found among street children in developing world. This example, among many others, shows that homeless youth and street children have to face different realities, although the causes of their different situations might to some extent be similar. The main reason for the runaways to be on the street often has to do with parental abuse, and in many cases parents rejecting the homosexual orientation of their children.

As much as for any middle class adolescent, the appearance of the runaways is a carefully orchestrated dress, which is designed to anger or embarrass their parents, in short to get back at them for being rejected in the first place. This is what makes them so different from the children of homeless parents who either live under a bridge or in a homeless center.

There are homeless youth who come from middle class families and many poor youth who do not runaway (Goering et al. 2002). Shaffner (1999) reports that as few as 10% of homeless youth in the US come from families on public assistance or families having unemployment problems. Up to one half of all families with runaway youth are from the middle or upper classes. Given the current economy in the developed world alone, these figures might no longer be valid, (but the point is not to assume that poor families have more psychopathology or are more abusive than middle or upper class families).[8]

According to another study of American runaway youth, "*most youth come from difficult backgrounds, those difficulties* ***cannot*** *(emphasis by authors) be assumed to include poverty or economic disadvantage*" (Cauce et al. 2000: 234).

Children in the U.S. living in a single parent female headed household are 50% more likely to be living in poverty (Menke 2000). Yet about two thirds of homeless youth in the U.S. are living in female headed families, about half of which have unmarried men in them (Hyde 2005). What the research suggests in the developing world is that leaving home is more related to poverty than abuse, whereas abuse/neglect is the major reason youth leave home in the developed world. This difference, as we will see, has significant implications for mental health for the two groups, particularly when gender is considered later in this chapter (Scheper-Hughes and Hoffman 1998; Aptekar and Ciano 1999).

Another way to distinguish homeless youth from street children is to apply an analytical reconstruction of experience from the Weberian perspective of the fictive "ideal-type". This can be accomplished by looking at how each child experiences the street. From this we can obtain a composite by accentuating one or several of his or her "points of view". This ideal-type (Weber 1922, 1968) reconstruction of experience enables us to identify typical ways of experiencing the street or typical street situations. When we do this, we show that while homeless youth and street children are both in street situations, these situations are not necessarily experienced in the same way. The incorporation of the actors' subjective sense of reality explains why the distinctions between homeless youth and street children cannot always be clear, and why, as a consequence, the term "children in street situations" is more inclusive as it allows them to participate in the definition of these situations.

Children in Street Situations

When the two groups, homeless youth and street children, share common characteristics, we will refer to them in the aggregate as children in street situations. The most obvious commonality is that both groups share the fact of the street being a significant part of their physical and psychosocial environment (Stoecklin 2008).

---

[8] At the turn of the 21st century, approximately 13 to 14 million children in the US were growing up in families below the poverty line. This is about one in five children under the age of 18 (U.S. Bureau of the Census 1999).

Personality and environment interact in such a way that what should be the focus of analysis is the relationship between a specific child and the street environment. Lucchini (1993) uses the perspective of the street career to highlight the progressive attachment to the street environment. This point of view casts light on the interactions which each child in the streets has with other social actors and gives importance to the children's subjective reconstruction of experience.[9]

In the same work, Lucchini (1993) makes a distinction between two types of competencies found with children in street situations, namely instrumental and symbolic competencies. Instrumental competencies are visible abilities: concrete know-how and performances. Children in street situations display such capacities in their multiple activities in generating income (from legitimate work to stealing and begging).

Symbolic capacities are invisible. They include long-term survival strategies which include inventive relationships in the street, the capacity for association and solidarity with friends, and a critical mind that evaluates the environment and creates opportunities by influencing the reactions of others. Symbolic capacities might be the reason why many studies show that street children are resilient, because they can be seen to have the ability to overcome adverse circumstances. For example, in most cases, children in street situations acquire autonomy not because they have been encouraged to do so, but because they find themselves in circumstances where only inventive ways of behaving can enable them to escape from abuse or poverty.

While resilience is linked to the children's symbolic capacities and to external resources in the environment (Rapin 2001; Cyrulnik 2002), there is a general tendency for the public to focus on the instrumental capacities, ignoring the competencies of children in street situations. This blindness is due to the fact that people only consider visible abilities, especially if they are shocking and deviant, and not the symbolic skills the child is using to cope. If these symbolic skills are exerted in deviant activities, it may well be because spaces to display them in socially acceptable ones are simply lacking.

Street situations are also evolving through the interplay between the individual's appraisal of him or herself in specific contexts, which helps to understand the different ways of experiencing street life. The essential stereotype of the "street child" should therefore be replaced in consideration of the several types of relationships to the street world that any child, as a social actor, may experience at some stage. This way we can get a picture of major profiles, derived from case histories, regarding the actor's choices and strategies related to personal and social dimensions.

For instance, Stoecklin (2000b) working in Bangladesh provides a six part description of street children's personality clusters; the hero, the hard worker, the ambivalent, the survivor, the isolated and the dependent abused. Each profile has specific characteristics, described mainly in key-words:

1. The "*Hero*": altruistic; virtuous; great sense of justice; good self-image; fights to defend others. These children see themselves as heroes because they have

[9] Another expression, children "*out of place*", is conveying the same idea: "*The emphasis should shift away from attempts to define street children towards analysis of their relationship with street environments*" (Ennew and Connolly 1996: 131).

acquired the ability to defend themselves, to develop work skills and to work in coordinated ways to save money, help others and develop solidarity despite adverse conditions in the street and a personal history of family violence.

2. The "*Hardworker*": strong willpower; important sense of solidarity; negotiation skills; under high pressure from adult competitors working in the same trade. These children see themselves as honest and loyal contributors to family income and would just like to live a normal life as street workers. They have a mixed image of themselves: as good and honest boys, but helpless, deprived and stigmatized as "*Tokai*" (street children). They tend to count on their own capacities to be recognized and want to achieve a position through their own efforts.
3. The "*Ambivalent*": neither positive nor negative image of self; often hides the truth and changes presentation of self; cannot make sense of the double-sided experience of street life; quite contrasted motivations. These children could as well become heroes, strong and proud, or isolated, abused and depressed. They have less control over things and depend almost completely on circumstances and external push and pull factors. They search for an identity. Deception and abuse have rendered them especially cautious when presenting themselves to unknown people.
4. The "*Survivor*": lost at least one parent; not happy to be on the street; marginal integration in peer group; working/earning on their own. These children feel sad and ambivalent, not satisfied with current activities imposed by fate or by violent relatives. The necessity to survive on a daily basis and a weak group integration prevent them from acquiring more elaborate social competencies; weak negotiation skills.
5. The "*Isolated*": absolutely no group insertion; usually newcomers with no or quite weak work skills; abandoned by parents or tortured and exploited by in-laws or elder siblings; usually fear and hide from officials (police); experience a very high degree of suffering. These isolated children are highly abused and assaulted by organized crime, the police and the general public. They feel apart from society; socially non-existent, rejected, neglected, a "nobody". They also want to become worthy citizens and respected workers (garment factory, teacher), but for now they see themselves as victims of society.

There are different types of abandonment; by family, community, State, and by any combination of these. There can be abandonment of one's self by losing hope (Veale et al. 2000). For example, in one study Montgomery (2000) shows how the State abandons the child prostitutes in Thailand. They are given no State support, but the children are not completely abandoned because they have good relationships with their families. Their parents do not see that allowing their children to be prostitutes is bad for their children or they see it as the only way to make enough money to survive. The importance of family looking after each other is the stronger value.

The children tell themselves, as part of their Buddhist tradition, that they were making "merit" for their parents, which will work toward negating any bad effects of prostitution in the next life.

But because the State does not provide any other means for them to earn an income, they could be considered abandoned by the State. Neither the State nor the free market offers them an alternative. This is getting to be more and more of a problem as the structural adjustments of the International Monetary Fund and other financial organization insist on austerity, which in effect takes away whatever safety net there might have been to help these children.

6. The "*Dependent Abused*": abused by relatives, including sexually; trauma and feeling of guilt/helplessness; highly dependent. The death of their biological fathers and poverty push these children to the street in order to survive and create a greater dependence towards their mothers. Street life is seen as absolutely negative, violent and destructive, while defence skills are limited. Cautiousness and fear, and absence of group insertion and protection prevent these children from acquiring work skills and the capacity for negotiation.

Thus, considering situations typical of street life instead of a stereotyped street "child" means that the term "street children" refers to members of a population described by reference to street situations, rather than by appealing to common characteristics of a collective group of youngsters (Cosgrove 1990). It is the "street" that is common to a diversity of children. The same applies to homeless youth. This raises a question: what amount of time spent in the street is required to be considered a "street child" or a "homeless youth"?

UNICEF uses a classification based on the contact between a child and its family. However, "contact with the family" is not as clear as it might appear. Does it mean the frequency or the quality of the contact? A child may have numerous contacts but of poor quality, and these contacts with the family may even be negative or abusive. If the regularity of the "contact with the family" is a criterion to define a normal childhood, children who spend more time on the streets would be seen as deviant simply on the basis of definition. This ignores the subjective meaning the child attaches to the quality of the contact with the family. Meanwhile, it is this subjective attachment, linked to affective and material expectations, which is more important for the protection and autonomy of the child. The family responses that are given to the child are subjectively perceived by the child who may consider, at some point, that the street offers better responses to his needs.

Many children in street situations suffer from a lack of affective and material response, but their identification to the family or to another group, for instance the peer-group in the street, will vary according to their own subjective evaluation of the situation. Poverty alone is therefore not the explanatory factor, even for street children (Fig. 2.4).

Children in street situations are not affected with the same intensity by similar events (poverty) or situations (homeless) because there are important differences between children, their environment and culture. This is why children with similar life conditions at home do not all take to the street. Otherwise many cities in the developing world would be literally invaded by children. From a psycho-sociological point of view, children in street situations represent a heterogeneous category (Lucchini 1993).

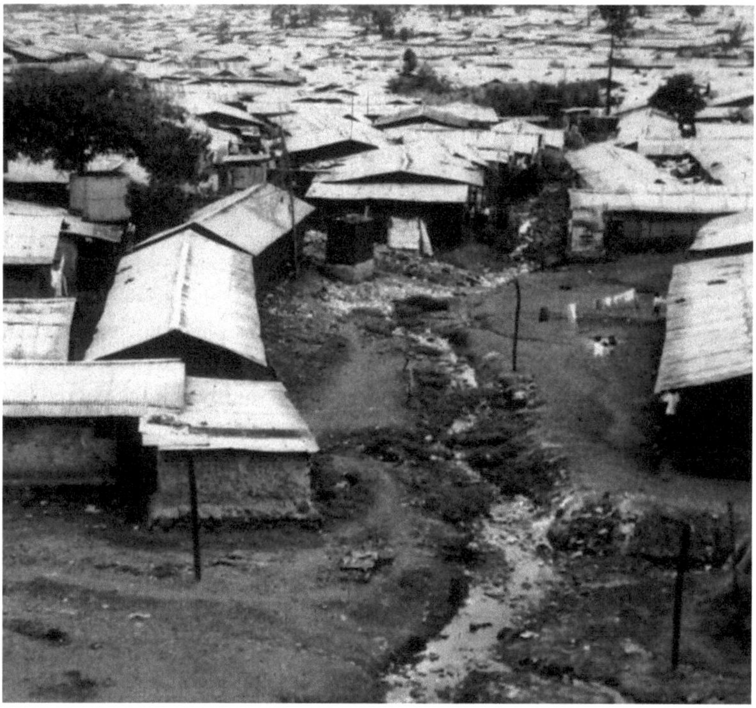

Fig. 2.4 Why do some go to the streets but not others?

Lucchini's (1993) perspective of the street career overcomes the static definition of street children or homeless youth. The choice to leave or stay home depends on numerous factors. These factors have not yet been isolated nor studied in a comparative and systematic way.

Yet, there are still many institutions (NGOs and government agencies) working with "children at risk" who make a distinction based on two criteria, the amount of time the child has spent on the street and the relations with parents or other responsible adults. "Children **on** the street" would be those who regularly return home and spend less time on the street, while "children **of** the street" would conversely stay mostly in the street and have few contacts with the family.

Lucchini (2007) criticizes the static notion of a single 'responsible adult' rather than dividing this responsibility among various people who do not necessarily live in the same place. At times, there is only a temporary responsible adult as when the child circulates from one domestic unit to another going back home daily without necessarily maintaining a relationship with a single adult. The on/off distinction of UNICEF (Taçon 1985) became widespread but according to Lucchini (2007) not operational, as between these two categories "children on the street" and "children of the street", made up of only two dimensions (spatial and social) there are a series of intermediary situations which raise important problems of a bifocal classification.

The majority of definitions given to 'street children' emphasize the amount of time spent on the street, but this criterion is insufficient to define who an individual street child really is, since instead of being either "on" or "of" the streets, the situation is gradual and evolving. Not only can children progressively become 'street children' (children of the street), but the reverse is also true: the child "of the street" may find new insertions in the community and gradually become a child "on the street". Then, one may ask: when does a child become or cease to be a street child? The criterion of duration of stay on the street is insufficient to answer this question.

Lucchini (2007) also identifies numerous other factors that influence the position of a specific child in the continuum between "on" or "of" the street. He groups them into five different categories: (a) Biological factors, such as age and gender: (b) factors directly linked to the family, such as family composition and organization, the strength of family ties, the economic situation of the family and the degree to which the family is rooted in the city (bringing up questions of migration); (c) factors directly connected to the street: the representation (the image) that the child has of the street, the contacts the child has had with persons who already have experience of the street, the presence of the child within a group or network of other children, the profitability of activities, police repression and violence among children; (d) factors connected to urban spaces: the significance of the distance which the child would have to cover from home to the street in which s/he practices her income generating activities, the speed of traveling between these two spaces, the nature of the urban space which the child has to cross to reach this place. This last issue has to do with the survival opportunities that the child encounters in moving within or towards the city centre; and (e) factors that we can term macroscopic, referring to the social, political and economic situation of the country.

These factors combine in multiple ways, and the different combinations influence the career of the child in a street situation. Some combinations may quicken or retard the street career. Other influences such as the child's insertion in the informal economy, shifting movements between the street, home and institutions, and the initiation rituals by peers to be accepted on the street or in the deviant underworld also come into play. This approach alters the simple divide between "children on the streets" and "children of the streets", and replaces it with a psycho-social and cultural complexity.

The model Lucchini (2007) proposes is called the Child-Street System (CSS) and captures the diversity of relationships that different children may have depending on several dimensions making up the child's subjective experience of street life (see Fig. 4.2. in Chapter 4). The children are considered social actors using symbolic elements (values, norms, motivations, images of self) when interacting with others. The CSS is useful to reflect how social interactions are performed and integrated, and the degree to which the dimensions are strong or weak. All of the dimensions are interdependent and therefore any change in one aspect affects the child's overall experience. This analytical tool has been used in interventions (see Stoecklin in chapter 4).

Other authors have also pointed out problems with the old nomenclature. There are, in essence, as Panter-Brick (2002) points out, four problems with the use of the term street child; it is too generic, obscuring differences (see also Raffaelli and

Larson 1999); it does not take into account the child's subjective life experience; it is judgmental; and it ignores the larger problem of poor working children. (See Moss et al. 2000 for information regarding the over individualized approach to solutions which leaves the social structural approach underutilized). In some cases, such as when a parent can no longer function as such due to illness, disease (HIV-AIDS), or injury (from war or work), it is the children, not the parents who are in charge of the household (Boyden 2003).

Invernizzi (2003) has worked on another not clearly defined boundary; that of children working on the street and **street** children working on the street. She begins by pointing out the many different ideas of childhood and the variety of experiences belonging to different childhoods. Her point is that what a child experiences as his or her childhood is bound up in gender, social class and ethnic tradition. Thus children become actors in their own drama of childhood. As they do so they become socialized. That implies, according to Invernizzi, an acceptance of certain standards and identities. This means that children learn what are the norms from which they can operate and what will happen to them if they do not take up the group's standards. But this is not all one way, the child also makes a mark on the groups' values, and the process, at least at times, can be contentious.

Invernizzi's work (2003) is based on an ethnographic description and interviews of girls and boys working on the streets of Lima, Peru. She defines the children's work as having a certain collection of social skills (like cooperating or competing) learned from a variety of sources including peers, parents, societal viewpoints, etc. While her data is based on children with parents and who are working but not living on the streets, the same framework could be used for street children. In fact the two groups, while separated in the extremes, are more likely to share similar working experiences. One example she uses is a girl who is selling sweets in the central market. At first she is looked after by her mother. Her mother tells her the hours she can work; how she will work, and how to negotiate with possible competitors. Invernizzi (2003) also looks at a group of boys shining shoes. The male shoe shiners do not have parents to organize their work, but they are under the direction of a non-related adult who is in charge of the area where the boys work. Both groups of young workers are being socialized through their respective work situations.

After talking about the work of children, she moves to the social context, pointing out that what is common among households of the urban poor is that women take over the role of men in income production. Men become angry and then, too often, there is domestic abuse. Also, it is not just the marriage roles that change, the children are also affected. It is in this context that she describes the neglected child. While the child does not have protection from a parent, he or she can find adults who will mentor them. Like the boys who are being supervised by a non-related adult, Invernizzi (2003) makes the point that the "neglected situation" is not necessarily abusive. She tells the story of a young man of poor circumstances who belongs to all of the categories that would define him as being at risk. He finds a mentor who helps him become a productive citizen. The examples she refers to show that children working in the street are quite diverse in circumstances and psychosocial functioning.

Fig. 2.5 Peer group support

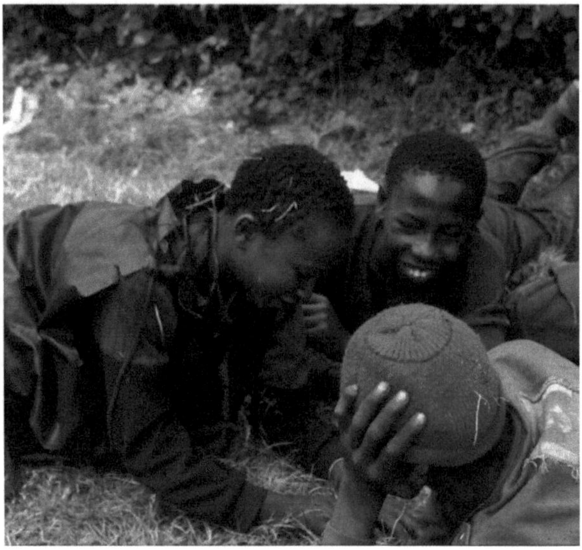

Yet, while there is diversity, there is also a pattern for all children working on the streets. This begins with being introduced to street work, the initial subsistence effort to learn the necessary skills, which is followed by enjoyment of the work and melding it into games and play. The child cements the new identity including looking for and obtaining, even from peers, recognition of their new skills, and finally as the child grows, he or she looks for ways out of street work into more substantial paying work that has a higher status and affords more opportunity (Invernizzi 2003).

What this research teaches us is that children's work is not just related to earning money, it also involves quite a bit of learning and becoming socialized, including the variety of personal skills that allow the children to get along with other people, to enjoy life with peers, and to grow into a responsible caring adult. It would be a mistake to only take the middle class view of child labor, that it is only exploitative as it takes time away from formal education.

At every stage and in all cultures, the relationship between peers becomes essential to consider. As much as any other factor that might determine their well being, their partnerships with each other are central. Those children in street situations who do not have friends fall by the wayside. Likewise, the children who can find meaning among peers will be able to find meaning in their lives (Fig. 2.5).

While the media suggest that the older children take advantage of the younger ones and the strong of the weak, in fact, as we show throughout the text, there are many factors that work against exploitation, such as the value of being young and appearing cute which leads to income and makes it unwise for the older ones to abuse them. The research that follows will show that the great majority cope and grow with each other.

Families of Children in Street Situations

The fictitious reality of a "normative family" is the middle class Western family that lives in a recognized, efficient, political State; with its children who are domiciled at home, are dependent on their parents for necessities, and who are nurtured at school and at home to succeed as adults.

Not all families that deviate from the norm produce children in street situations, but most of the children we are studying will be missing at least one of the factors that make up the normative family; that is, they will lack a parent or adult guardian who is nurturing, or a home to live in, or will not be living in a political State with benevolent enforceable laws for children.

While these new reasons for children in street situations are increasing worldwide, and while some are parentless, most do have parents. For those who are parentless, only some will be homeless for any significant period of time because most of them will be fostered, or will live in refugee camps. Among the stateless youth who are parentless and homeless, some are working and receiving an education and nurturing. None remain members of normative families.

Nor are all street children on the street solely because of psychological reasons. They are there because they are poor and being on the street is one way of coping with poverty or with conditions at home, and gaining access to other income generating sources.

Roma children, for example, are excluded from being street children, because as the UN definition of street children states, street children are not being adequately protected and supervised by a responsible adult (Thompson et al. 2002). The international norms make the distinction between the separated minor[10] and the unaccompanied minor[11]; both are separated from their parents, but the separated minor is nonetheless accompanied by another adult member of his or her family, whereas the unaccompanied minor is completely alone or simply accompanied by an adult who is not a parent (Stoecklin et al. 2013). Roma children are usually with their parents, and when they are not they are most of the time with another adult parent, and thus should be considered "separated children" rather than "unaccompanied children".

The Roma are among the most impoverished groups in Central and Eastern Europe. From 80% to 90% of the Roma in Bulgaria and Romania live below national poverty lines. Because of limited education, a low level of skills and discrimination in the

[10] Separated minors are "*children are under 18 years of age who are outside their country of origin and separated from both parents, or their previous legal/customary primary caregiver. Some children are totally alone while others may be living with extended family members*" (Separated Children in Europe Programme, http://www.savethechildren.net/separated_children/about_us/separated_children.html).

[11] According to General Comment Number 6 of the UN Committee on the Rights of the Child, "unaccompanied children" (also called unaccompanied minors) are children, as defined in article 1 of the Convention, who have been separated from both parents and other relatives and are not being cared for by an adult who, by law or custom, is responsible for doing so" (http://daccess-dds-ny.un.org/doc/UNDOC/GEN/G05/438/05/PDF/G0543805.pdf?OpenElement).

labour market, in some Roma settlements not a single person is regularly engaged in formal employment (UNICEF 2006). Yet there are no Roma street children. They meet the criteria for poverty and they meet the standard for being social outcasts viewed pejoratively by the public. But the Roma families are tightly knit (UNICEF 2006) which is why their children are not considered street children. The children of the Roma illustrate that while poverty is a necessary condition of being labeled as street children, it is not a sufficient condition.

Likewise, in Nepal, poor children are expected to migrate and work in the city streets and live on their own as if they were street children, but they are expected to return to their families, hopefully with something to show from their efforts. These children cannot be called street children because they are not homeless or parentless (Panter-Brick 2002).

In Latin America, as many as 80% or 90% of street children have home ties (Scanlon et al. 1998). In Colombia, nearly two-thirds of street children have ties with family (Felsman 1981). A similar percentage of homeless children on the streets in Istanbul give status to their families (Kidd et al. 2007).

After having been on the streets for more than 4 or 5 years, street children in the former Soviet Union retained close family ties (Naterer and Godina 2011). This study was from a non-random sample of 68 street children. The children were living in four groups, in four different geographic locations in the city of Makeevka. The authors interacted with the street children and took daily field notes, conducted interviews and applied an open ended questionnaire. They gathered information about children's lives, their family backgrounds, how they related to one another, and their future goals. Sixty eight children were interviewed. A more structured interview was used for demographic information. The authors, after having the children grow accustomed to them, used video equipment and kept a video record of the children's everyday lives. Before analyzing the data, it was triangulated by using at least three methods, mostly a combination of participant observation, visual notes and interviews.

Their findings suggest that the determination of street children status is not just related to time on the streets, it also has a very vital family and collegial (peer) component, and this can only be understood with reference to a particular culture.

Their results indicate that the majority of street children in Makeevka had two living parents, but that their parents did not have a lot of authority over them. Matchinda (1999), studying street children in Yaoundé, Cameroon, wanted to investigate the family situations that prompted street children to leave home. She weighed two main factors; poverty and family discord. Two hundred and ten street children were sampled from a population of 900 street children by using purposive sampling. The main tool for data collection was questionnaires. The results indicated a significant positive correlation between home-rearing patterns and children in the street. There was also a significant finding with the level of family income and children running away from home. The author concluded that in spite of the society wide economic crisis, poverty could not be considered as the major factor responsible for children abandoning the home for the street. What was the key variable in nearly two thirds of the sample was authoritarian parenting.[12]

Olly (2006) studied street children Ibadan, Nigeria. He collected qualitative data from Focus Group Discussions (FGD) and quantitative data from in-depth interviews (IDI) with 169 youths (89.3% male). The sample was obtained through a snowballing technique. The mean age of participants was 18.4 years. Contrary to the above study, in neighboring Cameroon the majority of his sample were on the street for financial reasons, not problems with parenting.

In many cases, these families were headed by women. The fathers were often unemployed, had alcohol or drug problems and even were imprisoned. In contrast to this, their peer relations were supportive. They exchanged information and provided help to one another.

The children worked on the streets by begging or by finding or buying waste material cheaply and selling it somewhere else for a profit. They parked cars and were guardians of goods in the market place. Like other street children from the former Soviet Union, they lived next to the heaters in the basements of large buildings.

They didn't save what they earned, most of it went to buying cigarettes and inhalants (their form of drug abuse), and playing computer games. Unlike other children who have been labeled street children, they did not give any of their income to their parents.

This might be because when they talked about why they left home, family violence and alcohol abuse were high on their list. The authors felt that they were able to cope by adjusting quickly to their new circumstances and because they came from urban backgrounds that favored quick acting skills. These children had developed their own urban culture, with each subgroup having its own physical space. In fact, the authors point out that they used space as an important part of their coping. They used the whole city, for begging and otherwise manipulating the concerns of the public for small children adrift from their families. They also begged and committed petty crimes such as stealing small items from stores or by skilled pick-pocketing. These items could then be fenced (sold illegally) for cash.

It is as if there is a huge sieve, labeled non-normative family, which brings in many children with a litany of major life stressors. But, by the time we get to the bottom of the sieve the numbers of children in street situations are few. So when looking across cultures for the reasons why there are children in street situations, it might be that the pertinent question is not why there are so many but why there are so few.

What we know is that in spite of the family circumstances of children in street situations, the image of an ideal family is rooted in their consciousness. Take for instance Brazilian street children who, according to Hecht (1998), never really break their maternal attachment. The children compare their lives to the moral life they believe their mothers would have liked for them to live had they stayed at home. Whatever the outcome, this suggests that they are certainly not parentless (Fig. 2.6).

[12] Matchinda (1999) recommended that interventions should focus on parenting skills, although means to supply basic needs could not be dismissed.

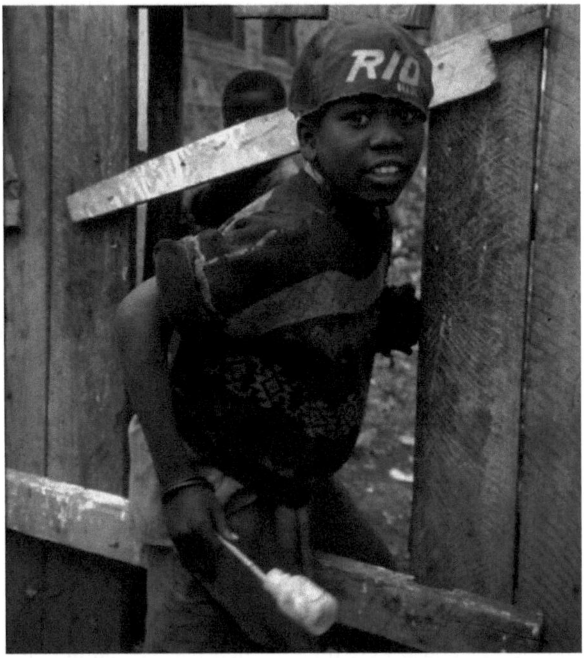

Fig. 2.6 A Brazilian street child

In Northeast Brazil, there is the well-to-do nurtured child who is protected and pampered and there is the child of the poor who is a nurturing child, called this because he earns something to help his family financially (Hecht 1998). Implying a psycho-dynamic perspective, Hecht (1998) shows that male street children define themselves in opposition to the acceptable social role of the nurturing child who helps his mother at home. Street children say they have no home, thus they have no mother; thus they help each other, rather than their mothers. When Indonesian street children were asked to draw their home, they often made reference to their mothers, as if she and home were the same (Beazley 2000).

Masondo (2006) found that South African orphans have come to believe in their deceased parents' ability to watch over them, suggesting that even though the parent may not be physically present, they experience a sense of security knowing that they are being protected by them. African life is permeated by the understanding that nothing happens without cause (Ozumba 2004). For example, most African societies hold that there is a causal link between misfortune, illness and death. What do African children in street situations believe are the roles of their parents in the case of their street lives?

Incarcerated street children in Caracas, Venezuela constantly thought about their mothers, feeling guilty about causing them pain (Marquez 1999). In fact the attraction of street children to their mothers was apparent even when these children were asked to leave home by their mothers so the other children in their family would have enough food. These children did not resent their mother's decision, they understood the need for it, and their mothers remained the central figure in their lives.

They felt proud and wanted their mothers to know that they were able to live on the streets and thus be independent, or better yet, earn enough to give something to their mothers.[13]

What Being Homeless Means to Children in Street Situations

The labels "homeless youth" and "street children" are, by the labels themselves, statements about home. Yet there is very little documented research on what being homeless means to children in street situations (Dufour 2000). Home obviously goes beyond the material aspect of having a roof and includes the value of social relationships, so it is closer to meaning the place where we can rely on others. This explains why some homeless youth would call "home" places that are seen as physically inadequate because of lack of "basic necessities", but which mostly because of peer support is "home" for them.

The low level of respect society places on homelessness can be seen in Beazley's (2000) work in Java where a person without a home is seen as a pariah, because there is no way to locate the homeless with respect to family, from which all definitions of personality stem. Castel (1994) uses the concept of disaffiliation to reflect the erosion of social ties of the individual with no work and no support, and thus no home.

Another way to seeing how the homeless view themselves is by using the French etiology of homelessness, "*itinérance*", which is associated with an itinerant life. In other words, more than being homeless *per se*, it is the peripatetic nature of being homeless that is how the homeless view their own lives. In the former Soviet Union street children are known throughout as *Bomzhi*, an acronym meaning, 'without a defined place of living' (Naterer and Godina 2011).

From time immemorial there has been an antagonistic relationship between the peripatetic and the sedentary (Berland 1982). Such terms as "precarious worker", "in need of public assistance", "detached", "mentally ill", "drug addict" which are used for children in street situations, correspond to sedentary points of view, but not the youth's subjective sense of being an itinerant. No matter how much they value and care about their families of origins, once they are on the street they will be judged by normative family values; to be sure the view will be pejorative and directed at them to include the "single mother" or the "deserting father", or the "evil step father". As de Queiroz (1996; p. 297) underlines, when a child in a street situation is shifting from one position to another, he or she has to make a subjective adaptation in order to keep a coherent self-image. This active reconstruction of a coherent self-image is a common feature with both street children and homeless youth.[14]

---

[13] There is always the danger that the children are telling the researcher what they think he or she wants to know. We talk much of this bias, called "*social desirability*", in Chapter 4.

[14] Bellot (2000) shows how much the public response to homeless youth misses the subjective reality of children in street situations.

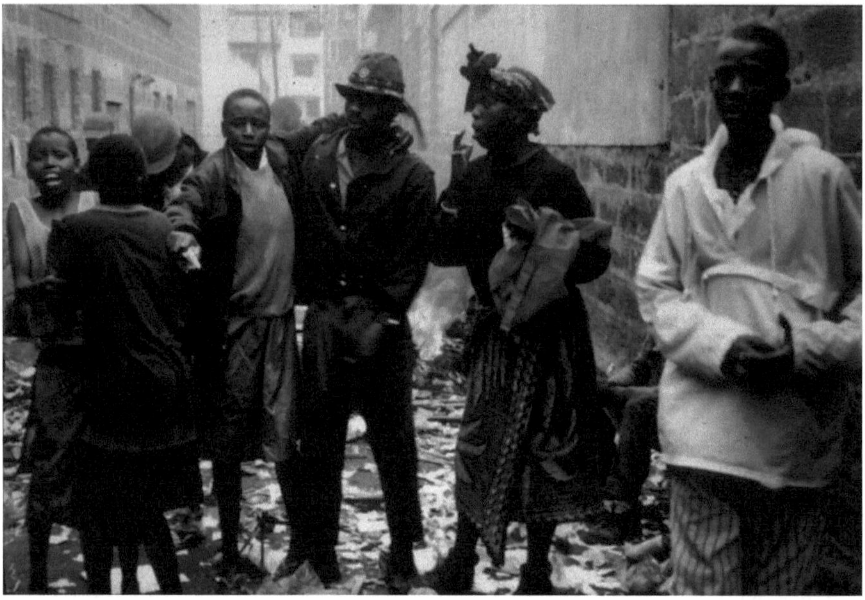

Fig. 2.7 A family of peers

Street children generally find a way to learn, but they have to find a way to live (food, shelter, basic medical attention). The streets often become their home. They have a home where they work, another where they sleep, another where they meet socially, etc. As we said, home is not just a physical space, it is also a mental category with a history of comfort and stress, and it is part of a place that grows over time to include more details and its own myth. In some ways street children see their "home" in contrast to their parent's home, which, not unlike other children, often is an illusion of brightness and well-being. They may be afraid to return home and face the possibility that they are not missed or appreciated, and possibly not even wanted as circumstances in their family home have changed.

As time on the street accumulates, street children form a family of peers who offer advice and friendship (sometimes good, sometime not so good, not all that different than the advice they might have received from parents). The street child's siblings are replaced by his or her peer groups who share these multiple homes of the city (Fig. 2.7).

The Street Career: Stages of Leaving Home

The stages of leaving home can be seen in a couple of ways. Conticini (2008) offers a cross-cultural phased approach to becoming a street child, (his primary data is from Ethiopia and Bangladesh, and his secondary sources come from several other countries). In the first couple of weeks of being a street child, the child learns whom to avoid and what to stay away from, as well as whom to rely on and where goods can safely be found. This process generally begins with observation, and continues as the newcomers starts to relate to one or two others.

When Conticini (2008) started work in Bangladesh, he took the train into town. On top of the train were street children windsurfing, that is, balancing against the wind generated by the speed of the train, standing upright and leaning forward, with their heads and their hands outstretched. He could see which children were new because the new children would watch others to see how it was done. Then they would try it and practice, eventually mastering the skill and having fun doing it; ready to move on to the next stage. In Latin America, children take the first phase in pieces, testing the waters and going back home and then testing the waters again. While in Ethiopia and Bangladesh, they jump in fully from the start. The second stage begins or the first ends when the child is accepted by a group of existing runaway youth or street children.

Shaffner (1999) has another type of categorization. He puts homeless youth into several categories. Pre-runaways still live at home but might be brought to the attention of authorities by a parent or a guardian because they are already showing sufficient problematic behavior. Two different groups of homeless youth live on the streets. There are situational runaways who have run away before, but do not report being abused, while justifiable runaways were abused or neglected. Chronic runaways have a history of at least three episodes of running. While most of this group report being abused or neglected, a smaller percentage did not.

Usually the process of becoming homeless is not the result of one episode, although a single episode can be the straw that breaks the camel's back. What this seems to be for American runaways (and for those from other developed countries), is the result of the long standing downward cycle of family dysfunction, particularly family violence, substance abuse, or a change of family make-up, and a new male in the house (Paradise and Cauce 2002; Barry et al. 2002).

In Canada, the psychological characteristics for the first time homeless and those homeless more than once showed more similarities than differences, and the need for services was as great for the first incidence as it was in subsequent episodes of homelessness (Goering et al. 2002).[15] The point being that the first time homeless were not a high functioning group who recently found hard times, they were like the long term homeless, who had many mental disorders. Paradise and Cauce (2002) studied American runaways and found that there was a positive correlation of homeless youth and adult deviance leading to contacts with the justice system and psychiatric care.

In her ethnographic participant observation study of runaway youth in America, Shaffner (1999) found that youth run away from home very reluctantly, even if there is severe family abuse. Essentially, while leaving home is not easy, staying at home is worse. There are intense and increasingly difficult scenes until leaving

[15] About 60% of the homeless become homeless again. The homeless came from poor homes with a history of mental illness and drug abuse and child abuse were common (Shaffner 1999).

home becomes the only way to release the tension. In spite of overt abuse, homeless youth want to have loving parents. They understand the moral duties of ideal children and while they don't really know what parents should be like, they use the ideal based on media presentations.

Homeless youth's feelings of not being wanted are not just from home. They occur in school and as they travel down the road toward running away. They come from the personnel of the variety of social service agencies they encounter whose edicts they must follow in order to receive help. They feel controlled, angry, and anxious about what is to become of them.

As the cycle continues and the youth feels further rejection, the expectation of the family caring for him or her is further reduced and the he or she feels less obliged to continue in the family's dynamics. The angry demeanor, the delinquent act, and the threatening gestures cover the hurt, but unfortunately these poses initiate more negative responses from adults, causing a downward cycle.

There is more than one way to look at the act of running away from home. Previously, we have talked about a decision to overcome the powerlessness of being a mistreated youth; and the consequent rebellion against the people holding abusive power. Yet only a third of homeless youth make this decision and leave home of their own accord. Another third are kicked out and about 20% are removed by the police or social services. The remaining few might come to a mutual agreement with their families that it is better for the child to leave (Paradise and Cauce 2002). At first it is difficult to know if a child is running away of his or her own accord or is being pushed out. In most respects, being a run away youth or a "throwaway" youth are two sides of the same coin.

It is not one act of abuse that causes American runaways to leaves home; some leave home because they perceive that parental demands are too high or that their parents are unfair (like blatantly disrespecting privacy or not being trusted). These runaways find it impossible to negotiate with their parents.

Since we are dealing with siblings in the same family, we must ask: Why do only some of these children become homeless, and if only some do, what are the characteristics that might differentiate them from their siblings?

Although it is less recognized as a cause of the children's move to the streets, sibling rivalry may account for more children leaving their homes than is commonly thought. In most research this information is obscured because when researches ask children if family problems caused them to leave home, the children do not understand that "family problems" includes problems with siblings.

If, as so many studies show, the major reason why homeless children ran away is abuse, then does it not suggest that it might be a wise move? Other runaways are exploring their independence or seek adventure (Roberts 2000). In a study of runaway youth in Los Angeles, slightly over 20% said they left home for the adventure. Many of them preferred to remain on the streets, rather than being in foster care or otherwise housed by the State. As one said: "*There is nothing like hopping a train and going wherever you want*" (Hyde 2005).

For street children, one reason for leaving home has to do with the variety of impacts of poverty. These children are often forced to sleep in the same bed as their mother and siblings and in the same room as their mothers' partners (Munyakho 1992). A major reason why girls leave home is because they can no longer sleep in the same room without the fear of being violated by a non-related man. They have something to worry about because, according to one study, more than 80% of street girls in Nairobi have been sexually abused (Onyango et al. 1991).

They found that 90% of street children in Nairobi went to school without anything to eat, 85% ate only one meal per day, and fewer than 10% of their parents earned more than the equivalent of $20 per month. Suda (1993) found that 75% of street children lived in a one-room house with no running water or indoor plumbing. Eighty percent of the street girls in Kenya came from homes with only a single room (Onyango et al. 1991).

In some cases, the streets are a better option. In a study in Sudan, street children said the streets afforded them a better chance at survival given that both the street and home were difficult, but there was less abuse in the streets than at home (Veale 1992). In Angola, a third of the street children chose to leave home for freedom or independence, or simply for fun and friends (Moberly 1999). Is it the thrill-seeking Tom Sawyers who run away, or the abused Huckleberry Finns? The two have quite different personalities.

The Street Career of Homeless Youth

We do know that the parents of 60% of runaway youth in America have alcohol and drug problems and half of all runaways have been abused at home (Flowers 2001). The overwhelming reason why American children flee is abuse, followed by neglect (Shaffner 1999). Poverty is far down the line.

Research in the United States (US) and Canada has extensively demonstrated that the majority of homeless youth come from homes with high levels of abuse, neglect and violence (Gaetz 2004a, b; Krabanow 2003; Tyler et al. 2004; Whitbeck and Hoyt 1999; Van den Bree 2009). Parental substance abuse is also a predictor of youth homelessness (McMorris et al. 2002).

There is no single composite of homeless youth coping strategies, but there are several coping styles laid out on a continuum (Roberts 2000). At one end are youth who aren't running away; they are able to cope and resolve conflict at home. Then, there are homeless youth who basically have a sound relationship with their parents, but feel over-controlled in one part of their lives such as dating. More girls than boys fall into this category.

Further along the continuum, there are homeless youth who are in chronic family conflict, and the behavior at home is escalating from yelling, to throwing things, and finally to hitting. Before homeless youth eventually enter this cycle of family breakdown and dependency, they are often involved in child welfare and protection services, or live in foster care or group homes (Eberle 2001). Homeless youth in the developed world rarely sleep rough. In desperate situations they can go to a hospital because hospitals are mandated by law to find places for them to sleep, even if on the floors in the hallways.

Dufour (2000) showed that homeless youth experience multiple relationship difficulties including: being unable to name significant persons in their parental network and having no filial feelings; having no privileged relations with their brothers and sisters, nor with their cousins; having no matrimonial alliances and living a solitary life; having no stable residence and not participating in domestic work in the places they are temporarily given shelter; eventually, not wanting any heritage from their parents (although they did not exclude the right to inherit).

Their heightened emotions are difficult to control. Many are likely to use drugs to reduce the pain. In addition to self-medication, another coping style is manipulation; hoping that their absence will hurt their parents. Finally, there are the "endangered runaways" who have been the victims of regular abuse. They leave to avoid being beaten and cope by using drugs that are stronger than alcohol and marijuana.

Among homeless youth, certain categories of are at special risk. About 20% of homeless youth in a five city study in the US claimed to be lesbian, gay, or bisexual (Whitbeck et al. 2004). When this subgroup was compared to straight homeless youth, they were at a greater risk for substance abuse, suicide attempts, and survival sex (Van Leeuwen et al. 2006).

Most homeless youth have histories of depression, family abuse and neglect, substance abuse, and suicide attempts Shaffner (1999). Shaffner reports that 17% of the girls were involved in prostitution, and two thirds of street boys and girls reported using glue the day prior to being interviewed.

An even more somber picture emerges from the results of the Seattle Homeless Adolescent Research Project (Cauce et al. 2000), probably the most cited research on American homeless youth. They found their homeless adolescent subjects not only had more than one diagnostic mental disorder; but one in ten met the diagnostic criteria for schizophrenia, and about a third tried to commit suicide. Slightly more than a fifth of American runaway youth in shelters attempt suicide (Shaffner 1999). Three quarters of the runaway youth in another study had one suicide attempt, and among those, eight out of ten tried at least once more (Van Leeuwen et al. 2006).

Using the Achenbach Youth Self Report test (Achenbach 1991), Stewart et al. (2004) noted the high incidence of mental disorders (about two thirds) and suicidal behavior among homeless youth in the US, Conduct Disorder being the most prevalent, followed by Attention Deficit Hyperactivity Disorder (ADHD), and depression.

Homeless youth in the US have depression rates between 19% and 39% (Solorio et al. 2006), which compares unfavorably to that of domiciled American youth (between 8% and 13%). The subjects of this study were under 17 years of age and had spent at least two nights away from home without parental and adult permission, but it was not clear where. It appeared that about half of the children were living in shelters and the other half on the streets. But later the authors say they had a hard time finding youth who were living on the streets and in the end suggest that the results be taken with this consideration.

In a study of the emotional health of homeless adolescents in Seattle, nearly a fifth met the criteria of PTSD (Post-Traumatic Stress Disorder), with a particularly high rate of hyper-vigilance and avoidance due to a nearly 80% rate of victimization, but the ages of the "adolescents" were between 13 and 21, a range that, by comparison to developing countries, goes into adulthood (Stewart et al. 2004).

Bao et al. (2000) studied social networks among domiciled and runaway adolescents in four American Midwestern States. Using a path model, they charted the effects of family abuse, which led to early independence and subsequent depression. They found that family abuse and leaving home early could be mediated by social peer support networks, but only if the support network was not deviant. If it was, then the peer pressure toward anti-social acts increased depression.

In a comparison of Canadian runaway and non-runaway youth on several factors related to mental health, Ayerst (1999) found that runway youth (although the gender makeup of her study is not mentioned) were more depressed; more engaged in self-destructive behaviors and exhibited a higher use of drugs and alcohol. Furthermore, they showed signs of poor problem-solving skills.

In a thorough study of homeless children and youth in the United Kingdom, Smeaton (2009) and a team of research assistants from the Railway Children Foundation demonstrated that many of the characteristics of these homeless children were similar to what was found in other developed countries. He refers to these children as "detached" and defines them as children and young people who are away from home or care for at least 6 months and who live outside of key societal institutions such as family, education or other statutory services, who do not have any formal sources of support, and who are self-reliant and/or dependent upon informal support networks.

Smeaton (2009) describes how they worked at keeping the role of the researcher to a minimum. He uses a grounded theory approach by first collecting data and then using the data to develop theories about what was happening on the streets. Thus they analyzed the data in two stages, first with the data from the fieldwork and then by applying a social science software package that developed categories of the data to identify themes and issues.

The results show that only 20% of the homeless youth grew up in poverty (as opposed to nearly 100% of street children). With few exceptions, the families of the detached sample were problematic and had no opportunity to get support from professionals. Many of the detached children were raised by single mothers, some never met their fathers. They were often lied to about the reality of their biological fathers, which was damaging. The children either idealized or were hateful to their absent fathers. When grandparents were involved, they were helpful to an extent, even though poor parenting was typical not only of the children's parents, but also of their parent's parents, making moral judgment of them more difficult.

Smeaton (2009) describes a great deal of violence. Mostly violence was from the youths' families, and then from peers and in some cases communities. The amount of violence the children perpetrated on others was considerably less, even though many of them carried knives and a few guns. About half of them said they were involved with gangs, but not organized gangs. The youth defined gangs to mean hanging out with a group of peers to increase their own safety and security.

Some children came to the streets because they were thrown out of their homes, some drifted to the streets because of the violence at home. The adult homeless community was at times a source of support, but more often a risk of danger. In addition to the violence they faced at home, the youth were not successful at school. More than half were asked to leave. They were not much more successful with alternative schooling.

When the children and young people discussed themselves, they talked about how the street set them free, and that they were different than other children. Once on the streets, the children had a variety of coping behaviors; the most rewarding involved being involved with other homeless children and youth. They learned where the safe places were, the behaviors which could enable them to survive without being incarcerated, and how to avoid danger. Some children and young people saw being homeless as completely negative, while others had positive things to say. There were children who saw the experience as a normal part of growing up. For those who had many of their peers involved, it was difficult to give up being homeless.

These children and youth were not perceived by the public as good examples of children. The differences between most people's experiences of childhood and their own were considerable. For example, there was no prolonged adolescence typical of the developed world that was available to the homeless children and youth. From an early age they were forced into adult like decisions, such as when to leave home, or find shelter, or how to care for money. As the children began to come of age (by 16), life changed. They became eligible for services provided to the adult homeless. Some of them took advantage of this, while others saw them as dangerous, or perhaps more importantly as a sign of a more permanent status.

Smeaton (2009) describes their future goals, having a family, a home, love, and a career, which were similar to what most of us want. While a few of them were headed in this direction, most felt it would be difficult to leave the streets. The experience of being away from home or caring adults either permanently or for long periods of time before they were 16 years of age, will not be forgotten.

It is hard to see how Smeaton (2009) found a remarkable amount of resilience, since she says this in spite of the widespread use of drugs among the youth (although she mentions that some of them were able to give them up). She adds that many of them had mental disorders, principally depression. A few attempted suicide. They had a lot of sex, although it is unclear how much of it was enjoyable, safe and desired. They were involved in many exploitative relationships.

Once on the streets, American homeless youth are prey to a variety of stalkers for sexual privileges or assault. Between a fifth and a third report some incidence of abuse and 10% report being raped (Whitbeck and Hoyt 1999).

There are a few studies which show homeless youth to be resilient. In an in-depth interview study, five female runaway youth in the United States, who had been exposed to chronic trauma and yet remained resilient, were asked what characteristics they thought were needed to maintain good mental health (Williams et al. 2001).[16] Some of the experiences they considered important were readiness to

[16]This study showed not only the difficulties of some research on the mental health of runaways, but also the problems in comparing the mental health of homeless youth and street children.

accept professional mental health help and long term treatment programs. These resilient American homeless youth were able to express their gratitude to mentors, and take pleasure in giving back to others. Nothing can make a person happy faster than making someone else happy.

Other specific examples included leaning problem-solving skills, and appreciation of what others are offering for help. One Native American woman mentioned that as soon as she discovered they would be accepting of her traditional religion, she felt she would be accepted.

Shaffner (1999) reports that some homeless youth (her study was only of girls) have good social skills and know how to please adults, if doing so is in their favor. They know that sociability is a good way to connect to other people. There was also the pride the resilient individual had in overcoming obstacles, which was expressed as personal determination to succeed.[17] The important factors identified in resilience studies of homeless youth are not only the identifying markers of their resilience (social and family support, intelligence, etc.) but also how they negotiate the stressful events of being homeless or on the streets.

For the great majority, who seem not to be resilient, one could ask which comes first, the mental disorders leading toward a difficult home life or a difficult home life leading to mental disorders. Or both, as Paradise and Cauce (2002) argue. They believe that the high incidence of mental disorders is the result of "individual vulnerability and environmental risk (p. 224)". On the environmental side, the authors note the family breakdown in the runaways early childhood followed by a series of negative interactions that build up over the years to the point where the adolescent is either thrown out of the family or leaves. It is not surprising then that homeless youth do not trust their parents, are not close to them, and do not see them as helpful. Nor, if this is the case, is it surprising that runaway youth report more depressive symptoms, suicidal ideation, and substance abuse than domiciled adolescents.

While the results on homeless youth seem conclusive, there still are many problems open to further research. In many of these studies it is difficult to know if the mental health problems reported were evident prior to family conflict and running away or were reactions to being on the streets. Nor do they take into account children who run away for reasons other than family discord. An interesting comparative study could be made between runaway youth without family discord and with family abuse. Also, the results of most studies assume that the reader knows the particulars in addition to the family dysfunction, such as prior mental health, but also the sibling order (the first to runaway in the family?), the communities from which they run away and the communities they run to.

[17] In the developing world there is often less of an emphasis on the individual's tenacity and more on the community. This might be a practicality due to limited options. The reader should note that when it comes to religious-run programs in the developing world, the emphasis is on adapting modern and western traditions, and incorporating in many cases the proselytizing measures of the religion.

The Street Career of Street Children

To understand the mental health of street children, we must first look at gender and child rearing expectations. To illustrate this, we take a concrete example. Consider pleasant, a 28 year-old mother of a street child in sub-Saharan Africa (Aptekar and Ciano 1999). Her life tells us quite a bit about different family structures and gender differences, which is important. We find it extraordinary that the term street children (and homeless youth) does not usually take into account gender, since there are important gender differences in the numerical ratio of male to female homelessness and in the different family expectations toward each gender.

Pleasant functions as the head of her impoverished household and copes with both poverty and culturally appropriate intimate relationships. We can see how her family is seen from the normative family context and what the gender differences are.

Pleasant has been married for 5 years by common law to a night watchman. They have four children (three boys and a girl), whom they supported together until her husband began to drift away from the family. This did not come as a surprise to Pleasant: "This is what most men do," she says. Pleasant has strong ties to other women in her neighborhood who have also been abandoned by their husbands. According to Pleasant, "This is how women live." The women help each other as any close group does, by providing material and emotional support.

By the time Pleasant's oldest son, Mbisa, has his sixth birthday, he is accustomed to playing with boys, including older boys in the neighborhood. His mother gives him plenty of time to practice being independent because Pleasant does not closely supervise his whereabouts. Within a year after his father left (and the household income dropped) Mbisa began to drift further from home and go into other neighborhoods to clean car windows, and find other sources of income for his family.

Pleasant is now working off and on as a domestic servant. She is showing her daughter, Dominion, how to take care of household chores at home. By the time Dominion is 7 years of age, she will fetch water, make fires, and cook most meals. It is unlikely that she will be drifting far from home.

While Pleasant and Mbisa are earning income, there is enough money to pay school fees for the two younger boys. After a short romance and a solid look by Pleasant into some economic facts about a man Pleasant knows from her upcountry community, the man moves in with Pleasant and her children. Their combined income allows Mbisa to return to school.

Pleasant, knowing the ups and downs of a woman's economic and romantic situation is aware that her new boyfriend will eventually move out (or that she will kick him out). This is as expected as the demise in the relationship with her common law husband had been. She knows what the economic implications of all of these changes will be. If the new man moves in, the two younger boys will be able to go to school, without his help they will have to leave school and go to work on the streets like Mbisa. She also literally prays that she will avoid complete financial destitution or the utter breakdown of her mental health because this could result in sending Dominion to work. (Some women do have daughters working in the streets, but they will most likely be supervised by an older child, and the mother will make every effort to see that her daughter is not abused.)

Pleasant and most women like her do not believe they are living in "broken" homes. Many believe they are better off without husbands whom they think are "too expensive to keep in drink, let alone food and clothes." Pleasant could say that even if her men wanted to work, they would be unable to find employment, because of the increasing opportunities in the informal sector for women and decreasing opportunities in the formal sector for men.[18]

Mbisa does not view himself as abandoned when his father left, because he expects serial partnerships between his mother and men. One advantage is that these children will not experience the emotional plight that comes from parents dissolving a marriage in a Western-style normative family. Instead like Mbisa, these children are accustomed to living in a family that included a series of men staying for short periods of time, some of them more benign than others.

More than three-quarters of the families in this Kenyan study began with a woman and man who were not legally married; they had children, and later separated. Subsequently, the man and woman formed unions with other partners. As a result, the children eventually belonged to three families: their biological families, their mothers' remarried families (usually common law marriage), and their fathers' remarried families (also common law).[19] These families as the research in Kenya shows are ubiquitous.

In the developing world, Mbisa's situation far outpaces his sister's. In Kenya, 91% of street children are male (Onyango et al. 1991); over 90% in India are male (Patel 1990; Verma 1999); in Zimbabwe, 95% of 520 children interviewed were boys (Muchini and Nyandiya-Bundy 1991), as were 84% of Angolan street children (Moberly 1999), and 76% of Ethiopian street children (Veale et al. 1993). Seventy percent Zambian street children (Mambwe 1997) were male, and nearly 100% of Sudanese street children in one study (Veale 1996) and 86% in another were male (Plummer et al. 2007). In South Africa, street children were, according to (Le Roux 1996), typically Black males. Virtually all the children living in the street in Turkey were male (Ataov and Haider 2006). All of the street children in Marquez's study (1999) in Venezuela were male. Nieuwenhuizen (2006) found between 10% and 30% female in her study in Bangalore, India.

In China the proportion of street boys grew with the progression in age (Stoecklin 2000b). There was a gender balance of children under 12, whereas the ratio is 1 girl to

---

[18] The diary of Maria de Jesus (1962) gives a gripping literary description of how one poor Brazilian woman in a similar situation learned that having men in her house was just too emotionally and economically costly. Peatrie (1968) provides a more scientific account of the same point of view in Venezuela. Similar findings come from a study of family life among the poor in Nairobi, where "*40 percent of the mothers ... felt that marriage spoils a relationship and gives the man too much power and control over the woman*" (Suda 1993, p. 113).

[19] It has been speculated, but not adequately supported by empirical evidence, that this type of family, unlike the extended traditional family, will lose its connection to the common community associated with traditional African kin (Erny 1981).

15 boys over the age of 15. This was also linked to strong differences regarding activities: while fewer than 40% of the boys were begging, this proportion rose to 90% among the girls. The begging children were accompanied mostly by a parent and any group of beggars and parents were always supervised by a "boss". There seemed to be a clear cut around age 12: above this age, the children are mainly unaccompanied vagrants and almost only boys. In this category, fewer than 10% of the children were selling things such as newspapers or train tickets on the black market, or scavenging.

In Haiti, because of the great numbers of female headed households from which street children allegedly come, Kovats-Bernat (2006) hypothesized that the streets might be for boys the natural place in which they grow into manhood, as one boy told him that the streets were kind to boys. In fact he defined street children (*timoun lari* in Haitian Creole) as only boys.

The gender ratio is particularly salient because across cultures girls are more likely to be abandoned and abused than boys (Kabeberi 1990; Korbin 1981). Thus if being a street child is the result of neglect or abuse, we would expect a high proportion of girls to be on the streets, which in fact explains the differences in the ratios among developed and developing countries. In the developing world, abuse is a less common factor to becoming homeless, thus the high percentage of boys. While in the developed world, abuse is the main factor of homelessness, thus resulting in a much higher proportion of girls (Shaffner 1999), between a third to a half (Cauce et al. 2000).

It might be that female street children have more problems than male street children, because they are raised to be at home and are found in the street only when they have received abuse at home.[20] While the street boys are raised for an early independence from their homes, so whatever reason why they are on the street it dovetails fine with their natural trajectory.[21] For homeless youth in the developed world of both genders abuse at home is at the heart of their running away.

Aptekar and Ciano (1999) are not the only ones to argue that street girls are taught by their mothers to cope with the vagaries of poverty by staying at home, and out of the streets. In Ethiopia (Aptekar and Abebe 1997; Heinonen 2011) found that girls once they were 8 years of age were discouraged from playing in the street due to fear that they would be bullied or sexually harassed and because it was conduct unbecoming for nice girls. In another study, Ethiopian mothers seldom approved of their daughters being outside playing and preferred them to be at home or in the neighborhood where they lived (Heinonen 2011).

In Brazil boys were expected to bring income into the house by working on the streets and coming home with money, girls were expected to stay at home and help

[20] Mtonga (2011) reports that in Zambia street girls were on the streets or returned to the streets because of abuse by a stepmother.

[21] Sometimes, within a country, the proportion of girls to boys on the streets varies according to local conditions. For example, in Muslim areas of countries that have groups of mixed religions (Nigeria for example), Muslim girls are very rarely found on the street as the presence of unaccompanied girls in that environment is socially unacceptable and so their families will not permit them to leave the home.

with the household chores (Hecht 1998; Scheper-Hughes and Hoffman 1998). Zimbabwe families did not send girls to the streets because they were fearful of sexual abuse (Muchini and Nyandiya-Bundy 1991). In Sudan, where street children were almost exclusively male, the influence of Muslim culture in Khartoum meant it was inappropriate for girls to wander unaccompanied in the streets (Plummer et al. 2007); the same in Ethiopia (Heinonen 2011). In Kenya, mothers expected the girls to help around the house from age five onwards. Asking daughters to act as surrogate mothers and nurses was common, even where there were several boys in the family (Kilbride et al. 2000). Again, in Sudan, where there is poverty and war, Plummer et al. (2007) report that the number of girls in the study was so small they could not even use them for measuring statistical significance.

Raffaelli (2000) studied gender differences among Brazilian street children, including a cultural analysis of how what they referred to as the cultural hypothesis of Aptekar and Ciano (1999) describes gender difference among street children. While the authors of this study discuss differences among male and female children, they are also point out some similarities that are relevant to street children. They say that in almost all cultures females are more likely to be closer to home, as women and girls are traditionally homebound because of child care, cooking and protection from the male environment found in the streets where males earn a living and participate in social activities. Thus, as mentioned above, Brazilian girls on the streets can be seen as out of their element (Rosemberg 2000).

From observational and anecdotal data, Rosemberg (2000) found that in Sao Paulo the male and female street children did different things during the day. The males played and worked more than the females, and the females begged more than the males.

Campos et al. (1994) working with a large group of investigators found that street girls are less likely to be hungry. They were also more likely to have benefactors who would physically look out for them and give them a place to sleep. According to the cultural hypothesis, the presence of girls on the streets violates cultural norms for female behavior, and thus street girls are more likely to be from dysfunctional families and exhibit psychological distress than their male peers (Aptekar 1994; Aptekar and Ciano 1999). From this point of view the "presence of boys on the street is thought to reflect a deliberate survival strategy by impoverished families who socialize sons into early independence in an appropriate male context—the street. In contrast, the presence of girls on the street is thought to reflect family dysfunction which has led to a breakdown in the socialization process. Thus, although boys and girls may share the common condition of being "on the street", they may be on distinct developmental trajectories, with homeless girls being at higher risk of negative outcomes than their male peers (Raffaelli 2000, p. 1432)".

As they (Raffaelli 2000) write, there is very little research on gender differences among street children, particularly in Africa. In addition to examining gender differences of coping capacities on the street and how well male and female street children are meeting their needs while on the streets, the authors discuss gender differences of the street children's views of their families of origin before going to the streets.

They gathered qualitative and quantitative data by using sentence completions and a semi-structured interview. Their sample was of 33 male street children from 10 to 17 years of age, and 33 female street children of the same age range. There was only a minimum difference between the mean ages of the two groups. They report that the subjects were fully engaged in the Sentence Completion test and that almost all of the responses were coded. The responses were coded by two independent coders and the few discrepancies between coders were resolved easily. The results are presented descriptively.

Both male and female street children said they left home to escape both family conflict and abuse. More females than males responded this way. Only three street children said they left home because of poverty. Particular questions about their parents had gender differences. More than two thirds of the girls wanted their father to change, which the authors report had something to do with the treatment by the father towards other family members. A third of the boys on the sentence completion wished their fathers were with them. One in eight specifically wished for a better life for their father, which by contrast was never mentioned by any of the girls. More of the girls slept in institutions than the boys, and fewer girls slept on the street. Boys were more likely than girls to have been victims of police violence, having to beg, being hungry and having committed petty crimes, like theft. In spite of these differences, about 75% of each gender said they were not alone when it came to having someone to help them. The same percentage of street girls and street boys were going to school.

Raffaelli (2000) believe that their study partially supported the cultural hypothesis of gender difference. On the one hand before and after leaving home the genders were not much different than one another, but there were differences in line with the cultural hypothesis in how they viewed their families. The girls were more likely to leave home because of negativity, either in the form of direct abuse or because of general family conflict. But the findings do not support Aptekar's and Ciano's (1999) results that girl street children had more psychological problems than male street children.

Aptekar and Ciano (1999) explain the different results by examining cultural factors. In Brazil, in contrast to Kenya, there are many programs, both governmental and non-governmental that help street children. Even though the female Brazilian street children are not following a typical gender path, they have found parental like care to help them in their daily struggles. They also point out their tentative data and therefore the difficulty of drawing conclusions from the study. Yet, as they point out there is plenty of data to make it clear that instead of using the label street children, there are both gender and cultural differences that should be taken into account, because it is likely that children in street situations of different genders and in different countries have widely different experiences.

In short, all over the developing world, boys are reared to go the streets (which is not what we would refer to as running away from home in the developed world) and girls are expected to stay at home and help out the family, although this depends on whether or not there is a man in the house.

The picture among homeless youth in the developed world is different. There boys and girls are approximately of equal numbers (Cauce et al. 2000). What do these gender differences across cultures tell us? They say that in the developing world, beyond poverty, most street boys do not run away from home without abuse. The boys, like the girls, are on the street because of abuse. In the developed world, both genders are raised to stay home; both boys and girls are likely to runaway if they have been abused at home and have no place to resolve their anger.[22] While there is a parity of males and females among runaways, their coping styles of not equally effective. Runaway American girls have lower self esteem and more depression than runaway boys (Maxwell 1992); evidenced by the fact that American female runaways are more likely to attempt suicide than males (Rotheram-Borus et al. 2003).

It is important to note that, according to the Shaffner study (1999), a third of American runaway girls came from two parent families, and another third were from single parent (female) families, and a third from families with a step-parent (step-father). She uses these numbers to debunk the idea that single mothers are the cause for girls running away from home, or that they cannot take care of their children properly.

As we have mentioned, gender differences, particularly with regard to how children are raised, play a large role in determining the mental health of street children. In Nairobi, Kenya, Aptekar and Ciano (1999) found that most (but not all) street boys were taught by their mothers to cope with the necessity of having to live in a very limited economic environment. They learned to become independent at a far earlier age than the dominant society deemed appropriate. Compared to other poor boys that stayed with their families, and to the brothers of street boys that remained at home, street boys were the more resilient. The less psychologically competent boys were unable to leave home and follow the expected cultural rules of male child development.

In Kenya, adolescent boys traditionally slept apart from their families in peer Groups. Thus street boys in Kenya can be seen to continue this tradition (Kilbride et al. 2000) as they huddle together at night while domiciled boys are leading a less traditional and more Western form of child development.

On the other hand, because girls were supposed to remain at home, when they became street girls it was because they had a more difficult relationship with their families of origin. Thus, Aptekar and Ciano (1999) found that the mental health of street boys was better than that of street girls. When compared to their domiciled sisters, street girls were worse off. That is, the girls who went to the streets had poorer mental health than their siblings who stayed home. The opposite is true for the boys who stayed at home. They were worse off than their siblings who went to the streets. Other authors have confirmed these results in Sudan (Plummer et al. 2007) and in Rwanda (Veale and Dona (2003).

[22] In a national study (Cauce et al. 2000) of American homeless adolescents, 60% of girls were sexually abused before leaving home (not quite 25% for boys).

In Colombia, Aptekar (1990) found difference in mental health among sub-groups of street children, but the majority of street boys were not psychopathological, nor otherwise delinquent and drug-abusing. Many developed adequate coping strategies, which allowed them to function at least as well as their poor counterparts who spent less time in public view.[23] Aptekar was not saying that street boys had the same mental and cognitive capacities as more affluent better educated and more supervised children in the West. But that the street boys had coping strategies that included finding a niche in the economic market, which gave them sufficient income to eat and clothe themselves. They found and took advantage of programs that served them, and were sufficiently informed about their physical health to stay reasonably healthy. They formed close friendships with their peers and, in many cases, belonged to strong communities. At the same time, they consistently maintained some form of connection to their families of origin.

The positive mental health characteristics of street boys also included their desire to learn and to have an education, their knowledge of how to survive, of having experienced the difficulties of life, yet having found ways to accommodate or overcome them. They were capable of a high level of self-management in organizing themselves in groups and had multiple friendships, and they were willing to work, and able to be creative in their recreation (Aptekar 1988; Ennew 1994).

Davies (2008) compared street children in northwest Kenya with poor children from the same town. The author says that while he doesn't want to belittle the lives of street children in any way. Instead of finding them physically and mentally unhealthy, he found that the street children in his study have a better quality of life than their siblings and peers who have remained at home. Certainly he finds that their standard of living is higher.

In fact, he thinks that the very street children who look so bad and whom the public pities, when compared to other poor children, are not "at risk children". He notes that only a small percentage of the children in his sample were rejected by their families and only a small percentage rejected their families. In choosing to be a street child, Davies (2008) believes the children have made a competent and informed choice, knowing both the good and not so good parts of being a member of that group. In fact, he thinks that being part of a street child culture breeds an activism toward self-preservation if not also toward social justice. They develop valuable skills and supporting friends. When he assessed the well being of street children, he notes that it might be that they need material help, such as access to health care, shelter, better food, etc. but they don't need to be separated from their peers (Fig. 2.8).

He does not advocate for providing social services that force street children to conform to the popular notions of what is considered to be an appropriate childhood. Asking them to do this would devalue their lives, rather than help them with their own coping strategies. Without long term studies of street children, which we do not have, there is no evidence to say that these children will not grow into

[23] The reader should note that this is an extrapolation and comes from the author's experience. For a review of street children in the developing world that includes the argument for street children being less benign, see Aptekar 1988, 1994.

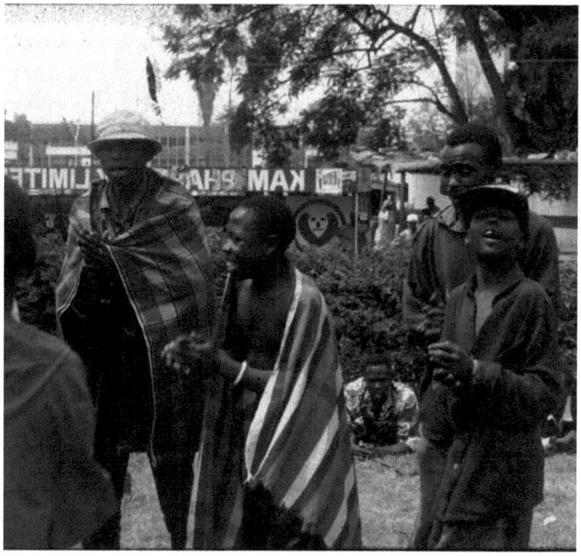

Fig. 2.8 Support from friends

productive citizens. Davies (2008) says the street children he studied were neither in crisis nor in need of immediate aid.

Essentially, his sample was male. When gender is not mentioned specifically, we can expect that the author is talking about males, if for no other reason that the population of street children is so dominated by males. Monteiro et al. (1998) used the Ericksonian model of human development to show that street children had the age appropriate characteristics of initiative, industry and positive identity. Felsman (1981) working in Colombia said street children displayed better mental health than their poor counterparts. Rizzini and Lusk (1995) claimed street children in several Latin American countries were able to organize and initiate behaviors to meet their needs.

Veale et al. (2000) found that it was not the street children in Ethiopia who were lethargic, self-doubting and uncreative. These behaviors were more likely to be those of the poor child counterparts than the street children who displayed more of the opposite behavior. In another study, Veale (1996) showed that street children had good internal locus of control (indicating a person who turns inward to understand their lives, rather than feeling the good was sent from God and the bad was due to someone else). It is generally associated with good mental health.

In a study of street children in Brazil, de Oliveira (2000) found that two-thirds of street children saw themselves in a positive light, with good self concepts. She measured levels of cortical, a neuro-chemical sensitive to anxiety and depression and found that the homeless street children were similar to middle class children. Dobrowolska and Panter-Brick (1998), also using cortical markers, found that Ethiopian street children had better cortical levels than working children living at home.

Kovats-Bernat (2006) over the years of his work in Haiti, found that in spite of the dangers of the streets, many street children loved the freedom. Some of them earned as much as 300% more than people doing minimally paid jobs.

After the demise of the former Soviet Union, orphans and other institutionalized children were able to break away from the institutions and go to the street where they found freedom and they were proud because of it. Again, it might be said that the stronger orphans were the ones who became street children not the other way around. Fujimora (2005) noted that Russian street children found food, shelter, and community, which in itself, she said, demonstrated their resilience. She reported on one boy, Kolya, who bought and sold flowers, earning more than his mother, and contributing to her well being. He even had excess to treat himself to a fast food hamburger. He saw himself as a survivor, not a victim.

Kerfoot et al. (2007) assessed the physical and emotional health of street children in Kyiv, Ukraine. The authors report that the numbers of street children in the Moscow area alone is around 40,000–50,000. This is greater than the number of homeless children there after World War II. The official statistics in the Ukraine estimate approximately 50,000 street children, a quarter of whom are in Kyiv. This is fewer than 1% of the 0–15 year olds in the population, a statistic which they use to show that the current number underestimates the true situation. They believe that this is the first study of Ukrainian street children using internationally recognized measures of psychopathology.

The sample consisted of 72 boys and 25 girls. After spending some time to get to know the children, the authors administrated questionnaires on psycho-pathology (Strengths and Difficulties Questionaire - SDQ) and depression (Mood and Feelings Questionaire - MFQ). The children were from 6 to 17 years of age, with an average of 12.8. Two thirds of the sample group were between 12 and 15 years of age.

A little more than a quarter of the subjects did not know and had no contact with their families, the rest maintained some contact. Almost all of them had families who were living in chronic severe poverty. Many of their families had alcohol related problems. The authors mention that the females were not evenly distributed among the three categories. And, males were significantly more likely than females to be disconnected or only partially connected to their families.

It is interesting that on three of the measures of mental health, substance abuse, delinquency, and early sexual experience, the partially connected group scored significantly worse than the other two groups, which the authors say means that the group that is on the street, but has some contact with families, had more mental disorders than the children living on the street but without any family ties, and more than the children who lived at home but spent their days on the streets. This is probably related to the problems of their families of origin mentioned above.

In a cross-cultural study, Blanc (1994) compared street children and working children in five countries (Brazil, Kenya, India, Italy and the Philippines). Their conclusion is that working children come from poor and stressed, but supportive families, while the families of street children are as poor but more violent and less supportive.

Typical health problems for street children (and homeless youth) center around the respiratory, digestive and urinary tract systems, as well as skin problems, bad teeth, sexually transmitted diseases, and whatever fall-out there is from smoking, drinking and abusing illegal drugs. Yet there is research that shows, when compared to their poor counterparts, street children have better physical health.

Two Styles of Development Among Street Children

Gamines and *Chupagruesos*

To understand more about the developmental stages of street children, it is important to distinguish two types of children found by Aptekar (1988) in Colombia,: the *gamines* and *chupagruesos*. This distinction is found in other developing countries as well.

He described the mental health of sub-groups of male Colombian street children based on psychological testing and ethnographic observation. About a third of his subjects in Colombia were quite resilient. These children were originally described by a French journalist who went to Colombia to write about the street children by their "spirit of rebellion". He called them *gamines*. In his view, the gamines were living in freedom from the demands of parents, much like the "Lost Boys" in *Peter Pan*, or like Mark Twain's character, Tom Sawyer.

Gamines, Aptekar says (1990), chose a life of partial misery with liberty rather than continue a life with total misery and no independence. He observed a pair of *gamines* who went every morning to the *El Paradiso* restaurant in Cali, Colombia where they washed the front sidewalk with a hose in exchange for leftover *sobres* (food) (Aptekar 1988). On one particular day, one boy put the plastic bag of *sobres* over his shoulder, and he and his partner went to a quiet side street, sat down in the shade and emptied the food, which was lumped together in a mass about the size of a small pillow. They ate some of it and traded the rest with a blind man for a few *pesos* and a couple of used cigarettes.

As they got on the bus that was going to the cemetery, they asked the driver to let them ride for free so they might ask for food, since, they said, they were starving. On the bus, one boy put on a pitiful expression and began to sing soulfully about the difficulties of having a sick mother whom he was trying to support. The song concluded with, "Would you give my mother a few *pesos* so she could go to the doctor?" He got a few *pesos*, enough to pay for their ride to the cemetery. Meanwhile, his partner lodged himself in the exit well, standing in the way of passengers getting off, offering them his hand so they might climb down more easily. Most of the passengers ignored him, some were indignant and made comments to the bus driver, a few found his performance amusing and gave him a coin.

Once at the cemetery, the two boys met a few older friends and gave them some of the bus money for a ladder which they carried over to an area where relatives were visiting a loved one's grave. As it was nearly impossible to place wreaths on the higher grave sites, they rented out the use of the ladder.

The quick wit and verbal interactions (and intellectual skills) of gamines were not typical of all the street children. The *chupagruesos* (*chupar* means to suck or absorb and refers to those who suck up to the bigger boys) coped with street life by becoming servile to the more powerful.[24] They were the lackeys to the more powerful children, and they tended to have more mental health problems. Luiz, (again from Cali, Colombia) not yet even a teenager, went to the street after his new stepfather started demanding he bring home a certain amount of money each day for his room and board. Once on the streets, Luiz was befriended by Jorge, an older street boy who made his living by shining shoes. He taught his trade to Luiz, but after a few weeks he demanded that Luiz, despite his fear of doing so, beg for money. After a while, Jorge taught Luiz how to help him steal a watch from a street vendor. As Jorge walked behind the vendor and got his attention, Luiz was supposed to grab a watch and run, but the man grabbed Luiz instead, which led to Luiz being placed in reform school, where his low status among his peers continued. In reform school, he ran errands for the more powerful kids, gave them food from his plate, and washed their clothes. In short, Luiz coped by being dependent on the more powerful. As part of the *chupagruesos*, he lacked the independence of *gamines* in their daily coping strategies.

Aptekar (1990) found that *gamines* and *chupagruesos* from the onset of their street lives developed very differently psychologically. At first they played together, but soon a differentiation between them occurred. Since the preadolescent children were more effective at soliciting alms, they were eventually asked to provide their services to the older children. Some of the smaller children responded to this demand by compromising their liberty and becoming dependent on the larger boys. Others refused, even if it meant fighting against the odds, and established themselves as independent.

The assumed abuse by the physically superior of the weaker has a natural check. The older children need the young ones because the image they portray to the public makes them more likely to get goods or money. While the older ones, as they grow bigger and stronger, will have to rely largely on crime. Sometimes only the gamines are strong enough to understand and take advantage of this dynamic.

The demands upon the *chupagruesos* by their older peers made it extremely difficult for them to break this submissive pattern. In their relationship with other street children, the *chupagruesos* formed sadomasochistic relationships with the larger boys, which often resulted in depression or regression to immature behavior. This in turn increased their submissive lifestyle.

This difference in the relationship of each group to authority is related to a universal motif of children that Bettelheim (1976) discusses in his book about fairy tales. This motif features a giant in conflict with an ordinary child who through wit overpowers him. This theme is common to all cultures in some form, since children everywhere fear and resent the power of people who rule over them. Children know that short of doing their bidding, they have only one way to get back at them; through outwitting them. It was through wit and cunning that the *gamines*

[24] *Chupagruesos* are more pushed than pulled into the street, while the *gamines* are more pulled than pushed (Aptekar 1990).

channeled their anger and learned to cope with their situation, while the *chupagruesos* were too afraid to express their pain.

As the two groups approached adolescence, they faced different problems. *Gaminismo* ended at puberty, when they became unable to continue with their petty robberies and still be *gamines*. These alternatives no longer provided the satisfaction of outwitting adults. With the increased experience and skill acquired with age, the same acts of mischievousness that once were thrilling became degrading. They no longer tested the *gamines'* intelligence and ability. As they grew older, they were compelled by their perceptions of themselves as haughty provocateurs to give up the small-scale mischief and become either full-scale delinquents or find a way to live outside the mainstream of society. However, escalating petty mischievousness into delinquent acts was unsatisfactory because it led to associations with gangs and the friendships and customs of that delinquent world. The ethos of the delinquent subculture was not to outwit authority, but to commit crime in order to gain wealth or power.

The motives of the *gamines* were different. Thus, *gaminismo* is a developmental stage which faces a nearly inevitable end as the child reaches puberty. This made adolescence for *gamines* a particularly difficult time because they had to give up so many of the acts that had brought them mastery and pleasure. The only way to maintain their hard-won sense of independence was to hide their haughtiness and accept poverty, a task which was not palatable to them. Having made one important life decision - to leave home at a time when most children were fully dependent on the decisions of their families - the *gamines* were forced by puberty to make another vital decision. One such decision was to become a small-scale entrepreneur. This allowed them to live outside of the mainstream and avoid being beholden to "bosses." If they could not do this, they would have to accept the servile life of a worker; that is, they became *chupagruesic*.

Chupagruesos also had difficult choices to make at puberty. Since they had not chosen to leave home, they lived with great emotional turmoil. As they approached adolescence, their problems were more related to gaining independence than losing it, to increasing self-respect rather than having to trim down excessive self-perceptions, and learning to live with their fears and lift their depression rather than curtail their grandiosity, as the gamines must. Paradoxically, the very servility which worked against them as small children on the streets helped them when they faced integration into adult culture. This style allowed them to be dependable and successful in menial jobs - the only kind of work available to them. Although the *chupagruesos* were thus more employable and able to avoid delinquency, they were rarely able to achieve the internal satisfaction experienced by the *gamines* who became small-scale entrepreneurs.[25]

What happens to street children as they get older? There are two different views on this question and not much hard data to support either one. In Brazil, Hecht (1998) notes that the lives of street children are short, they end up in prison, are killed or go insane (although he also notes that many 20 year olds say they are younger because

[25] Scheper-Hughes and Hoffman (1998) refer to the *Moleques*, who are the Brazilian street kids known for their charming but cunning entrepreneurial skills.

this generally affords them better treatment by the police). Raffaelli, (2000) reported particularly for street girls that they either die from abortion or STDs, or that they disappear (presumably into sexual slavery) or commit suicide.

Yet, Barker and Panter-Brick (2000) say that Nepalese street children pretty much return to normal poor working men and women. Aptekar (1988) reported that many Colombian street children became small scale entrepreneurs, finding something cheap in one place and selling it dearer in another.

Nieuwenhuizen (2006) found that in Bangalore, India the boys older than 15 years of age tended to leave the street. She offered several possible reasons. She found that the younger boys were better educated, and had more opportunities. They could more easily resolve their family situations. The older boys expressed an interest in returning to their rural origins.

Street children have their own order of development. Essentially, when they reach the size that suggests a social menace they are no longer street children, but thugs that scare the populace.

Comparisons of Street Children and Impoverished Domiciled Children

There are several studies which make comparisons between street children and their matched impoverished counterparts. If the street children fare better, one could argue that street children are not victims, but are the more resilient of the poor. For example, Wright et al. (1993) studied about 1,000 children, divided into two parts, one was made up of working children living at home. The other group was made up of street children not living at home. They were surprised to find that the street children had somewhat better nutrition and physical health than the street vendors.

Perhaps the most forceful comment based on a comparative study (in Jakarta, Indonesia) between street children compared to other poor children living at home showed that the street children had, at times, more financial resources than their poor counterparts and were not less healthy or underweight than their counterparts at home (Gross et al. 1996). This might well indicate that the street children worked better in their groups of peers than poor families, or it might mean that the street children had more resources due to having more social services (Gross et al. 1996).

In Northeast Brazil, "…street children do experience hunger at times. But most street children are probably better nourished than their siblings at home" (Hecht 1998, p. 54). In Nepal, street children suffer from less severe malnutrition than children from the countryside (Barker and Panter-Brick 2000). Also in Nepal, (Panter-Brick et al. 1996) slum dwelling kids were better nourished than rural children.

Panter-Brick has a long history of excellent public health studies in Nepal where she has made several physical health comparisons between homeless street children and both urban and rural poor children (Panter-Brick et al. 1996). In one study, she reports that one of her comparisons was directly between street children earning money by begging, foraging for food, and finding some items and reselling them, while the comparative group did the same thing, only at night they slept alone. The homeless kids (she reports on boys) were less deprived. In 2001 she used a finger prick sample of blood to determine the body's ability to ward off pathogens. While she mentions several possible sources of error in the data, she showed that homeless street children experienced significantly less ill-health than children of rural areas (Panter-Brick 2002). Both in Nepal and another study she conducted in Ethiopia, she showed that while middle class children did better than poor children, among the poor children the homeless did no worse than the ones who stayed in their families. She points out that the major British medical journal (British Medical Journal) in an article by Scanlon et al. (1998) reported that when street children are compared to children of comparable backgrounds they do as well.

They compared the physical health of street children and their matched counterparts living at home. They found that while street children suffered more physical trauma such as cuts bruises, sprains, etc. they had better nutrition than their counterparts. Some the advantage might come from begging and thievery, which is directed at food or means of obtaining food. They also cite evidence to show that the adults who help street children feel they are helping the children with low self-esteem, without the will power to succeed, and without discipline to achieve goals. However, the street children they are talking about aspired to many careers, have had experience in working toward their goals, and were adept at achieving them.

Aderinto's (2000) qualitative and quantitative study comparing 202 street children and 201 non street children in Nigeria (Lagos and Ibadan) using case studies and questionnaires found that street children had larger families (due to polygamy) with marital discord and little education, but the bottom line is poverty. The two samples that were compared were of street children and secondary school children living at home. Some of the school children were also working after school. The street children had left homes and lived on the streets.

Before the final study, a pilot was used to identify where and how to get in touch with the street children. The author found, for example, that during the workday they could not collect data, while they could do so early in the morning or late in the evening. They were only able to collect data during the workday if they, in essence, paid the street children for their time.

The pilot study also helped to refine the questionnaires that were to be the main instruments for data collection. There were two questionnaires, one for the street children and the other for the control group of secondary school students. Finally, Aderinto (2000) had 17 case studies with audio recordings to provide verbatim accounts of what street children said. There are also comments regarding how the sample was obtained, including the difficulty of getting access to street children, in contrast to the easy access to the school-going children.

The results indicated that 90% of the street children were male. He explains the gender imbalance in three ways. First, by differences in socialization, he believes girls are more supervised than boys. Secondly, he states that there are girls on the streets, but they are not there for long, in part, because they are more likely to get attention from their extended families than boys. The author notes the contrast; there are significantly more girls in school than boys.

The age range for the street children was from 8 to 18, but the majority of them were 14 and over. There was a difference in educational levels. Only 1 in 20 fathers of street children had any tertiary school education, while more than a quarter of fathers of in-school juveniles had a tertiary education. More than two thirds of the mothers of street children had no formal education at all. In contrast only one in five of the in-school sample had mothers with no formal education. There were also differences in marital patterns. Nearly two thirds of the fathers of street children were in polygamous marriages. Fewer than a third of the fathers of in-school students were in polygamous marriages. Religious affiliation between the two groups was not significantly different. This finding is not in line with the Plummer et al. (2007) study in Sudan which shows that Muslims are underrepresented.

What was significant in Aderinto's study (2000) was how many of the parents of school-going children were living together (80%) as compared to a very small percentage of the parents of street children. The street children worked. Thirty-eight percent were porters at the markets. Another third worked as bus assistants (a highly prized job), and the remaining street children washed cars. Getting any work was very difficult and conflict among the children was pitched.

More than two thirds of the street children said they left because their parents did not meet the expectations of what the children thought they should have. This included not having enough food and lack of support for getting work. Almost no street children said they left because their peers were on the streets. They left home because of the family disruption caused by polygamy. Since most of the fathers of street children have little education, are in low income producing jobs, and have more than one wife and a large set of children to support, there simply is not enough money to go around. The socio-economic situations for the urban poor are already dire enough. Street children, perhaps the strongest in their families, go out and provide for themselves. Indeed for many single parents, the only way to feed the family is to have children work. While he says that there are some similarities with school-going children in this regard, the burden of this problem falls more heavily on the mothers of street children.

Ninety-seven children were recruited and interviewed using a semi-structured psychosocial interview schedule; psychopathology was measured using the Strengths and Difficulties Questionnaire (SDQ) and the Mood and Feelings Questionnaire (MFQ). The results indicated that 70% of street children had significant scores for behavioral and emotional difficulties on the SDQ, and 74% had significant scores for depression on the MFQ. Current health problems were reported by 78%, with 43% described as persistent or severe. Two thirds of the children in this sample were not homeless but had chosen life on the streets in preference to permanent residence with their families. While there were high rates of physical and emotional problems in this population of street children, many were still connected to their families, emphasizing the importance of developing different approaches for street children, not all of whom need family counseling.

Landfried, Herman, Huang and Huang (2008), in a paper describing their project for street children in La Paz, Bolivia, compared at risk youth with street children. They found that school attendance, problems with the police, and physical abuse separated the two groups.

Davies (2008) did some comparison between street children in Western Kenya and poor domiciled children. He found that street children had a higher standard of living than domiciled children. In part this is because street children keep themselves in the public view, thus drawing more than their fair share of aid.

The males in his study found and exploited several economic opportunities. They cultivated relationships with small business owners. With them they negotiated odd jobs like cleaning their shops or their shop fronts. They ran a variety of errands and became part of the informal economy doing labor that others didn't want to do. Importantly, slightly more than half of the boys in this study not only had an economic relationship with a small scale entrepreneur, they had also developed a personal relationship. They also developed personal relationships with restaurant owners that led to getting leftover food items before they were thrown away.

They found other sources of income, always including scavenging for something they could find cheap and sell dear (from plastic bottles to charcoal). They carried luggage from train and bus stations and carried food during market days. Through this type of work, not only did they make money, but they cemented friendships. Most of the children who did this had a schedule, a routine and well thought out plans. It was not uncommon for street children to save their money for something special they wanted to buy.

Begging was less common that is assumed. It was not very profitable. Theft, was not considered righteous work, and Davies (2008) did not see much if any of it. It might be that in his case the town was small enough to make getting away with it unlikely.

What was common was sharing, and it had a code of behavior. If someone earned money it was his (or hers), and was usually not shared but used for buying something special or in case of an emergency. What was shared were clothes, food, and music if there was a means to listen to it. Not only did the sharing allow for spreading the wealth, but it built friendships and a system of reciprocity. All of these scenarios, from how they find and keep work, to sharing experiences and goods, are indicative of good mental health.

Looking further into the many studies that show street children with good mental health, at least as compared to their poor domiciled counterparts, two possible explanations come to mind, the differences of family abuse and gender differences. We have shown that family abuse for runaway boys and girls is higher in developed countries. As we will see, looking at gender, we find that abuse to runaways happens to both genders, while only to females among street children.

As street boys were resourceful, street girls are often victims. Aptekar (1988, 1989a) found that Colombian street boys by age 10–12 were able to maneuver the legal system. Each time they were arrested, they gave authorities a different name, which meant that with each offense they were given the light sentences afforded first offenders. When compared to other poor Kenyan boys, street boys worked and played in a far larger geographical area (Suda 1993). In their expanded geographical terrain, boys made many entrepreneurial deals; finding things cheap in one place and selling them dearer in another. This was not only their daily survival, but it took considerable cognitive skills (Aptekar 1989b, 1990). They often earned more than their mothers, and maintained contact with them; often earning sufficient money to share some of it with them (Kovats-Bernat 2006).

They were also aware of the importance of making peace with social workers so that their medical needs could be met when they were ill or injured. They knew where the programs were that served them, and were able to get food and shelter when needed (Aptekar and Ciano 1999).[26]

What we have are two large data sets from many countries that tell us that homeless youth in developed countries are having many mental health problems while street children in the developing world are resilient (those that break down the genders favor resilient boys).

There are studies that show street children with poor mental health (Ahmadkhaniha et al. 2007; Mathur et al. 2009; Sherman and Plitt 2005; Njord and Merrill 2008; Thabet and Matar 2011). Among Chinese street children in Shanghai (Cheng 2006), most suffered from hunger, cold, illness and psychological uncertainty. The rather harsh conditions, constraining the child to immediate survival strategies, with almost no compensation in terms of peer-group sociability, were, according to the author, an illustration of how psychological satisfaction can be reached only when physiological needs are met. It was the lack of satisfaction regarding basic needs that explained their low self-esteem and their corresponding low subjective well-being (Cheng and Lam 2010).

Most studies that show poor mental health come from reports by NGOs or other organizations seeking funds by preying on pity. And, to be fair, it can be difficult to ascertain the level of mental health. Kilbride et al. (2000) for example show, in Kenya, that it can be a mistake to equate street skills with good mental health. This is a proposition that might contradict many of the studies quoted above. Also, in most of these cases mentioned above, the gender divide is not clear. If more women were added it might reduce the overall functioning. Sometimes the results are not clearly presented. For example, Nieuwenhuizen (2006) said half of the street boys in Bangalore, India cut themselves; and she reported that a national report found the same for street girls. Going on to explain that while the street boys were aware of sexually transmitted diseases (although their terminology was not sophisticated), they were often forced into sex. Evidently, in spite of cutting themselves and being forced into sex, "the majority of children are in reasonable psychological shape and most of them are in better shape than their companions from comparable socio-economic status who live at home (p. 50)".[27] It is difficult to know how to respond to these contrasting images.

[26] It has been assumed that while street boys (and homeless boys) earned a livelihood in both legal (trading, begging) and illegal ways (stealing and fencing), female street children (and female homeless youth) become prostitutes. Thus it wasn't surprising that American runaway girls used sex as a way to get by and it was almost a necessity for girls as stealing or selling drugs were for boys (Paradise and Cauce 2002).

[27] Another problem is that there is a lack of deep structure to studies, even the ethnographies. Most mental health studies of both street children and homeless youth rarely look deeply into a child's life, including how street children love and show fear.

Another methodological problem with the above studies of the mental health of street children is that they are not clear about the time period studied; is it before or after they leave home? And, if both the good and the poor results are accurate, does it mean that there is a bimodal distribution of mental health?

A well planned study of street children in Jaipur, India suggests that abuse of all street children is high, but that when the abuse is examined in terms of type and severity and adjusted for gender, age and experience on the streets of the street children, a more nuanced result follows (Mathur et al. 2009).

The authors note the importance of understanding street children in India's context. There are 11 million children on the streets of India. It is, as the authors state, the county in the world with the largest number of children in difficult circumstances.

The study began by mapping the city of Jaipur, India for numbers of street children and then dividing the city into six zones. Then highly populated city centers and market places and other places where street children congregate such as the railway and bus stations were identified on the map. The study followed a type of sampling based on the snowball technique which meant that the street children were identified by another street child or someone who was familiar with them as workers. The authors were able to identify 478 street and working children in these areas. They added demographic information and from this they chose 200 street children of varied ages, incomes and geographical working areas.

Before administering the interview protocol to the children, it was evaluated by academics and those who work directly with the children. Based on the feedback received, the protocol was finalized and the authors conducted a pilot study with a group of 20 street children. Before implementing the final interview schedule, the authors gave themselves plenty of time to get to know the children and they state that they gained a level of rapport. In part this was possible through working very closely with specific cases often involving those who might have been sexually abused.

It is very helpful to the reader that the authors are clear about who is in their sample. They included working children but not children who begged. The final sample consisted of 100 boys and 100 girls. They were split equally into two age groups; 10–14 and 14+ –18 years old

The authors clearly explain their questionnaire. The categories of abuse included general abuse and neglect statements and included such items as the degree of parental care, the opportunity for education and the presence of a hygienic environment. There was a section on abuse related to health. In that part of the questionnaire the authors asked about the overall health of the child, including access to basic necessities such as clean water and adequate shelter, cleanliness and access to health services. Another category was verbal abuse from home, peers, while on the streets, at work, and from the police. Physical abuse was defined as being beaten (not just being hit once) under various circumstances including related to alcoholism and from various sources such as at home, from peers, the police, and while in the streets. Finally, they assessed for depression and suicidal ideation.

The authors coded four categories from 1 to 4; mild, moderate, severe, and very severe. The demographic information included socio-economic level, age, gender, religion, family background, income and place of residence, such as with family or in an institution, or on the streets. The article has both descriptive statistics, such as frequencies and percentages, and inferential information from t-tests and correlations.

The results indicate that the greatest areas of abuse were verbal and psychological. Boys were significantly more likely to be abused than girls. It was also significantly (.01) shown that the higher age children were more likely to be abused than the children in the younger group. Because the older group included children 14+ to 18 years of age, they would be more physically developed than the younger group of 10–14 years of age. This indicates that abuse is higher among the older children, and thus it would seem that the abuse has less to do with family than with societal reactions to having adolescents on the streets. Further results bear this out. For example, another significant positive correlation (.01) was related to income; the higher the income, the higher the abuse. Thus once the children were making money and older, they were met with severe reactions from the public, not least of which must have come from those in competition with them for income-earning opportunities.

It is also relevant to look at the various forms of abuse the older and higher income boys faced. At work they were continually exposed to unhealthy and unsafe working conditions, there were cases of cruelty in work their work settings, and they worked without written contracts.

The results indicate that as street children spend more time on the streets, thus getting older and earning more, they feel more abused by working conditions and from the public's response to them. The picture is less of family abuse than one of economic and social injustice. While Mathur et al. (2009) carried out the study to examine the prevalence, types and intensity of abuse in street children, what the study shows, in part because of its methodological sophistication, is that from the point of view of the majority of the street children in Jaipur, India, the major cause of abuse is not from their families, as would be assumed by the concept in the developed world, but from the societal and economic factors that we have mentioned which are associated with homeless children in the developing world.

Comparisons of Street Children and Homeless Youth

In addition to gender differences, there are other comparisons to be made between homeless youth and street children, particularly developmental differences, which bring in two new and related topics: 1.)- extended adolescence in the developed world versus a shortened adolescence in the developing world, and 2.)- differences regarding the power of the State to control child rearing in the developing and developed worlds.

Street boys rarely begin street life before they are 5 years old, yet many are in full control of their lives by 10 or 12 (Aptekar 1988). Aptekar (1992) reports seeing many Colombian street children who were so small they should have still been dependent on their mothers for many of their basic needs. They often weighed less than 70 pounds (32 kg) and were no taller than the tables at restaurants where they were routinely seen begging successfully for food from the patrons. But they developed many friendships, found programs available to serve them, and in many other ways acted much older.

The ages of male street children are comparable in other parts of the developing world. For example, The UN Committee on the Rights of the Child (2006) reported from Morocco that nearly 30% of street children were under 10 years of age and nearly 40% were between 10 and 14 years of age. In the study of Nairobi, Kenya, Aptekar and Ciano (1999) found the average age in a random sample of street children to be 12.58, (and a standard deviation of 2.15). In Ethiopia (Veale et al. 1993), the average age of street children was 10.7 years old. (The average age of beginning street life for boys was 9.96 for boys and 10.47 for girls).[28]

The age of onset for homeless youth in the developed world is later than it is for street children and lasts well into what we would consider young adulthood. The lives of street children end when they begin to take on the secondary sexual characteristic of men.

In the US, the average and modal age for runaway youth is 15 (reported in Shaffner 1999). In the Seattle Homeless Adolescent Research Project (Cauce et al. 2000), the age of entry into the study was 13. In the Johnson and Tyler (2006) study of American runaways, to be included a subject had to be between 19 and 21 years of age. This study was part of a longitudinal study that was specifically looking at the transition into young adulthood, which they say typically includes youth over 18 years of age.

In the developing world people this age would be considered full-fledged adults. Although there are age statutes that determine entry into adulthood, in the developing world they are far less likely to be applied by the State than in the developed world, because the State is stronger and likelier to enforce laws to get them off the streets.

Being an adult in the developing world has far less to do with the State and more to do with behavior. By the age of 17, almost all poor children are for any practical purposes adults. In Caracas, Venezuela, Marquez (1999) noted that around the age of maturity, a child is often not taken to a "rehabilitation center" for youth, but sent to adult prison. In the developed world youth and adults are for the most part separated when incarcerated, but not so much in the USA which is not a signatory to the UNCRC, because it does sometimes adjudicate children under 18 as adults and may imprison them in adult facilities, although this is rare.

Street children have a unique developmental life span. Essentially once they reach the physical appearance of adolescence, they are viewed as dangerous adults rather than as pitiful or bothersome children or youth. They are tolerated by society only when they are seen as pitiful or cute, but once they look menacing they are no

[28] When war is a factor, ages change. For example, in post conflict Rwanda (Veale and Dona 2003) the mean age was 14.2 and nearly half the Rwandan sample was over 15 years of age. While Hecht (1998) points out that in spite of being called "street children", most of the kids on the streets were adolescents, since adults were treated worse in the justice system, it was far better to be an adolescent for as long as possible. He knew of many 20 years olds who remained "street children" for years.

longer even given a fair shake, particularly by a society that fears the independence of poor people.[29]

If the children are small in size, yet independent of adult authority, they challenge society's concept of a child as innocent and in need of family protection. This makes people feel uncomfortable, because small children who are independent are incongruent with the notion of childhood. It is so much easier to grant these small children the status of helpless and dependent children, no matter how independent they may be, than to change the age of entry into adulthood (an example of cognitive dissonance, more on this later). This helps explain why small children are paid to clean the windows they had just dirtied, and may be described as cute, just at the moment they are picking someone's pocket.

Once the street children get big enough to appear menacing, their economic options are reduced. While children can beg, adolescents cannot. They must pick pockets or take purses, and then before long as they become older, they will be introduced to intermediaries working for drug dealers or forced into survival sex.

In fact most work that might be available to street children is sporadic or rare, dangerous, physically difficult, or boring. For example, working in the dump, which has also been a mainstay of employment for street children has many hazards to health because of pollutants and safety issues. Since scavenging involves carrying materials from the dump to another place, they are open to being robbed along the way.

The most likely successful business activity for street children is to find something cheap in one place and sell it dear in another. The urban slums of the developing world favor small scale entrepreneurs. In nearly every poor household one can see some form of nascent capitalism, selling something, offering tailoring services, or providing beauty care, etc. Street children grow up with this so when they take to the streets they are not new to self-employment.

The problem is that, as they stake out a geographical area and a kind of work that becomes effective, it will be taken over by an older child or an adult. This is the case in Mexico City where shoe shining, window cleaning and hawking newspapers, all activities once done primarily by street children, are now adult work (Aptekar personal observation, 2011).

While street children can hawk some items that require little capital, they can rarely apprentice with an artisan. If they look acceptable to foreign tourists, and they rarely do, they may work as informal tour guides, but this is atypical and not reliable income. They can do odd jobs such as carrying or cleaning things, but this is not consistent, as well as being hard work and boring. It is also open to abuse such as not getting paid. They can help their parents in their work, which is good if they have parents and if they work.

Since all of their work is either very competitive, dangerous or offers little financial reward, there is a tendency with age (although difficult to assess the time) to

[29] Heinonen (2011) notes that the conflict that befalls Ethiopian street children is that they have two developmental periods at the same time. Dependency, blind obedience and total deference to parents and all adults were associated with the ideal child and childhood. This was a heavy task to achieve for the street children she worked with since they were expected to be self-sustaining in the street, but instantly turn into dependent, malleable and voiceless children when at home.

look toward higher paid unlawful jobs such as working in the drug trade, or being carriers of illegal items. Then there is petty theft, which does not have a future and is dangerous.

Yet, the degree of criminal activity that street children engage in is not clear. Kovats-Bernat (2006) believes that few street children are involved in criminal activities and those who are involved tend to be the older boys. Nieuwenhuizen (2006) said that the longer street boys in Bangalore, India are in the streets, the more likely they are to use drugs including alcohol, glue and cannabis, and to be involved in criminal activities.

But once the law is broken, particularly if street children are older and appear menacing, the repercussions can be serious. In the Strengths and Difficulties Questionnaire (SDQ), the older street children face more serious repercussions than the younger ones from breaking the law (Marquez 1999). The police pick them up and hand them over to the adult justice system whereas the younger ones are treated like child delinquents. The point that Marquez is making is that developmental progression for street children is not just physical, but also social and political, and that the reason for this is that the public views them differently according to their age; from vulnerable children to delinquent adolescents to adult criminals.

Conclusion

In this chapter we showed that there were multiple definitions of non-domiciled youth. We divided them by homeless youth in the developed world and street children in the developing world. The origins of homeless youth are related to abuse. They are older than street children, more likely to come from middle class families, and roughly equal in number by gender. Street children are poor, but the boys usually are not abused while the girls usually are. We showed that street boys generally carry out culturally appropriate roles of coping with poverty by finding income generating sources in the streets. A newer vision of street children must include those who are victims of war, natural disasters, and statelessness. Many live in child headed households.

To find a way to understand all of the different dynamics, we introduced the concept of the Child-Street System (Lucchini 1993), which placed less emphasis on the child's characteristics and more on their reactions to the street. Six examples of different adaption strategies were offered: hero, hard worker, ambivalent, survivor, the isolated, and the dependent abused.

The career of street children and homeless is explained from leaving home to being fully engaged in street life. Gender is a key difference in this process. Almost all street children maintain family ties. At first they observe and find another newcomer to relate to. They soon learn whom to avoid and what to stay away from, as well as whom to rely on and where goods can safely be found. At some point the child is accepted by a group of existing runaway youth or street children.

Once on the street, the street children and homeless youth must cope with difficult circumstances. There are conflicting results on how well they do with some research suggesting that they fare poorly (particularly true for the homeless) and others that they do at least as well as the siblings they left behind (street boys). Gender considerations favor the mental and physical health of boys over girls.

References

Achenbach, T. (1991). *Manual for the youth self report and 1991 profile*. Burlington: University of Vermont Department of Psychiatry.

Aderinto, A. (2000). Social correlates and coping measures of street-children: A comparative study of street and non-street children in South-Western Nigeria. *Child Abuse & Neglect, 24*(9), 1199–1213.

Ahmadkhaniha, H., Shariat, V., et al. (2007). The frequency of sexual abuse and depression in a sample of street children of one of the deprived districts in Tehran. *Journal of Child Sexual Abuse, 16*(4), 23–35.

Aptekar, L. (1988). *Street children of Cali*. Durham: Duke University Press.

Aptekar, L. (1989a). Picaresque tragedies: The 'Abandoned' children in Colombia. *Phenomenology and Pedagogy, 7*, 79–92.

Aptekar, L. (1989b). Characteristics of the street children of Colombia. *Child Abuse & Neglect: The International Journal, 13*(3), 427–439.

Aptekar, L. (1990). Colombian street children: Gamines and Chupagruesos. *Adolescence, 24*(96), 783–794.

Aptekar, L. (1992). Are Colombian street children neglected? The contributions of ethnographic and ethno-historical approaches to the study of children. *Anthropology & Education Quarterly, 22*(4), 326–349.

Aptekar, L. (1994). Street children in the developing world: A review of their condition. *Cross-Cultural Research, 28*(3), 195–224.

Aptekar, L. (2004). A global view of street children in the third millennia. In B. D'Souza, E. Sonawat, & D. Madangopal (Eds.), *Understanding adolescents at risk* (pp. 1–29). Mumbai: Multi-tech Publishers.

Aptekar, L. (2010). *In the lions mouth: Hope and heartbreak in humanitarian assistance*. Bloomington: Xlibris.

Aptekar, L., & Abebe, B. (1997). Conflict in the neighborhood: Street children and the public space. *Childhood, 4*(4), 477–490.

Aptekar, L., & Ciano, L. (1999). Street children in Nairobi, Kenya: Gender differences and mental health. In M. Raffaelli & R. Larson (Eds.), *Homeless and working youth around the world: Exploring developmental issues: New directions for child and adolescent development*, Number 85 (pp. 35–46). San Francisco: Jossey Bass.

Ataov, A., & Haider, J. (2006). From participation to empowerment: Critical reflections on a participatory action research project with street children in Turkey. *Children, Youth and Environments, 16*(2), 127–152.

Ayerst, S. (1999). Depression and stress in street youth. *Adolescence, 34*(135), 567–575.

Bao, W., Whitbeck, L., & Hoyt, D. (2000, December). Abuse, support, and depression among homeless and runaway adolescents. *Journal of Health and Social Behavior, 41*, 408–420.

Barker, R., & Panter-Brick, C. (2000). A comparative perspective on children's "careers" and abandonment in Nepal. In C. Panter-Brick & M. Smith (Eds.), *Abandoned children* (pp. 161–181). Cambridge: Cambridge University Press.

Barry, P., Ensign, J., & Lippek, S. (2002). Embracing street culture: Fitting health care into the lives of street youth. *Journal of Transcultural Nursing, 13*(2), 145–152.

Beazley, H. (2000). Home sweet home? Street children's sites of belonging. In S. Holloway & G. Valentine (Eds.), *Children's geographies* (pp. 194–210). London: Routledge.

Bellot, C. (2000). La trajectoire: un outil dans la compréhension de l'itinérance. In D. Laberge (Ed.), *L'errance urbaine* (pp. 101–119). Ste-Foy: Editions MultiMondes.
Berland, J. (1982). *No five fingers are alike*. Cambridge: Harvard University Press.
Bettelheim, B. (1976). *The uses of enchantment: The meaning and importance of fairy tales*. New York: Knopf.
Blanc, C. (Ed.). (1994). *Urban children in distress: An introduction to the issues*. London: Gordon and Breach.
Boyden, J. (2003, Spring). Children under fire: Challenging assumptions about children's resilience. *Children, Youth, and Environments, 13*(1). Retrieved August 25, http://cye.colorado.edu
Campos, R., Raffaelli, M., Ude, W., Greco, M., Ruff, A., Rolf, J., Antunes, C. M., Halsey, N., & Greco, D. (1994). Social networks and daily activities of street youth in Belo Horizonte, Brazil. *Child Development, 65*, 319–330.
Castel, R. (1994). La dynamique des processus de marginalisation: de la vulnérabilité à la disaffiliation. *Cahiers de recherche sociologique, 22*, 11–27.
Cauce, A., Paradise, M., Ginzler, A., Embry, L., Morgan, C., Lohr, Y., & Theofelis, J. (2000). The characteristics and mental health of homeless adolescents: Age and gender differences. *Journal of Emotional and Behavioral Disorders, 8*(4), 230–239.
Cheng, F. C. (2006). The street children's street life and the victimizations against them: An ethnographic study. *Youth Studies, 9*, 1–9 (in Chinese).
Cheng, F. C., & Lam, D. (2010). How is street life? An examination of the subjective wellbeing of street children in China. *International Social Work, 53*(3), 353–365.
Conticini, A. (2008). Surfing in the air: A grounded theory of the dynamics of street life and its policy implications. *Journal of International Development, 20*, 413–436.
Cosgrove, G. (1990). Towards a working definition of street children. *International Social Work, 33*, 185–192.
Cyrulnik, B. (2002). *Un merveilleux malheur*. Paris: Odile Jacob.
Davies, M. (2008). A childish culture? Shared understandings, agency and intervention: An anthropological study of street children in northeast Kenya. *Childhood, 15*(3), 309–330.
de Benitez, S. (2011). *State of the World's street children: Research* (Street children. Series 2). London: Consortium for Street Children.
de Jesus, M. (1962). *Child of the dark: The diary of Carolina Maria de Jesus* (trans: St. Clare, D). New York: Dutton.
de Oliveira, W. (2000). *Working with children on the streets of Brazil: Politics and practice*. New York: Haworth Press.
de Queiroz, J.-M. (1996). Exclusion, identité et désaffection, dans. In S. Paugam et al. (Eds.), *L'exclusion. L'état des savoirs* (pp. 295–310). Paris: La découverte.
Dobrowolska, H., & Panter-Brick, C. (1998). How much does life style matter? Growth status and cortisol variations in Ethiopian children. *Social Biology and Human Affairs, 63*(1), 11–21.
Dufour, R. (2000). Trois vilains petits canards. Etude sur la filiation de parenté et la désaffiliation sociale. In D. Laberge (Ed.), *L'errance urbaine* (pp. 137–159). Ste-Foy: Editions MultiMondes.
Eberle, M. (2001). *Homelessness – causes and effects: Profile, policy review and analysis of homelessness in British Columbia*. Vancouver: Housing Management Commission.
Ennew, J. (1994). *Street and working children – A guide to planning* (Developmental manual #4). London: Save the Children.
Ennew, J., & Connolly, M. (1996). Introduction: Children out of place. *Childhood: A Global Journal of Child Research, 3*(2), 131–145.
Erny, G. (1981). *The child and his environment in Black Africa: An essay on traditional education*. Nairobi: Oxford University Press.
Felsman, K. (1981, April). Street urchins in Colombia. *Natural Histories,* 41–48.
Flowers, R. (2001). *Runaway kids and teenage prostitution: America's lost, abandoned, and sexually exploited children*. Westport: Praeger.
Fujimora, C. (2005). *Russia's abandoned children: An intimate understanding*. Westport: Praeger.

Gaetz, S. (2004a). Safe streets for whom? homeless youth, social exclusion, and criminal victimization. *Canadian Journal of Criminology and Criminal Justice, 46*(4), 423–455.

Gaetz, S. (2004b). *Understanding research on homelessness in Toronto: A literature review.* Toronto: York University and Wellesley Central Health Foundation.

Giannini, R. (2011). ODUMUNC 2011 – Issue brief for the UN General Assembly Third Committee: Social, Cultural, and Humanitarian (SOCHUM) – *The abolition of modern day child slavery.*

Goering, P., Tolomiczenko, G., Sheldon, T., Boydell, K., & Wasylenki, D. (2002). Characteristics of persons who are homeless for the first time. *Psychiatric Services, 53*, 1472–1474.

Gordon, R. (2004). Criminal organization, street gangs, and wanna-be groups: A Vancouver Perspective. In J. Schneider & N. Tulley (Eds.), *Gangs* (pp. 55–76). Aldershot: Ashgate.

Gross, R., Landfried, B., & Herman, S. (1996). Height, weight, a reflection of the nutritional situation of school-aged children working and living on the streets of Jakarta. *Social Science & Medicine, 43*(4), 453–458.

Hagedorn, J. (2006). The global impact of gangs. In J. Short & L. Hughes (Eds.), *Studying youth gangs* (pp. 181–192). Lanham: AltaMira Press.

Hecht, T. (1998). *At home in the street: Street children of northeast Brazil.* Cambridge: Cambridge University Press.

Heinonen, P. (2011). *Youth gangs & street children: Culture, nurture and masculinity in Ethiopia.* New York: Berghahn Press.

Huang, C., & Huang, K. (2008). Caring for abandoned street children in La Paz, Bolivia. *Archive of Disabled Children, 93*, 626–627.

Hyde, J. (2005). From home to street: Understanding young people's transitions into homelessness. *Journal of Adolescence, 28*, 171–183.

Invernizzi, A. (2003). Street working children and adolescents in Lima: work as an agent of socialization. *Childhood, 10*(4), 319–341.

Johnson, K., & Tyler, M. (2006). Trading sex: Voluntary or coerced? The experiences of homeless youth. *Journal of Sex Research, 43*(3), 208–216.

Kabeberi, J. (1990). *Child custody, care and maintenance.* Nairobi: Oxford University Press.

Kerfoot, M., Koshyl, V., Roganov, O., Mikhailichenko, K., Gorbova, I., & Pottage, D. (2007). The health and well-being of neglected, abused and exploited children: The Kyiv Street Children Project. *Child Abuse & Neglect, 31*, 27–37.

Kidd, S., Miner, D. W., & Davidson, L. (2007). Stories of working with homeless youth: on being "mind-boggling". *Children and Youth Services Review, 29*(1), 16–34.

Kilbride, P., Suda, C., & Njeru, E. (2000). *Street children in Kenya: Voices of children in search of childhood.* London: Bergen and Garvey.

Korbin, J. (1981). *Child abuse and neglect: Cross cultural perspectives.* Berkeley: University of California Press.

Kovats-Bernat, J. (2006). *Sleeping rough in Port-au-Prince: An ethnography of street children and violence in Haiti.* Gainesville: University of Florida Press.

Krabanow, J. (2003). Creating a culture of hope: Lessons learned from street children agencies in Canada and Guatemala. *International Social Work, 46*(3), 369–386.

Kufeldt, K., & Nimmo, M. (1987). Youth on the street. *Child Abuse & Neglect, 11*(4), 531–543.

Le Roux, J. (1996). Street children in South Africa: Findings from interviews on the background of street children in Pretoria, South Africa. *Adolescence, 31*(122), 423–431.

Lucchini, R. (1993). *Enfant de la rue. Identité, sociabilité, drogue.* Genève/Paris: Droz.

Lucchini, R. (2007). "Street children": Deconstruction of a category. In: I. Rizzini, U. Mandel D. Butler, D. Stoecklin (Eds.), *Life on the Streets. Children and Adolescents on the Streets: Inevitable Trajectories?* (pp. 49–75). Sion: Institut International des Droits de l'enfant.

Lutjens, S. (2000). Schooling and clean streets in socialist Cuba: Children and the Special period. In R. Mickelson (Ed.), *Children on the streets of the Americas* (pp. 55–65). New York: Routledge.

Mambwe, A. (1997). Stress and coping strategies amongst street children in Lusaka. *Journal of Psychology in Africa, South of the Sahara, the Caribbean and Afro-Latin America, 2*, 24–33.

Marquez, P. (1999). *The street is my home: Youth and violence in Caracas*. Stanford: Stanford University Press.

Masondo, G. (2006). *The lived-experiences of orphans in child-headed households in the Bronkhorstspruit area: A psycho-educational approach*. Masters Mini-dissertation. University of Johannesburg (full text: ujdigispace.uj.ac.za).

Matchinda, B. (1999). The impact of home background on the decision of children to runaway: The case of Yaoundé City street children in Cameroon. *Child Abuse & Neglect, 23*(3), 245–255.

Mathur, Me., Rathore, P., & Mathur, Mo. (2009). Incidence, type and intensity of abuse in street children in India. *Child Abuse & Neglect, 33*(12), 907–913.

Maxwell, B. (1992). Hostility, depression, and self-esteem among troubled and homeless adolescents in crisis. *Journal of Youth and Adolescence, 21*(2), 139–150.

McMorris, B., Tyler, K., Whitbeck, L., & Hoyt, D. (2002). Familiar and "on the street" risk factors associated with alcohol use among homeless and runaway adolescents. *Journal of Studies on Alcohol, 63*(1), 34–43.

Menke, E. (2000). Comparison of the stressors and coping behaviors of homeless, previously homeless and never homeless poor children. *Issues in Mental Health Nursing, 21*, 691–710.

Moberly, C. (1999). Creating policies which address the "voluntary separation" of children in Angola. In A. Schrader & A. Veale (Eds.), *Prevention of street migration: Resource pack* (pp. 36–50). London: Consortium for Street.

Monteiro, J., Campos, M., & Dollinger, S. (1998). An autophotographic study of poverty, collective orientation, and identity among street children. *Journal of School Psychology, 138*(3), 403–406.

Montgomery, H. (2000). Abandonment and child prostitution in a Thai slum community. In C. Panter-Brick & M. Smith (Eds.), *Abandoned children* (pp. 182–189). Cambridge: Cambridge University Press.

Moss, P., Dillor, J., & Statham, J. (2000). The 'child in need' and 'rich child': Discourses, constructions and practice. *Critical Social Policy, 63*(20), 233–254.

Mtonga, J. (2011). On and off the streets: Reasons why street children escape institutional care and their survival on the streets. Unpublished Master's Degree. Trondheim: Norwegian Centre for Child Research (NOSEB).

Muchini, B., & Nyandiya-Bundy, S. (1991). *Struggling to survive: A study of street children in Zimbabwe*. Harare: UNICEF.

Munyakho, D. (1992). *Kenya: Child newcomers to the urban jungle*. New York: UNICEF.

Naterer, A., & Godina, V. (2011). Bomzhji and their subculture: An anthropolitical study of street children subculture in Makeevka, Eastern Ukraine. *Childhood, XX*(X), 1–19.

National Runaway Switchboard. (2001). *News and research*. Available on line: http://www.nrscrisisline.org/news.asp

Nieuwenhuizen, P. (2006). *Street children in Bangalore, India: Their dreams and future*. Antwerp: Het Spinhuis Publishers.

Njord, L., & Merrill, M. (2008). Characterizing health behaviors and infectious disease prevalence among Filipino street children. *Journal of Adolescent Medical Health, 20*(3), 367–374.

Olly, B. O. (2006). Social and health behaviors in youth of the streets of Ibadan, Nigeria. *Child Abuse & Neglect, 30*, 271–282.

Onyango, P., Suda, C., & Orwa, K. (1991). *A report on the nairobi case study on children in especially difficult circumstances*. Florence: UNICEF.

Ozumba, G. O. (2004). African traditional metaphysics. *Quodlibet Journal, 6*(3), 1–5. (Full text: www.Quodlibet.net/articles/ozumba-africa.shtml)

Panter-Brick, C. (2002). Street children, human rights, and public health: a critique and future directions. *Annual Review of Anthropology, 31*, 147–171.

Panter-Brick, C., Todd, A., & Baker, R. (1996). Growth status of homeless Nepali's boys: do they differ from rural and urban controls? *Social Science & Medicine, 43*(4), 441–451.

Paradise, M., & Cauce, A. (2002). Home street home: The interpersonal dimensions of adolescent homelessness. *The Society for the Psychological Study of Social Issues, 2*(1), 223–238.

Patel, S. (1990). Street children, hotel boys and children of pavement dwellers and construction workers in Bombay – How they meet their daily needs. *Environment and Urbanization, 2*, 9–26.
Peatrie, L. (1968). *The view from the Barrio*. Ann Arbor: University of Michigan Press.
Plummer, M., Kudrati, M., & Yousif, N. (2007). Beginning street life: Factors contributing to children working and living on the streets of Khartoum, Sudan. *Children and Youth Services Review, 29*, 1520–1536.
Raffaelli, M., & Larson, R. (Eds.). (1999). *Developmental issues among homeless and working street youth: New directions in childhood development*. San Francisco: Jossey Bass.
Raffaelli, M. (2000). Gender differences in Brazilian street youth's family circumstances and experiences on the street. *Child Abuse & Neglect, 24*(11), 1431–1441.
Rapin, A. (2001). Entretien avec le neuropsychiatre Boris Cyrulnik. *Sciences Humaines.com, vol 45*.
Rizzini, I., & Lusk, M. (1995). Children in the streets: Latin America's lost generation. *Children and Youth Services Review, 17*(3), 391–400.
Roberts, A. R. (2000). An overview of crisis theory and crisis intervention. In A. R. Roberts (Ed.), *Crisis intervention handbook: Assessment, treatment and research* (pp. 3–30). New York: Oxford University Press.
Rosemberg, F. (2000). From discourse to reality: A profile of the lives and estimates of the number of street children and adolescents in Brazil. In R. Mickelson (Ed.), *Children on the streets of the Americas* (pp. 118–135). New York: Routledge.
Rotheram-Borus, J., Song, J., Gwadz, M., Lee, M., Rossem, R., & Koopman, C. (2003). Reductions in HIV risk in runaway youth. *Prevention Science, 4*(3), 173–187.
Scanlon, T., Tomkins, A., & Lynch, M. (1998). Street children in Latin America. *British Journal of Nutrition, 316*, 1596–1600.
Scheper-Hughes, N., & Hoffman, D. (1998). Brazilian apartheid: Street kids and the struggle for urban space. In N. Scheper-Hughes & C. Sargent (Eds.), *Small wars: The cultural politics of childhood* (pp. 352–388). Berkley: University of California Press.
Shaffner, L. (1999). *Teenage runaways: Broken hearts and "Bad attitudes"*. New York: Haworth Press.
Sherman, S., & Plitt, S. (2005). Drug use, street survival, and risk behaviors among street children in Lahore, Pakistan. *Journal of Urban Health, 82*(3), 113–124.
Smeaton, E. (2009). *Off the radar: children and young people on the streets in the UK*. London: Railway Children.
Smollar, J. (1999). Homeless youth in the United States: Description and development issues. In M. Raffaelli & R. Larson (Eds.), *Homeless and working children youth around the world: Exploring developmental issues* (pp. 47–58). San Francisco: Jossey-Bass.
Solorio, M., Milburn, R., Andersen, S. T., & Rodriguez, M. (2006). Emotional distress and mental health services use among urban homeless adolescents. *Journal of Behavioral Health Services and Research, 33*(4), 381–393.
Stewart, A., Steiman, A., Cauce, B., Cochran, L., & Hoyt, D. (2004). Victimization and post traumatic stress disorder among homeless adolescents. *Journal of the American Academy of Child and Adolescent Psychiatry, 43*(3), 325–331.
Stoecklin, D. (2000b). *A baseline survey of the street children of Chittagong City in Bangladesh*. Aparajeyo-Bangladesh / Terre des hommes. Dhaka: Aparajeyo-Bangladesh.
Stoecklin, D. (2008). Ecoute et participation des enfants en situations de rue. *Enfants en situations de rue. Prévention, intervention, respect des droits* (pp. 53–65). IUKB/IDE.
Stoecklin, D., Scelsi, M., Antony, E. (2013). Statut et carrière des mineurs séparés en Suisse: objets d'intervention ou sujets de droits? Revue Suisse de Sociologie.
Stonge, J. (2000). The education of homeless children and youth in the United States: A progress report. In R. Mickelson (Ed.), *Children on the Streets of the Americas* (pp. 66–76). New York: Routledge.
Suda, C. (1993). The impact of changing family structures on Nairobi children. *African Study Monographs, 14*, 109–121.
Taçon, P. (1985). *A UNICEF response to the needs of abandoned and street children*. Geneva: UNICEF.

Thabet, A., & Matar, S. (2011). Mental health problems among labor children in the Gaza strip. *Child: Care, Health and Development, 37*(1), 89–95.
Thompson, S., Pollio, J., Constatine, J., Reid, D., & Nebbitt, B. (2002). Short-term outcomes for youth receiving runaway and homeless shelter services. *Research on Social Work Practice, 12*, 589–603.
Tyler, K., Whitbeck, L., Hoyt, D., & Cauce, A. (2004). Risk factors for sexual victimization among male and female homeless and runaway youth. *Journal of Interpersonal Violence, 19*(5), 503–520.
U.S. Bureau of the Census. (1999). Poverty in the United States, 1998. In *Current population reports series*. Washington, DC: U.S. Government Printing Office.
UN Committee on the Rights of the Child (CRC). (2006). *UN Committee on the Rights of the child: Concluding observations, Morocco*, 17 Mar 2006, CRC/C/OPSC/MAR/CO/1. Available at: http://www.refworld.org/docid/45377ed80.html. Accessed 4 May 2013.
UNAIDS. (2002). www.unaids.org/barcelona/presskit/childrenonthebrink/introduction.pdf
UNICEF. (1986). *Children in especially difficult circumstances*. New York: United Nations Children's Fund (UNICEF).
UNICEF. (2006). *The state of the world's children 2006: Excluded and invisible*. New York: UNICEF.
Van den Bree, M. (2009). A longitudinal population-based study of factors in adolescence predicting homelessness in young adulthood. *Journal of Adolescent Health, 45*(6), 571–578.
Van Leeuwen, J., Boyle, S., Salomonsen, S., Baker, J., Hoffman, A., & Hopfeer, C. (2006). Lesbian, Gay, and Bisexual homeless youth: An eight-city public health perspective. *Child Welfare, 85*(2), 151–170.
Veale, A. (1992). Towards a conceptualization of street children: The case from Sudan and Ireland. *Trocaire Development Review, DR1992*, 101–120.
Veale, A. (1996). *An empirical and conceptual analysis of street children in Sudan and Ethiopia*. PhD dissertation, University College Cork.
Veale, A., & Dona, G. (2003). Street children and political violence: A socio-demographic analysis of street children in Rwanda. *Child Abuse & Neglect, 27*, 253–269.
Veale, A., Aderfrsew, A., & Lalor, K. (1993). *A study of street children in four regional towns in Ethiopia* (Report for UNICEF in conjunction with the Ministry for Labor and Social Affairs, Ethiopia). Cork: University College Cork.
Veale, A., Taylor, M., & Linehan, C. (2000). Psychological perspectives of 'abandoned and abandoning' street children. In C. Panter-Brick & M. Smith (Eds.), *Abandoned children* (pp. 131–145). Cambridge: Cambridge University Press.
Verma, S. (1999). Socialization for survival: Developmental issues among working and street children in India. In M. Raffaelli & R. Larson (Eds.), *Homeless and working children youth around the world: Exploring developmental issues* (pp. 5–18). San Francisco: Jossey-Bass.
Weber, M. (1922, 1968-english). *Economy and society*. New York: Bedminster Press.
Whitbeck, L., & Hoyt, D. (1999). Nowhere to grow: Homeless and runaway adolescents and their families. *Youth & Society, 22*(1), 109–125.
Whitbeck, L., Chen, X., Hoyt, D., Tyler, K., & Johnson, K. (2004). Mental disorder, subsistence strategies, and victimization among gay, lesbian, and bisexual homeless and runaway adolescents. *Journal of Sex Research, 41*, 329–342.
Williams, N., Lindsey, E., Kurtz, P., & Jarvis, S. (2001). From trauma to resilience: Lessons from former runaway and homeless youth. *Journal of Youth Studies, 4*(2), 233–253.
Wright, J., Kaminsky, D., & Wittig, M. (1993). Health and social conditions of street children in Honduras. *American Journal of Disabled Children, 147*, 279–283.

Chapter 3
Group Dynamics of Children in Street Situations

Children in Street Situations: Intragroup Behavior

In the last chapter we defined children in street situations and explored various demographic data about them. In this chapter we somewhat artificially divide them socially, into their intra and intergroup dynamics. This helps us answer some important questions about their alleged behavior (gangs, sex, and sub-culture) and their origins including the role of cultural and historical factors.

Street children in Colombia were organized into two groups; the *galladas* and the *camadas* (see Chapter 2 and Aptekar 1988). The *galladas* consisted of 20–25 children who associated with each other primarily for economic reasons. The children stayed together as a group in order to divide the labor that could make them all more successful than if they acted alone or in smaller groups. As is the case with most business partners, they rarely associated outside of work.

The leadership of the *galladas*, as well as the majority of its members, had been on the streets for a long time and had adopted a somewhat delinquent lifestyle along with the associations such a style brought. As in Kenya, (Davies 2008) the oldest and usually most ruthless street boy ruled the roost, becoming the leader inside the group and the contact between the group and the outside world, usually through those adults who fence material from the street children.

Although the *galladas* were composed mainly of adolescents, there were some pre-adolescents who helped bring in the goods. In addition, there were a few adults who helped integrate the children's economy into the larger culture. The *gallada* was integrated into the poor urban subculture.

The ultimate authority of the *gallada* resided with the adolescent *jefe (chief)*, who maintained his power and prestige by physical prowess, intelligence, and the ability to "fence" the products of his labor. The *jefe* not only had to learn how to control his *sub-jefes* and members, but also had to acquire the appropriate skills for dealing with the established criminal element. This gave him and his *gallada* access to more lucrative goods and a place to cash in what they had. The *jefe* knew how to cultivate and maintain friendships with adults such as street vendors, restaurant

L. Aptekar and D. Stoecklin, *Street Children and Homeless Youth: A Cross-Cultural Perspective*, DOI 10.1007/978-94-007-7356-1_3,

Fig. 3.1 A "*Camada*"

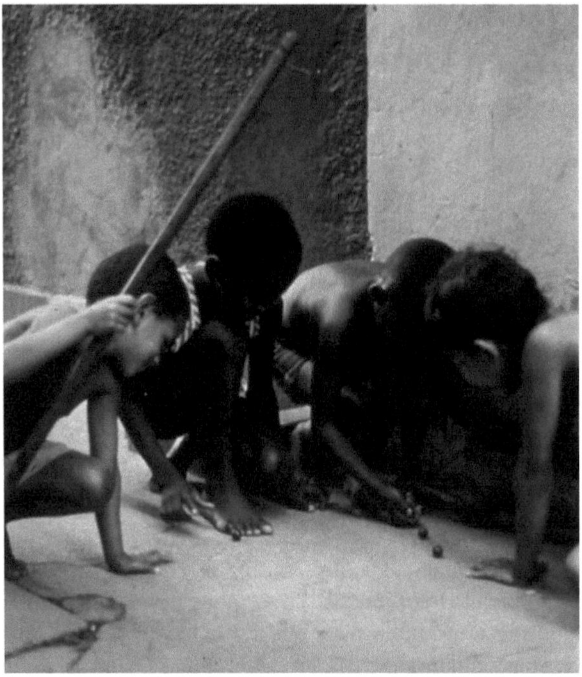

owners, and taxicab drivers, all of whom occasionally fenced his materials, even if they were not fully committed to a criminal existence. These skills cemented the *jefe's* power over the group, since they relied on him and his connections to bring them what they needed and wanted. The *jefe* was the bridge between the street children and the subculture of urban poverty.[1]

There was quite a difference between the way the pre-adolescent *chupagruesos* and the *gamines* (see Chapter 2) responded to the *galladas*. The *gallada* was suited for the *chupagrueso*, who learned quickly what was expected of him. He was reliable to those whom he saw as having power, and did what was necessary to stay in their good graces. The *chupagruesic* style helped maintain the integrity of the hierarchy and method of doing business. However, the *gamine* used the *gallada* only so long as it helped him. He had little respect for authority *per se*, and maintained his allegiance to the powerful only so long as it served him better than he could do on his own, or in another *gallada*.

In comparison, the *camadas* were composed of small groups of two or three pre-adolescents who shared intimacies and camaraderie. These groups were different from the *galladas* in that they were more like family and friends than business partners (Fig. 3.1). Davies (2008) calls their relationship symbiotic; each member bringing complementary skills that make the group stronger (in Davies' case, Kenya). The children in the *camadas*, or as Davies calls them, "dyadic-apprenticeships

[1] Not all authors found a similar hierarchy. Davies (2008) for example saw no formal hierarchy among the street children in a small town in North Western Kenya.

(2008, p. 317)" were in the middle childhood developmental stage, a time when friendships consist primarily of two-person, same-sex dyads.

The *camadas* existed not for economic or pathological reasons, but because, as Sullivan (1953) suggested, this is the time of psychological development when such friendships are most needed. By forming chumships[2] they were able to deal with the demands of street life in a rather healthy manner. In fact, chums were nearly synonymous with *camadas*. The problem was that chumship ended at puberty when, as Sullivan noted, "lust" for the opposite sex pulled the relationship apart. One pre-adolescent, for example, began puberty and an interest in friendship with the opposite sex earlier than his companion, which made his chum extremely lonely at times. As a result, he sought out another chum, one who was younger. When that did not work, he joined a *gallada* and became an isolated and marginal figure which only added to his loneliness. This phenomenon occurred often, because it was rare that the breaking of a chumship was simultaneous.

Davies (2008) noticed a similar social formation in his study of street children in northwest Kenya. In this case he found that there were dyadic relationships that were essential to becoming a group member. The dyads were same sex groups of two. One was a more experienced leader who had been at one time the new initiate in a dyad, and whose job it was to help the less experienced member of the dyad. Learning from the older child, the younger member developed a strong personal attachment to him. Davies says the relationship was not exploitative. He described it as symbiotic. In the dyads food was shared, they slept together in the same place, and they played together. They appeared affectionate with one another, hugging and holding hands. They took care of each other when one was sick and recognized each other as special partners.

It is through the dyads that children are incorporated into the culture of street children. Thus the smaller children new to the street are not left to fend for themselves. They have an enjoyable and structured way to become part of the group of street children. This takes time. Most of the children are living at home at the beginning, but as time progresses they slowly leave home to join the group.

Davies (2008) says that it is through the learning experience that goes on in the dyad that the subculture of street children is built and renewed. He asks if this dyadic life in the subculture of street children is not, given the options that these children face, a better choice than being demeaned as part of the urban poor. Most street children see themselves as being a members of a valued street children subculture.

With the passing of chumship came the demise of the *camada*. Like flowers in bloom, the *camadas* were intense, but ephemeral; beautiful but carrying the seeds of their own destruction. Because of these developmental differences, the internal dynamics of the *camadas* were different from those within the *galladas*. There was less formal organization in the *camada*, less delinquency, and the *jefe* was less

---

[2] A chum is a good friend, pal, or buddy. The term comes from British student slang for a dormitory roommate (chamber fellow). Sullivan (1953) referred to chumships as a unique developmental period of pre-adolescence when boys played with boys and experienced their first love outside of the home. He felt it was a necessary developmental stage needed to later have a healthy heterosexual love relationship.

important. Since the pre-adolescent children usually were fairly successful in getting food, by relying on their youthful image and thereby posing less of a threat to the public, they were able to secure their basic needs. Thus, they had less reason to obtain goods that had to be fenced. This reduced their level of delinquency and dependence on a *jefe*. Because the pre-adolescent children in the *camadas* came together more for personal than for business reasons, their relationship with each other was more intimate, resulting in less hierarchy and formal organization.

The *gamines* moved among *galladas*, frequently residing in any one *gallada* only as long as it served their economic needs. *Chupagruesos*, on the other hand, needed the *galladas* for both personal and economic reasons, and they often found themselves deeply attached to a *gallada,* or a particular *jefe*. When the *chupagruesos* reached puberty, they were particularly hard hit by the change; they had not been able to enjoy their chumships in their *camadas* as a result of needing to attach themselves to the *jefes* in the *galladas.*

The *camadas* were composed only of pre-adolescent children; the *galladas* were run by adolescents, but also included pre-adolescents. The pre-adolescents joined the *galladas* in groups that corresponded to their chumships. Typically, at the end of each day's work, a group of chums who were in the same *camada* left the larger business arrangement of the *gallada* and went to their pre-arranged private spots to sleep. In the morning they rejoined a *gallada,* either to work, as in the case of the *gamines,* or for personal and economic reasons, as in the case of the *chupagruesos.* When the pre-adolescent children wanted the older children to help them integrate into adult society, they also turned to the *galladas.*

Marquez's (1999) discussion of social groups of street children in Venezuela begins with the *Huelepegas*, the glue sniffers, who are ubiquitous (seemingly in all developing world cultures) and whose identification includes the carrying, if not caressing, of a bottle, from which they sniff intoxicant. In Venezuela they are the dirtiest and the youngest (between 9 and 13 years of age) and always on the move to avoid police and bullies. Their favorite activity, besides inhalants, is playing video games and bathing in the public fountains. One *Huelepega* described himself like a floating beer can found in the middle of the ocean. The video games provide them with a small entrance into the global economy and technological sophistication.

Marquez (1999) also notes the importance of their friendships; sleeping together for warmth, but also for the pleasure of touching each other. Because they are so young, they are pitied, seen as dependent and in need of support, like all children. But because they are drug abusers, they are also looked upon as delinquents.

There is also an inevitable decline of public acceptance as they grow facial hair, look stronger, and appear less pitiful and more menacing. By this stage, they become interested in heterosexual activities, having more money and increased safety, and perhaps use more drugs. Those who grow into delinquents, particularly those who become involved with smoking *basuka* (the residue of purifying cocaine, something like crack cocaine), often become involved with the drug trade (Young and Barrett 2001).

At this time, they graduate from being *Huelepegas* into being *malandros* or *monos*. These are the adolescents running in the streets. The distinction is in skin color. The darker skinned *monos* (monkeys) come from the shanty towns, and are trying to make an impression by showing they have money. Thus they are the ones who have a modern haircut and who are dressing as they imagine the hip youth in American cities do, i.e., with baggy pants hanging below their hips. They also listen to working class *salsa* music, thus separating themselves from the children living in the barrios, who are considered common criminals. The *malandros* are the leaders who have secured enough resources to dress like the television heroes that the children in the barrio admire. By doing so, they indicate that they are more successful and less common than the *monos*.

The *Malunde*, a group of street children in Johannesburg (Swart 1990), had a complex set of rules for reciprocity in groups. Each person knew who owed whom what, and if the person in debt did not eventually pay off, they were excluded from the system of friendships. Altruism did not exist. Money was lent with the idea that it would be paid back in full. Food lent or shared was expected to be paid back in full either with equal kind or money. But begged food had its own sense of rules (as it did among the Ethiopian poor, see Aptekar 2010). It was to be shared without incurring the demand to be repaid.

Illness held a very high valence among groups of street children. It was perhaps, (along with bereavement) the time that the group acted most as a family by being counted on to help. This was the only time they shared valuables without counting on getting something in return, in short, the closest to true altruism.

Stoecklin (2000a) distinguishes two types of groups in Shanghai according to several themes that appeared through interviews and that can be considered as indicators of the way the children make sense of their experiences. The "beggars" (*taofan*) are constantly confronted by violence from the supervisors if they do not bring in enough money. They do not experience the full range of street life where harsh conditions are compensated by a high level of autonomy, as is the case for the second group, the "vagrants" (*liulang*).

Being exploited together with their parents, the beggars develop a familial solidarity strategy, whereby the strict control by adults reduces their strategies to the question of how to maximize the income and minimize the risks of being kicked or beaten by passers-by who treat them with hostility. They resolve this dilemma mainly by asking other migrants to help them by giving them some small money, or look for coins lost under the seats of taxis that just brought some passengers to the train stations. They rarely ask the Shanghai residents for money, as their reaction is violent.

The vagrants, on the other hand, have a lot of autonomy. They develop defiant attitudes to challenge the social reactions toward them. The vagrants are more targeted when it comes to repression by the police. They are sent to deportation stations in order to be repatriated in their rural hometowns. The vagrant children are often caught because they correspond to the Chinese official definition of the "street child" (*liulang*): "a child below the age of 14, who left home without parental supervision, without a definite destination, and without any legal method to make a living" (Tao Zhiming 1995, p. 9).

Meanwhile, the official response of sending them back home or to reeducation schools didn't address their main problem. As Cheng (2008) demonstrates, initially coercive parenting and/or the lack of parenting (not poverty) are the main causes of children entering into street life. Out of the 49 street children examined in his study, 32 linked their choice to leave home with the neglect, abandonment, or abuse they suffered in their families. To authorities, the problem is that these children are illegal wanderers; to the children, the problem is that they were mostly confronted with violence at home. The public's reaction, ignoring their harsh experiences and concentrating on their visible and possibly threatening behaviors, reinforces their feelings that their sufferings are not acknowledged.

Chinese street children, (like most across the globe) use the street space in different ways than do members of rule-abiding society, provoking a reaction against them as they are seen as "outsiders". Once labelled as such (in China the term *waidilaide* – those who come from outside – is frequently used to speak of the floating population), street children tend to accept this label and begin to view themselves as different from "mainstream" society. Thus they start what Becker (1963) calls a career of secondary deviance. Being caught by the police, or stigmatized by passers-by, is a crucial experience leading to crime as a reasonable way to respond to rejection and to adapt to the new identity one is labelled with.

As the official response and the social reaction are not addressing the root causes of children surviving in the streets, these children are denied the means of carrying on a normal everyday life. Any "outsider" denied the means to carry out daily routines most often turns to illegitimate means to make a living. This is how children who were victims of violence at home may end up involved in "criminal" activities that are functional not only to survive but also to maintain a coherent identity: they enter into and actively elaborate a deviant subculture. This affiliation with an organized group provides street children with moral support. Thereby they develop a self-justifying rationale, in turn defining dominant rule-abiding members of society as illegitimate and ridiculing them. This can be illustrated with the following example:

Three boys, Tong, Chang and Xiang, smoke cigarettes and shout and laugh at some tea and egg sellers; they make noise in order to attract attention. A little while later, they have met two girls and smoke another cigarette with them. The boys seem particularly proud to show themselves as being tough guys. Suddenly, Tong points his cigarette at an old beggar who was approaching: he wants this old beggar woman to leave this place which he apparently considers as being their own space. What is interesting here is that Tong takes on the role of Shanghainese passers-by who are generally rude to beggars. In fact, Tong proves his ability to identify these symbolic, stereotypical reactions and by over-dramatizing them, he ridicules the Shanghainese and provokes a social reaction (Stoecklin 2000a).

The differential treatment of beggars and vagrants is due to the discretion of the police.[3] As the vagrant children want to be independent, and consequently refuse the "protection" of a patron, they are caught in police round-ups. With the unpredictable character of police arrest, the vagrants are not in a position to constitute fixed

[3] The "bosses" who exploit the little beggars and their parents are also in a position to bribe the police.

territories. Thus routine activities and sociability are limited and peer groups are all the more important on a short-term basis.

Also, because of police round-ups, the links between peers are fragile and actually only groups with fragile and changing peer relationships can be seen. This helps explain why street children have survival strategies that are linked to their capacity to establish a reputation as someone who is courageous and free. The problem is that while their provocative attitude is a defense strategy, they are made to be seen as delinquents.

The confrontations they receive from these social reactions become central elements in their lives. Thus (like the example of little Mogadishu below) when these children smoke cigarettes, they are "on stage." They look at themselves and they take on the attitudes of others toward them. In order to compensate for the degradation of self, the vagrant children incorporate the repressive characteristics of the street as part of their presentation of self and as part of a collective identity. This actually happens only if the children have sufficient competences to distance themselves from dominant norms, which is not the case with the smaller beggar children.

Even if the two types of children experience a deviation from dominant social norms (children have to stay at home and go to school), only the elder ones, the vagrants, subjectively distance themselves from these norms and experience a positive redefinition of their identities. It is only when the children have access to and develop peer-group sociability, collective identity and strategic competences that a child can spare some time not dedicated to immediate survival activities. The construction of this relative satisfaction contributes to the motivation of staying in the street. Therefore, the social determination of a street child's personality seems to be quite important in the Chinese context. Likewise, the differences between vagrant and begging children cannot be understood without considering the cultural factors influencing behaviors in the street. The marginalizing effects of the one-child policy for the "out-of-plan" begging children and the repression of street life for all children impose clear limits to their autonomy.

Is There a Subculture of Children in Street Situations?

Our hypothesis is that children in street situations (both street children and homeless youth) are a subculture of childhood that is by contrast different from the dominant societal view of childhood.[4] They are essentially an urban phenomenon

[4] It should be noted that not all authors think that street children are a subculture. Heinonen (2011) points out that in Ethiopia groupings of street children had cultural values quite in line with what is socially acceptable: "*They judged and valued each other's qualities or defects with the same conventions and social expectations used by mainstream society*" (p. 111).

organized for survival.[5] They share a lifestyle which is behaviorally distinct from the larger populace of children. Some of their activities, such as begging or buying discarded or uncared-for items cheap and selling them dear; or using and selling illegal drugs, are seen by the larger culture as pejorative. Children in street situations share on a daily basis their food, cigarettes, drugs, and they take care of one another when one of them is injured or sick. And in addition to earning money in common ways, they often spend it to define themselves in relation to the dominant adolescent culture in their society. For example, in some cases they have enough for buying new clothes but they don't because it would violate their subcultural standard, which in the case of street children is to look dirty and disheveled (Davies 2008), and in the case of homeless youth, is to dress in counter-culture attire to stand out from the larger youth culture. A similar situation exists for those homeless youth who have enough money to buy clothes or to get tattooed and pierced so that they can be contrasted to their domiciled peers while they shabbily mimic the world-wide youth culture of entertainment. As Smollar (1999) points out, homeless youth in the USA form a group of self-support that offers them a sense of connectedness, but alienates them from the larger society.

In Davies (2008) own words, he finds that street children in Kenya developed their own subculture from their interactions with main stream society. I quote:

> *"In terms of street children, majority experiences of childhood ('normal' childhood) are contrasted with the observed behaviors of 'street children' (that is children who are unable to comply, or for whom it is undesirable to comply [by remaining at 'home'], with ideas of acceptable childhood behavior) and new modes of interacting with these children are developed. These new modes of interaction often marginalize 'street children' in various ways, such as denying them equal status (i.e. a belief that as abnormal children, or even abnormal humans, they lack the needs of normal children) or embodying them with characteristics or abilities that may, in reality, be beyond (or strain) their actual physical and/or emotional development (i.e. seeing them as tough, resilient, self-sufficient and dangerous, etc.). In this manner, the dominant pattern of practice, what we might term the dominant discourse or hegemony, is able to conceptually accommodate street children through denying their needs (p. 313)".*

He goes on to build his case by showing that street children are not passive recipients of the dominant culture. Street children engage the mainstream culture, even though it is often in reaction to the pejorative attitudes of the main culture. As he says, the formation of street children culture results from having certain behaviors and beliefs that can only be understood in relation to the wider society. Therefore he says street children have their own subculture.

What Davies sees as central to street children subculture is their incorporation of the dominant and negative view of them held by mainstream society. In the process of adapting the enemy's viewpoint, the street children, by acting out these stereotypes, are in effect participating in painting the picture of themselves as outsiders. He believes they do this because it gives them a certain freedom. At least in the circle of how their otherness is defined they are free to act; by living within

[5] While they are usually found in the capital city, they are also in district capitals and even small towns. See Davies (2008) for the street children of Mukutano, Kenya.

acceptable dimensions they insulate themselves from the negative view of mainstream culture. This is why, he says, they wear a unique style of clothes that identifies them as street children and develop their own argot to communicate among themselves but also to be identified as street children.

In fact they have adopted, by accepting and broadcasting the accepted society's view of them, a subculture that by definition is anti-mainstream. They threaten dominant culture because their very existence is a challenge to mainstream mores.

In fact, Davies (2008) goes further in saying there is more than one subculture of street children, although they may share the above characteristic of existing within the context of the larger and accepted mainstream culture. As a large subculture, the street children of northwest Kenya, called *chokrra*, meaning garbage pickers, by the public, are clear about their characteristics; they don't go to school, they scavenge, beg, steal, sniff glue and are not clean like us. Like, most generalizations there is some truth to these, and like other generalizations, they obscure the differences. As we have shown in a variety of the literature presented, and as Davies finds in this study, the lives of street children are not the same. Some live at home, others do not, some are orphans some have full families, some are permanently outside of their homes of origin, while others never leave them, etc.

Davies (2008) presents the idea that street children cannot be defined in relationship to living or working on the streets. He defines them as having a clear intra-group structure with a shared culture which is always malleable through their own continual interactions with mainstream culture. Thus he argues for groups of subcultures of street children.

The same can be said of homeless youth, whose peer relationships are an essential element of their subculture (Schaffner 1999). In supporting each other, they look out at "others", the mainstream culture, and point out how they are different. This is one of their strategies which allow homeless youth to come into adulthood (Paradise and Cauce 2002). Through a system of sharing, they learn to improve their self-esteem, and separate themselves from the problems of their families of origin (Schaffner 1999).

Similar to their support for each other is the importance of siblings among homeless youth. Given the trouble of family life, siblings either support each other by acting as buffers to their parents, or they turn against each other as a way of taking out their anger. In one study, sibling relationships among homeless youth went from love to hate, from being uninvolved to very protective. But more times than not, in the long run they supported each other (Schaffner 1999). Older siblings felt guilty when they ran away because it meant abandoning their younger siblings at home in such bad situations. The point is that this "on-again/off-again" cycle of sibling and family ties, with its concordant guilt and anger, is a normal part of their subculture.

Homeless youth have many coping mechanisms beyond just peer support and help from siblings. They share an ability to make quick decisions, a flexibility in dealing with problems, and an unusually developed sensitivity to adults. These unique strengths are part of their subculture.

But in spite of the variety of subcultures, Davies (2008) claims there was only one culture of street children in his study and that is was unanimously clear to the children and to the public who was and was not a street child. There were 42 street children; 4 were girls and 38 were boys. Their ages ranged from 6 to 18 years old, with a mean age of 12.5 years. They had a clear leader, *kichwa* (in Kiswahili, this means 'head'), who was the oldest and biggest and with the important role of being the contact between his group and various groups that his group would be in contact with such as police and local employers.

When street children and homeless youth gather together they identify each other as being of a common element that differs from the general population. They have their own argot, which is widely enough spoken that the public knows of it. The words are taken from the *lingua franca* and are modified by pronunciation, by reducing the number of syllables, by dropping a prefix or a suffix, or by giving the word another meaning, making it different enough from the lingua franca that it is beyond being easily understood by the general populace.

The street language found in the Ukraine by Naterer and Godina (2011) shows how the vocabulary of street children is a cohesive force for the group, while also a force toward isolating them from the public. Their slang is vulgar and taken from Russian vocabulary, truncated, modified in composition and pronunciation and concatenated into new, subcultural words.

Lucchini (2007) shows several reasons why street children are a subculture. These include the acceptance and the initiation of neophytes into the group; the rules of cooperation and, eventually, of solidarity that guide the relations between the children; the sanctions and rewards that connect these rules; the mediation of conflicts within the group; the relations with people outside the group (adults and children); the basis of trust and, therefore, the social ties on the street; and also the representation of justice for the child on the street. This applies also to homeless youth.

Both homeless youth and street children are also subcultures in other ways. They use physical space with its own rules of behavior and typically a predictable public response. Thus different activities may have separate physical areas. One important category is public space, which are the places in the city where children in street situations conduct business on their own (begging, picking pockets, and other illegal activities). These behaviors in the public space define who they are in comparison to the social norms of society.

Naterer and Godina (2011) saw groups of between 5 and 15 Ukrainian street children coming together for specific reasons and uniting with some of the same or with different street children if the situation called for it. They cite such factors as weather, the local political situation, and the pressure from police.

They note some very specific ways in which the subculture of street children differ than other subcultures. More commonly, subcultures have a commercial element. The image of street children is based on looking pitiful. What the authors point out is that the street kids have plenty of money to buy clothes that are not ragged. They have the money to buy new clothes. Yet they don't. Only by dressing in dirty and old clothes can one become a member of the subculture of street children.

The authors discuss the fact that in most cases subcultures reflect the values of the subculture in comparison to the dominant culture. Most subcultures have a wide choice of "costumes" to choose from in the commercial marketplace. Indeed many styles are the result of market forces. There is a relationship between the desirability of a particular subculture which is dependent on the desirability of its specific image in the society. The authors point out that these street children (and homeless youth) are in this respect deviant. They cannot and do not go to the market place for their icons because their image cannot be reduced to a set of stylistic garments or hair styles.

Like other subcultures, street children and homeless youth receive their definition partly by what they do, or claim to do in the case of those who just dress the part, and society's attitude toward them. These feelings are based on subcultural norms and mores. Thus outsiders might see street children as helpless victims, while the researcher who knows them better knows of their manipulative skills, and to their peers they are seen as friends or foes. What is unique is that all of this is indeed part of their survival skills. Unlike gangs who are delinquent and deviant, street children are for the most part deviant and not very delinquent.

The difference between deviance and delinquency is explained by sociologists in terms of an attitude or behavior that violates a social or cultural norm (deviance) and an act that violates a legal norm (delinquency). Becker (1963) has shown that many people may be deviant without being delinquent. This is also the case with street children.

Probably the most important part of the subculture of children in street situations is the importance of solidarity. Solidarity is the basis for the collective identity of street children and homeless youth.

Naterer and Godina (2011) define solidarity in a collective sense and point out three spaces where it is manifested; on the macro, meso and micro levels. They refer to the macro level to include not just single groups of street children, but the collective of street children in the city or even beyond. They introduce the Russian word *Guliat*, which not only has the manifest meaning of roving or strolling that is common to the word in the dictionary, but is also used by the subculture as a collective self-identification that is a construction of common values, ways to communicate with each other, and their code of friendship. The use of the word is particularly poignant when used by different groups of street children, thus if one group member is talking to a member in another group and uses this word, it establishes solidarity between groups.

The use of this word is really an acceptance of a code that indicates accepting reciprocity (and obligation). By sharing this, they come together to fend off outside forces which might be detrimental to all, such as a particularly broad police sweep.

A lower level of solidarity, which they refer to as the meso level, includes two forms of subcultural identity; assimilation and integration. The authors suggest that the more time a child spends on the streets, the more they integrate into the subculture by accepting all forms of the subculture, including its norms, language, image and attitudes. It is the most experienced kids who are in charge of subculture. They are at the center of the group, while newcomers are at its periphery. The core group finds it harder to change their subculture and accept a more mainstream way of life, while the newcomers can more easily do so.

The reason for this is that the support the group gives to its new members builds up over time, so that by the time the experienced children are in the core of the group and they are less likely to give it up. Some of these support activities take place even before a child becomes a fully fledged member of the street group.

It begins by giving emotional support to compensate for the loss of family, and in providing a new social support network, which includes new social roles, and a new form of hierarchical authority. Over time, this forms a new family support system. The authors show that in one of their groups there was a clear family-like structure that included a mother and a father (both played by boys) each with his or her own gender related roles. The children turned to the father for advice and protection. He was also the one who made the important decisions for the group. The mother was in charge of the "house". She balanced the budget, bought the food, took to the doctor those that needed medical attention and gave emotional support for those in need of this kind of caring. The group thus made itself into a family providing for needs that asked for attention now that the children had left their families.

We cannot speak of the behavior of subgroups of street children without discussing how they provide physical support for one another. This involved protection against the police, gangs, or anyone from the public. In spite of the rough play of bigger children toward smaller ones, the support they feel from the group, against physical abuse from the outside, helps to build group identity and solidarity. Thus, in spite of being treated very badly at times within the group, weaker group members can expect to have food shared, smoke cigarettes when they are available, use inhalants and have some money to spend. They can also get help when they are sick or injured, if even only to walk the child to the emergency room. All of this builds group solidarity.

Once a child is part of the group, he or she has more opportunities to earn money. As a group member, he or she is more likely to be able to get hand outs from vendors who make deals with the groups that are mutually profitable. A group of street children might guard a vendor's assets allowing him to leave the premises without worrying about them, in exchange for clothes, food, etc. The vendors might even employ the children at low wages.

The group of street children that lives in a particular marketplace also prevents street children who are not members of the group from participating in any of the economic activities at "their" marketplace and keeps them out of there.

The predominance of interactions with people outside of their groups is based on economics. The fact is that there are not only similarities within different groups of street children but also between groups of street children and the community. As the authors say, street children have similar interests and motives, and they tend to respond to similar problems in a similar way.

They believe that street children, in their groups develop a sense of community whereby they establish over time concrete rules about how to mobilize and organize resources to benefit the whole. They learn to surrender their individual needs to support the needs of the group. Of course, this is not felt equally among all group members. It is strongest among the core members. What is at the heart of this is the fear of being excluded. Not unlike those who pledge to any established groups, there is an initiation stage, which can be painful. The authors show that while there is support in their daily activities such as begging, sniffing glue or playing, there are demands made upon the initiate in other areas of group life. They are often the victims of psychological and physical abuse and even rape by other group members. These behaviors, like being hazed to enter a fraternity, are accepted because the fear of being excluded is more than the fear of being abused at the moment. For the children who accept the abuse and move on to become members, they have entered a sacred pact with the group and can be assured of a place in the family. As we note in the section on drug abuse, the sacredness is most easily manifested in the consumption of intravenous drugs.

The Use of Public Space and Intragroup Dynamics

Comparing homeless youth with street children in their use of public space is helpful to our hypotheses of the differences among children in street situations, between the genders and for various degrees of abuse. It is also relevant to our discussion of intra and intergroup behaviors. We will discuss in more detail that space often defines how the children react to each other; the level of intimacy for example is related to space. Also, they use the public space as a form of theater to get back at the public which devalues them. This is how we describe, for example, their public use of drugs in places where they are easily seen.

We believe that street boys in the developing world were taught to find in the urban environment any possible niche that might help their economic condition (Aptekar and Ciano 1999).[6] They started to be independent and to perform at an early age in a manner that was strikingly similar to the children of nomads. Like the children of other peripatetic groups, street children move between parked cars, through crowded buses, or among restaurant patrons and waiters, swarming the stationary community who view them with awe, envy, and disdain. Street children were obliged to learn how to be extremely sensitive to understanding and influencing the reactions of their audiences. Many of their behaviors are a result of the financial potential the children had as performers; a skill learned as a part of child training.

In fact street children do a variety of work. They pick up paper and sort through garbage dumps, often providing a public service that no one else is doing. They hawk items that require little capital. Some of what they do, such as begging, is dangerous and really productive only for the youngest. They scavenge to find something cheap in one place to sell it dearer in another, which is good work for them, but has its limits because only so many things can be carried and they may be stolen. We know that they sometimes engage in petty theft, which obviously does not have a future.

More middle class work is not available to them, such as apprenticing with artisans or working as a guides for tourists, although they are often seen trying this

[6] Raffaelli (2000) suggested that while this hypothesis is correct with regard to family, many girls do better than boys on the streets.

angle without adult supervision with varying degrees of success. They are sometimes asked to do odd jobs like carrying or cleaning things, but the income is not reliable, and the work can be hard and boring, and they may not get paid. Of course many of them work to help their parents, but this is work without pay.

Being more abused and less trained for this peripatetic lifestyle, homeless youth occupy the shadows of the streets, and have little ability to roam and earn money. They rely more on the State, and those few who can be found outside of the State's control are more likely to associate with the long term homeless adults. Homeless adults might be able to offer some street advice, but their status in society is so low that by association homeless youth do themselves little service. As they connect with the adult homeless, they demonstrate to the larger society how little competence they have and of how little worth they are.

On the other hand, street boys flaunt their early independence, demonstrating to the public in cultures where the vast majority of people, in order to make ends meet, have more than one job and thus more than one boss, the independence that the public does not have. Because of their numbers and strategic presence they are able to manipulate public opinion, often (and perhaps surprisingly) by behaving in a way that encourages society to view them pejoratively. They actively act out the very behaviors that society condemns them for having. In the end, this gives them two advantages. It makes them stronger as a subculture of childhood with its own identity, and secondly by focusing the fear society has of them, they are likely to be left alone out of fear, thus inadvertently becoming freer from the image of a protected domiciled childhood (Aptekar and Abebe 1997; Davies 2008; Scheper-Hughes and Hoffman 1998).

Antonio and Roberto, two children of about 11 years of age, whom Aptekar (1989a) followed as they left their day program to begin their nocturnal activities, went to the Sexta, an avenue of fashion in Cali, Colombia where their disordered and disheveled dress produced menacing looks and rude comments from the middle-class shoppers with whom they mingled. Ignoring these comments, they approached a young and rather affluent couple who were dining at an open-air restaurant. The couple tried to ignore them. The boys, hoping to be paid to leave the diners alone, stayed close by. Finally, the man who was dining told them in a loud voice to leave. When they didn't, he called the waiter for help. Half-heartedly the waiter told the boys to go. The waiter then took the opportunity to ascertain whether the customers were willing to pay an additional *propina* (tip) for the extra service of an undisturbed dinner. Not getting a definite response, the waiter disappeared inside the restaurant. The two boys, engaged in their normal style of work, were now in full charge. While Roberto approached the table from one side and distracted the couple's attention, Antonio came from the other direction and grabbed a piece of meat off the man's plate. Running and laughing, they appeared like any other 11-year-olds as they receded into the darkened street. As they had eaten lunch at Bosconia only a few hours before, they were not hungry, so they traded the meat to a vigilante for the safety of sleeping in the building he was protecting. Roberto and Antonio, and the children whom Aptekar (1990b) refers to as *gamines*, are not submissive like other poor children in Colombia, nor for that matter as poor people are supposed to be.

Instead, they are haughty and cunning. He saw them earn their livelihood in a variety of clever ways. They collected Popsicle sticks left over from a vendor in El Centro, washed them, and sold them back to be reused.

Two other 12-year-old street children (also a small *camada*), received a bag of leftover food each day from a concerned restaurant owner who thought they were starving. Regularly, they dumped the mess on the ground, and after eating the sweets, traded the rest to a street vendor for cigarettes. At a meeting with representatives from UNICEF, Aptekar watched 28-year-olds pick the pocket of a potential patron at the very moment she was telling the directors of the program how cute and adorable these children were. He saw others dirty car windows while the owners were shopping; then when the owners returned, they would clean the windows and be paid for it. The boys antics became enviable and worthy of a few coins. At the same time, for the minority of higher social class onlookers who are more financially privileged and less beholden to others for survival, the boys were seen as a threat to their privileged position—a position which was jeopardized by the increased democratization and rising meritocracy in the civil politic.

These boys lived in the collective private space where other street children in small groups live. Aptekar has seen others like them in the harsh Ukrainian winters living in the heating tunnels under large buildings. In these spaces they live like cats in their den, some jockeying for power and favor, others relaxed and cajoled. It is the one place that they can act without reference to society at large.

In between the two extremes is a semi-public space, which is also where they work. In contrast to the public space where they are acting with reference to society at large, or the collective private space where they can shed the public's reaction, they develop a personal connection to adult society either in a business relationship with adults whom they work for as middle men, or with an individual adult who acts as their benefactor. The semi-public physical space includes shopping areas, bus stops, bars, and restaurants. In the chapter on programs, we learn this might include spaces to meet with a street educator in the case of street children or a social worker in the case of homeless youth. But, it is also within this semi-public space that they learn to be on guard against potential intruders who might jeopardize their opportunities with adults. This space is also the realm of the older children.

Among street children, elder status depends on time on the streets (or time away from home). It does not depend on chronological age. The groups use space to define social status; the leaders are at the center, and the periphery is for the recently arrived. One of the older children acts in the role of the "boss". He has control over the group's activities and a large share of females. Another older boy is like a mother in that his role is to care for the injured or those in need because of emotional problems.

Naterer and Godina (2011) saw the use of the public space of the Ukrainian street children they studied as essential to their coping skills. They divided the children's use of space into public space, collective private space and semi-private space. As mentioned before, the children use the public space of the whole city to manipulate public opinion by begging and using it for minor, income-earning delinquency.

The authors identified what they referred to as a collective private space which was where they lived, in the heating ducts under large buildings. It was here that they felt safe and enjoyed the benefits of their friends. Also, in their privacy, they were able to get away from being a public persona, an important element of relaxation that people who have homes take for granted.

In their case, in public their role was as a victim and this was accepted by their peers as normal and respected behavior. But, in the space they shared collectively, immaturity or weakness was frowned upon.

Another category of space which the author's referred to as semi-private space, were the densely populated sections of the city such as the marketplace, bus stops, and shopping malls.

It was here that they socialized and carried on most of their economic activities such as being porters, or caretakers of goods for small business people. To do this they had to be seen as mature and trustworthy. It was here that they developed their meaningful relations which often endured over time.

The problem was that when outsiders such as other street children or criminal elements that wanted to use them infringed on this space, there were conflicts.

The authors reported that when there was conflicts they could be resolved fairly easily without physical violence, although there was often a lot of vocal abuse.

On the one hand the children want peace to survive; on the other hand they know what they need to survive and will defend their space to do so if necessary. Street children are aware of the importance of good social relations on those three levels, for their survival depends on the groups in collective and public space, and they defend these relationships fiercely. The authors found that most physical fights were fought over the territory of other groups of street children. While violence for this reason is fairly common, it was not limited just different groups of street children, it was done against anyone who might be disrupting their social order and their group solidarity.

Comparisons of Group Behaviour Between Children in Street Situations and Gangs

One question that we routinely see is: are the delinquent gangs found in the developed world similar to the groups of street children or homeless youth? The words thief and thug help to describe the difference between street children's associations and gangs. We believe it is important because it shows that children in street situations do not relate to each other as gang members do. This offers an important insight into their subculture, their mental health, and makes a strong case that the public view of them is erroneous.

Male street children of the *gamine* subset are likely to take advantage of events by cunning rather than by power. *Gamines* incorporate much of what is thievery into their entrepreneurial skills. And, the line between good business and thievery has its cultural differences.

Gangs in the developed world have a clear line of authority and an accepted organizational structure. Certain behaviours are tolerated, other condoned, and some not allowed. In contrast, among children in street situations the group is considerably less formal. Rules are not clear; the informal organization does not spell them out so neatly. Rules of entry and exit are less important; and sometimes non-existent. Social roles within the group are fluid and less hierarchical.

As Heinonen (2011) points out, there is no professional literature on gangs in Ethiopia. Her interest in them came about as an offshoot of her interest in street children. Yet, from the onset of her work, she noticed groups of boys sleeping in the streets, apparently oblivious to what was happening around them. She later identifies these groups as *borcos* (gangs). She notes that they looked and acted differently than street children. Street children when they were on the streets were constantly moving, alert and in active pursuit of goals, usually income related. The *borcos* were lethargic and indifferent to their surroundings. She came to learn that the gang members were homeless by choice overwhelmingly because they were abused by their families. Even though they knew where their families lived, they did not want to be with them. Some came from fairly well-to-do families.

The public's view of the *borcos*, by which they meant a person living in the street and likely to be addicted to drugs and deviant behavior which was uniformly pejorative. She was constantly warned to stay away from them. Yet, she says that she never found them dangerous, although they were deceitful.

Unlike gangs in the developed world, these *borcos* were not organized around a common ethnicity, nor did they have much group alliance. They lived away from their abusing families as homeless children in disparate parts of the city. They did not sleep for long in the same place, because they were constantly bothered by the police. As a result of this, they gave little weight to where they slept and this is why she would see them the midst of traffic, on sidewalks, or in roadside ditches. Not all of the gangs were alike. One of the four gangs she studied had a semi-permanent place and was cleaner and better adjusted than the others, whom she described as unkempt, unwashed, and barefoot and dressed in filthy tattered rags.

The gangs were different than unemployed youth who lived at home but hung out on the streets, and were cleaner and better dressed than the *borcos*. Because they looked better and lived with their families, and in spite of having no job prospects, the police seldom harassed them. All of the gang members had been badly abused by their respective families, mostly in line with the values of *yilunta* (honor, shame, family pride) which sanctions parents to verbally and physically discipline their children. This can be passed on to stepmothers, uncles and half-siblings as well as stepsisters and stepbrothers.

Unlike the dominant view that youth gang members are supportive of one another and have strong affective relationships, the gang described by Heinonen (2011) had a highly unstable society. The members had contradictory concerns. They wanted both their personal freedom, and to be part of a group. The compromise that was reached was to belong to a loose organizational structure[7] that made few demands on their freedom. They kept their freedom to leave and come back to the group. They also wanted to spend their own money on what they wanted. Because most

[7] R. Lucchini (1993, p. 80) also refers to the notion of the near-group, developed by Yablonsky (1979), when saying that the organization of the near-group is adapted to members who come and go rather than really belong to the group. This is especially the case for more peripherical members of the near-group.

gang members wanted to belong but to be free, the usual ethic of reciprocity was difficult to follow, and thus did not always provide each gang member with the supportive companionship system he sought.

This could be seen in the rules for entering and leaving the group. There were no formal initiation rites to get into a gang, nor were there rules for leaving. As she says, it is only difficult to get into a group if someone in the group did not want you. And after someone left he could easily go back in as long as he had no scores to be settled or debts to be paid.

The degree to which a person would submit to an initiation depended on how much the initiate was willing to take from one or two members of the gang. According to Heinonen (2011), newcomers were easily and quickly able to get out from under an exploitative relationship. If not, they voted with their feet as soon as the situation became unbearable.

There were some internal rules of behavior regarding how they lived together. Stealing from other gang members was not accepted. Informing the police, family members or any outsiders about the whereabouts of a missing comrade was an act of betrayal. A member had to help another member who was sick or injured, or loan money for food, or support the group if they were attacked. For failing on any of these accounts, a person could be ostracized, beaten, thrown out, or all three.

While there was no clear leader in the group, all gangs that she studied had a special child who was liked by all as a mascot. Likewise, the most admirable behavior amongst group members was the behavior most closely associated with masculinity as described by the rules of *Yilunta*. Thus one member was feared and admired because he was self sufficient, he didn't need to talk much to be seen as powerful and apparently fearless of life's demands. Such a person would be a warrior when fighting other gangs. In fact, members judged each other by the same expectations of mainstream society, which also used the rules of *Yilunta*.

Heinonen (2011) points out that street children living at home have some feeling of being productive and useful in their families, and have a family and community upon whom they can rely, even if for nothing more than emotional support. After all, when they are living at home street-related activities bring in income for school expenses, clothes and even food for the family. It is not surprising that they feel better about themselves than homeless street children.

There are very few among the homeless children who can find a satisfactory life unless they are in a gang. The pain they felt that led them to leave their families in the first place, including having no socially supportive relationships at home, makes it very unlikely that they would go back into family life.

> "*In contrast to street children living with their families, homeless children lacked the reciprocity expected of close relatives and friends that goes along with the nature of social support and social network available within the family unit. The vast majority of home-based street children attended school part-time; none of the homeless children I knew attended any kind of educational institution. Street children living at home could count on some form of continuity in their lives. They had someone to provide them with emotional support and with a place to sleep, and on whom they could rely for help and affection* (Heinonen 2011, p. 130)".

Hecht (1998) found that in Brazil street children rarely form gang alliances. They had different origins. Gang members were more likely to come from the *barrios* and *favelas*. Even though it is easy to lump the group behaviour of street children into the larger social group of poor urban children living in poor communities, this connection is not always viable.

Both Aptekar (1988) and Hecht (1998) found that in Colombia and Brazil there were no initiation rites and no penalties if they get out of the group. Hecht defines this as a loose forming alliance, held together without force, showing that street children do not live under or accept power structures. As one street child said to him, "chiefs are for indians (p. 45)".

The idea that gangs replace families has it proponents and critics. Hecht (1998) argues that Brazilian gangs as a community fell far short in providing the support than an ideal family might, but the comparison is problematic, because the members of the gangs did not have ideal families, far from it. The street children Hecht studied, did not, according to him, function as a family. Their home life was unsatisfactory, and their group did not replace it with a better alternative. The children did not feel a continual sense of belonging, nor did they have their emotional needs met. Hecht is saying that the subjects in his study grew up in abusive homes and in the group remained in abusive relationships. While this might be true of the *gallada*, we think it is not true of a *camada*; quite the opposite.

In the peer relationships found among the *borcos* of Addis Ababa, friendships within groups took the form of needing someone to come to your aid if needed for protection or to provide sympathy after a bad day. What Heinonen (2011) mentions as the violence within the gang is smaller children being forced to give goods or money to larger ones, or even made to steal from their parents and bring the goods back to the group. If they did not hand over what was expected, the older boys would beat them. There are seemingly incompatible positions on this, but in the end, the children play rough and fight and are also very close to one another.[8] This is why she found that when a child put his faith in another group member and was let down, or in any way betrayed, he became very distressed, more so than she encountered in any other situation. As if it were a family.

Swart's study (1990) of the *Malunde*, street children in Johannesburg, South Africa, Aptekar's study (1988) of the *galladas* and *camadas* in Colombia, Sharf et al. (1986) study of the *strollers* in Cape Town, South Africa, and Glazer's historical study (2000) of *Bo-Tsotsi* in Soweto, all point out that the street children's affiliation is positive at least to the degree that it provides group support against a hostile society and the police.

In some senses, the movement from *camada* to *gallada* is a move from group to gang. The street children came from the *camada* to the *gallada* with a mixed expectation. They wanted to belong, but they also did not want to give up their autonomy. This might be why the initiation ceremony is minor. On the first night, a group member befriends the initiate, who remains for some time under that

[8] It is interesting to note that Heinonen (2011) found that a couple of the group members came from less than abject poverty. They were the only ones to use their own names. They said they did this to get back at their family who had abused them. The difference was between abuse and poverty as reasons for entering the gang.

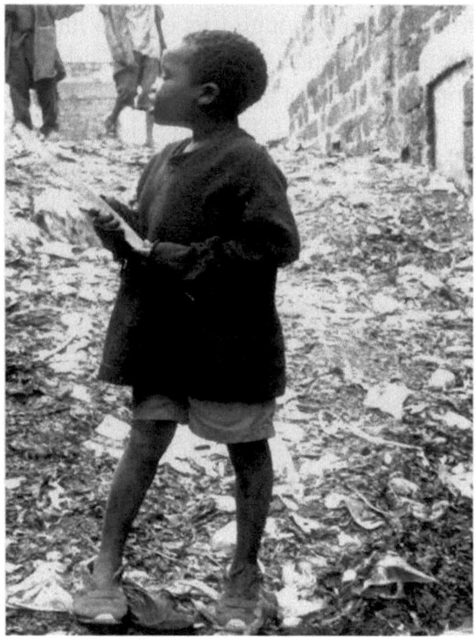

Fig. 3.2 There is value in being young

person's power. While the initiate might call his sponsor a friend, and they might be friendly, the relationship can become abusive, and certainly will contain an element of co-opting.

What kept the abuse to a minimum was that the initiate had the option of using boots to vote. Many did. Some came back and tried again with another sponsor, or went to another group; a few remained outside of the system. There were other factors that kept abuse at bay. For one, the smaller kids, looking pitiful and being able to succeed at begging, had a card to play (Fig. 3.2).

For the homeless youth, the roles within the groups are related to the dysfunctional families they come from. The homeless youth subculture looks like family, but not a family based on love or interacting for the purpose of personal growth. It looks more like a family in desperate straits, trying its best to keep together, which means being clear about who's in and who's out. It is not common that these groups and delinquent gangs come from the same origins, nor do they share personalities or group structures. In a study in four Midwestern States (Kevin et al. 2003) about the extent of gang involvement and membership in a sample of homeless and runaway youth, the authors found that about 15% of the sample was made up of gang members.

It might be difficult to ascertain the extent of gang involvement. Research on street children might not indicate if they are engaged in crime. Nor should street children and youth violence be equated. There is youth violence from street children and there are street children who are not violent.

In the 1990s and the few years of the 2000s, the number of gangs across the country increased, but the number of violent crimes decreased (Sullivan 2006). He heuristically defined groups of people working toward a similar end as a group. There is permanency of members, and cliques, which are diffuse in nature but enduring over time. While there is no ritual membership, they engage in several activities over time and see themselves as an entity. Finally, there are named gangs, which have clear internal organizations, rituals for membership, and operate together for many goals. Street children can be found in all three, but are much less likely to be in the 3rd group, whose primary purpose is too easily associated with violence.

Homeless youth in the developed world have a cycle of estrangement (they are "*not one of us*") and public fear (they are "*out of control*") (Hutson and Liddiard 1994). The public's "need for security" is on the political agenda in many western democracies. For instance in France, new laws have been adopted in 2007 and 2008 (retention law and security against the recurrence) which are meant to prevent delinquency, based on a political discourse of danger. This has given psychiatrists a major role in detecting potential threatening individuals (Martin 2011), including claims of *potential* (italics from authors) violence of drug-induced, maladaptive behavior which supposedly can occur at very young ages.

One problem is that homeless youth are associated with the apparently irrational behaviors of elder homeless people, such as the Sans Domicile Fixe (SDF) (without fixed homes) in France who refused to accept shelters and even sometimes individual flats that were offered to them. While the homeless youth preferred the adjustment to street life as opposed to the feeling of being imprisoned, the public was left with the idea they were irrational or crazy.[9]

The public negative response to homeless youth and street children, seeing them as threatening, can in effect increase their affiliation to gangs. Gang affiliation leads toward more violence.

Magazine (2003) in an ethnographic study of street children in Mexico City made a distinction between *bandas* and gangs. *Bandas* are large groups of street children, without a defined territory or any specific income generating purposes. For income generation, they work in two or threes. At the end of the day, the two and three gather together to share their wealth in a way that Magazine connected to a gift economy. This means that one of the members of the *banda* receives something, often a drink of *pulque* (fermented Agave Cactus sap beverage), and they become mutually dependent. This strengthens the *banda's* organization and help's in distinguishing their *banda* from others.

While crime defines the gang, it was only opportunistic among groups of street children. They talk of the difficulty of stealing and the consequences if caught which might include being beaten to death, and even the fear and loneliness that jail has for them. They admit that if they see something on the ground that is not theirs they would take it.

If there is violence, it occurs within the group and concerns unpaid debts, or fighting to show ones masculinity. These fights are often situational. That is because of a third party looking on, it is necessary to fight to maintain pride. Being aggressive is at times the only way to save face. This became more evident when girls were involved.

[9] In fact, Zeneidi-Henry (2002) showed that the shelters for the "*sans-abri*" ("without dwelling") are administered in a way that was felt as a control over one's body and freedom.

Sexual Behavior and Group Dynamics

To almost all concerned, the mention of girls on the street brings up images of sexual exploitation. This perception offers us a good deal of information about the relationship between society and street girls. We will see that sexuality among children in street situations is often more related to group dynamics than it is to love or friendship *per se*.

A major issue for female children in street situations is the question of sex and prostitution. Kovats-Bernat (2006) reported from Haiti that as female street children entered puberty they were perceived (and evaluated) in sexual terms. If they were not considered attractive by men, they were shunned. If they were not shunned, they got pregnant because they could not insist on having their partners use condoms. They were also victims of rape.[10] It is no wonder that unlike the street boys, we never met a street girl who liked being on the streets.

In a study of four American states, Johnson and Tyler (2006) found that one third of their sample of American homeless girls traded sex for money or goods. But to get to this number they defined trading sex as not always actually trading sex. They included having been propositioned to trade sex and refused, or having friends or acquaintances who had traded sex for favors. Given the expanded definition, it is surprising why it wasn't more than a third of the sample, and it is difficult to know what percent actually did have sex for money. In a survey of literature on this topic, survival sex among American runaway girls varied between 7 and 46% (as reported in Van Leeuwen et al. 2006).

Johnson and Tyler (2006) found that it was not only the girls in their study of American runaways who traded sex for money. The incidence for runaway boys might even have been higher if, because of the stigma, they did not underreport. Among American runaway youth, more time spent on the streets led to more risky behaviors and being in more risky situations which led to both more victimization and more opportunities for sexual exploitation. The authors noted that the younger a girl or boy was when they went to the streets, the fewer coping skills they had and the greater the chance of sexual abuse. The more female runaways used drugs, the higher the incidence of sexual victimization. Seventy five percent of runaway youth of both genders have sex while intoxicated (possibly not much different than the general population). Those young women who traded sex were five times more likely to be victimized by a stranger, while males who traded sex were six times more likely to be victimized by a stranger. A male acquaintance was the most likely victimizer for a girl runaway, while a male stranger was the most likely victimizer for a male runaway.[11]

[10] It should be said that it was very difficult to talk to street girls about their sexual history (Kovats-Bernat 2006).

[11] In spite of these differences, there are no significant differences when it comes to the mental health profile of first-time homeless and long-term homeless.

Aptekar and Ciano's (1999) ethnography of street children of both genders in Nairobi (Kenya) showed the family circumstances of street girls and how they were treated by their male counterparts in the streets. Aptekar reported that one evening he and one of his female ethnographer colleagues stopped to talk to several street boys who were at the end of a deserted alley near an open sewer just outside the city center. Here they lived in two shacks they had constructed from rubble. To enter they had to bend low to pass through the doorway. They found that two of the occupants were female. Jocylyn, who appeared to have just reached puberty, lay covered in rags, a jar of inhalant in her hand. Through glazed eyes, she barely greeted them. The next day, they returned to the site and were able to take her to a center that serves street girls where she had received good treatment before. When they arrived at the center, none of her peers, some of whom she knew, greeted her.

Jocylyn had been raised in Mathare Valley (one of the poorest area of Nairobi) by her mother and had three older brothers. When sales of her mother's illegal beer were good, Jocylyn's brothers went to school while Jocylyn stayed at home to help out with chores and business. Because her mother was not always present, she was abused several times by men who came in to buy beer. Over time, she began to make friends with older boys, one of whom she liked enough to accept his invitation to live with him in the alley.

Before long, she was in a similar position as she had been at home. Because many of the boys found her attractive, they paid to enjoy her company, and with nowhere to turn, she tried to find refuge in inhalants. The path that Jocylyn appeared to be traveling was not an uncommon one for street girls. By the time they became young adults, the Kenyan street girls studied by Muraya (1993) and Suda (1993) were following in their mothers' footsteps, having many children, often by different men. While this had historical and cultural precedent, in which men assume responsibility for all of their children and wives, this was no longer the case according to Kilbride et al. (2000). Most of the men did not regard them as legitimate wives and therefore the women and children were unworthy of continual financial support. A similar finding comes from Venezuela (Marquez 1999).

It was common for the leaders of groups of male street children to take several street girls as "wives." Each boy saw that his "wife" was not bothered by other boys, from inside or outside the group, and that the girls got enough to eat and were taken care of. In return, the boys received the sexual privileges of husbands. Although some of the girls on the streets exchanged sex for money on a limited basis, none of the girls in Muraya's study (1993), the most complete study of Kenyan street girls, was living solely by prostitution.

In Nairobi, Aptekar and Ciano (1999) found that the "husbands" were content to let their "wives" live with the dual roles of wife and part time prostitute. Whatever else the street girls were learning in these male groups, they were learning the cultural status of women, the same status they witnessed as children in the homes of their mothers.

It would have seemed just as developmentally appropriate for the girls to be deeply committed to same-sex friendships in groups as the boys were (see Aptekar 1988, 2004), based on the psychological value of prepubescent street children of both sexes to play with same-gender friends. However, neither Aptekar and Ciano (1999) nor Muraya (1993) found a strong unisex group structure among the girls unless special circumstances warranted, like for example if a girl was in need of immediate medical care. Many girls seemed to cope only as appendages to boys, even though the boys did not provide the support they needed. Indeed, the very liberty that the boys allowed the girls in their dual roles as "wives" and as sources of income via sexual favors illustrated the lack of care they gave them. Yet the girls accepted this, evidently feeling unable to conceive an alternative possibility.

If, as was assumed, boys were expected to bring income into the house, and thus go to the streets to do so, while girls were expected to stay at home and help out with household chores, street boys and street girls would relate to their families of origin differently. Indeed, we found that almost all the groups of street boys in our study remained connected to their mothers. In fact, the boys often contributed part of their income to the parent. (To learn how the same is true of street children in Latin America, see Aptekar (1988, 1992), Ennew (1994), and Lusk (1992).) One of the street boys routinely took a 3 hour bus trip to give his mother half of what he had earned during the week. This was common knowledge among his peers, and he was given high status for his behavior.

In contrast, the groups of girls were not connected to their families of origin. For example, Muraya (1993) found that two-thirds of Nairobi's street girls severed family ties completely. Aptekar and Ciano (1999) found that street boys were eager to make friends with outsiders and establish close sibling-type relationships with other boys. In contrast, street girls remained distant, even after considerable time spent with Kenyan women experienced in working with street girls (including the women working in their study).

Many Kenyan girls were raised in female-centered homes, and if they ended up on the streets, it was often because they were abused or had conflicts at home. On the streets, the coping strategies of their mothers failed to protect them. Whereas, boys were taught by their mothers from an early age to survive on the streets and rummage to supplement the family income, girls did not get such training, which contributed to their vulnerability in this harsh context. Partly as a result of this situation, our findings suggest that street girls may suffer from more mental health problems than street boys (Aptekar and Ciano 1999).

On the other hand, even if they are forced to have sex, street girls did not always see themselves as prostitutes, because selling themselves for sex was a way to make money, not, from their point of view, a way to define who they were (Kilbride et al. 2000).

The media was likely to accuse street girls (and homeless girls) of having children for financial reasons, because begging could be more lucrative by having a child involved. They pointed out that, as for the rest of us, a street girl having a child also brings personal satisfaction, affords a way of being important, gives a loving relationship, and opens up wider views of life's possibilities. The street girls with babies turned to their families for help or they banded together with other street girls in a group to support each other.

Heinonen (2011) saw that in the mixed gender gangs she studied in Addis Ababa, the girls who were sexually active were both victimizers and victims. When they had sex with the boys it was voluntary. Yet, they were under pressure to prostitute themselves for the good of the group. The girls did not join the gang for adventure or because of poverty, but to escape abuse at home. They were angry and depressed.

She reported that the girls, by prostituting themselves, brought in the main source of income for the gang. The males begged for food from the wealthy homes. They also protected the girls when they were having sex. At the same time, the girls were also responsible for washing clothes, buying groceries and cooking. The head man had the power to distribute wives to those he favored. If the girls complained or if boys complained, they would be beaten by the leader or his henchman. The membership of the group changed constantly.

When one of the girls was punished, it was usually the other girls who would beat her. They would hold her down, slap and scratch her face, and abuse her private parts, all in front of the boys. One girl remarked that the worst was seeing her friend (male) watching and laughing. When asked why the girls did not form their own gangs, they said it was too scary, particularly at night, and also the boys would find them and hurt them.

On the other hand, some research shows that the vast majority of girls who are living on the street do not turn to prostitution. Stoecklin and Chuard (2003) observed that only a small minority of the girls interviewed in Madagascar openly claimed that being involved in prostitution is a good choice. In fact, they are more likely to be victims of sexual abuse. While there is no scientific or ethical justification in classifying them as professional prostitutes, the media often follows other agendas than scientific and ethical ones.

Lucchini (1994) showed that the survival strategies of the street girl are incompatible with the exercise of professional prostitution. Yet he also showed that street girls are still stigmatized as if they were prostitutes. He thinks part of this is because of the social perception of female sexuality.

Rosemberg (2000) noted the exaggeration of the numbers of girls who were supposedly prostitutes. She says that one estimate is that 20% of Brazilian girls between 15 and 20 were engaged in prostitution.

Drug Use and Group Dynamics

While children in street situations use a variety of drugs, from inhalants to heroin, their use is symbolic, that is they use drugs more than for getting high, they also use them as a way to claim of identify with their subculture, or as Scheper-Hughes and Hoffman (1998) believe, as a regressive reaction of the street children to comfort themselves.[12] Davies (2008) found that sniffing glue was not only used for

[12] Diversi et al. (1999) express the more psychological position in their study of Brazilian street children. They stress that Brazilian street children use crack cocaine as a practical means of reducing hunger and fear.

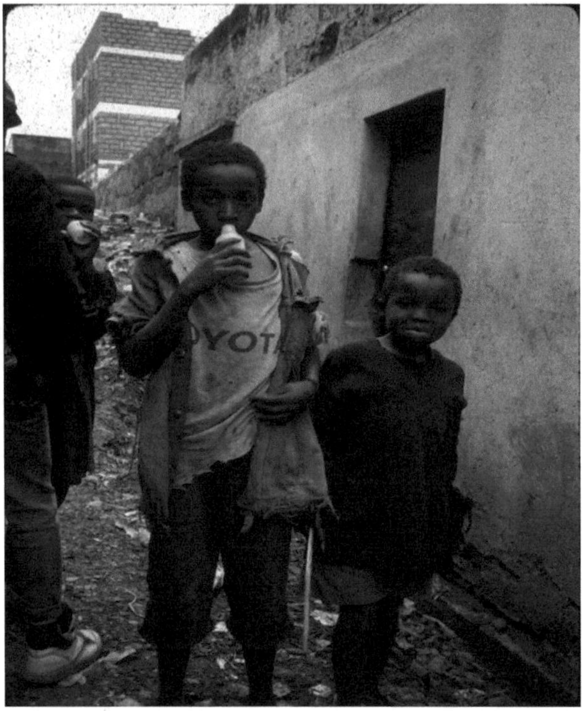

Fig. 3.3 Sniffing glue

pleasure but was part of the group-culture. There were several group-imposed rules. For example, children knew that they didn't have to sniff glue, but they did so to be a part of the group did (Fig. 3.3). By participating in the intoxicated behavior associated with the use of glue, such as being loud and seemingly out of control and thus dangerous, the children seemingly lost status with the general public, even as they gained status within their group. But there was more to this. By acting intoxicated, they not only contributed to the pejorative opinion of them, it allowed them to show their anger at the society that put them down. What Davies (2008) brings to the table is the fact while the group of street children encourage this, they do not allow anyone to regularly become over-intoxicated or to be overly ridiculed his or her peers. If this happened, they took the glue away.

Davies maintains that sniffing glue is part of their way of getting back at a society that devalues them. The group's behavior works because it plays to the fears of the public. The key to understanding the children's drug behavior is to know that the positive value that the children give to drug use is only partly related to the intoxication the drug provides. By apparently accepting the description the public has of them, such as, among others, drug abusers, they become involved in an "in-group joke"; based on scaring those who are mean to them, giving their detractors, if you would, a little of bit of what those detractors give to them.

This description is similar to what Aptekar and Ciano (1999) noted while seeing street boys consume drugs in Nairobi. It was common to see them inhaling publicly.

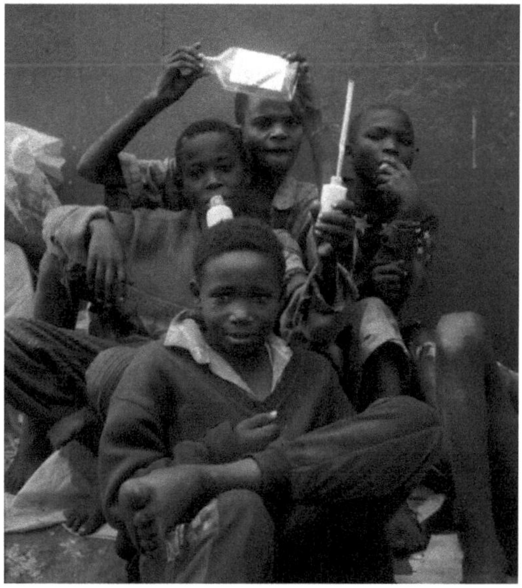

Fig. 3.4 Public display of substance and alcohol use

Held in low esteem and being illegal, why did they not consume drugs more privately? Usually, studies indicate that street boys use inhalants to kill hunger, or to forget the tragedy of their lives, to self-medicate fear and depression, to provide strength to live in difficult circumstances, or as indications of a pathological need for immediate gratification. But none of these would necessitate they consume them in public view (Fig. 3.4).

One evening, Aptekar was visiting street children in the "Little Mogadishu" section of Nairobi (Aptekar and Ciano 1999). There were about a dozen boys on a small island of trash in the middle of a busy roundabout inhaling glue. Around them sped a steady onslaught of traffic. He observed them through the traffic, as did other pedestrians. All he could see were many pairs of eyes peering over noses covered with paper bags or shirt-sleeves. Of course, as he watched the boy's eyes, the boys were also watching him.

It was then that he realized the most impressive phenomenon was not the one or two who had obviously overdosed even though these would be the boys most likely to be presented in the press and most likely to leave a lasting impression on most observers. The most impressive aspect was that, as every street boy in the group was inhaling, every passer-by was watching. Each group eyed the other as if they were shopping in a market filled with exotic goods. Being interwoven like this started Aptekar thinking that the effect of using the drug might be less important to the boys than the role it played in consolidating their subculture.

Knowing that the boys were very adept at manipulating public opinion (Aptekar 1992), it was no accident that every passer-by saw the boys using the inhalants. In fact, if they had wanted to advertise their consumption they could not have developed a better strategy. It was very much like what happened in their traditional culture where initiation into adult roles was held in full public view of all the elders in the community. Only by staring down the pain of circumcision in front of one's parents and elders, does a boy become a successful initiate. As the pedestrians and the people in cars and buses watched with disdain, the boys shared in inhaling glue and simultaneously building subcultural solidarity. Could not their public consumption of inhalants be a way of declaring their uniqueness in earning adult status for their own subculture? Could it be that at the same time they were staring down the adults watching them, they did not realize how they would be responded to? Most likely they knew very well what the reaction would be.

If the emphasis was placed on observing the boy's coping skills, and not on sensational accounts of drug abuse, we would find that most of the boys who use drugs do not succumb to them. Indeed the alleged inevitable connection between street children and drug dependence is more of an accusation that serves to diminish the children's capacities than it is a culturally free statement of their mental health (Aptekar 1988). Before drawing conclusions related to the use and misuse of inhalants by street boys, the sociological in-group perspective should be fully considered.

Such a symbolic use of drugs was found among Ukrainian street children who inject *baltrushka*, a mixture of flu medicine, vinegar and water up to six times a day, and although it is not habit forming, they could not resist taking it, nor could they avoid participating in the elaborate ceremony around it, because it is a ritual with the purpose of insuring subgroup solidarity (Naterer and Godina 2011).

Children used a dose of 4–10 ml, four to eight times a day. The poignant fact is that *Baltushka* does not produce any direct physical addiction observable from withdrawal symptoms among users, but does result in high levels of social dependence. Street children who have been using the substance on a regular basis report that while they can quit its consumption at any time without having any withdrawal crisis or other side effects provided they are alone, they cannot resist the temptation when they are in the group.

They take it as a ritual. And they do so only in structured social events for this purpose. There are rules that are followed for preparation and consumption. There are special tools to get the drug ready to use and a special vocabulary is used during this time and while it is being consumed. It is clear that taking this drug has more to do with the cohesion of the subculture than it does with getting high.

Are There Children in Street Situations in All Cultures?

Groups of street children are found in various degrees in different cultures, making it hard to understand the relationship between the State and street children. Yet, in order to look into the origins of street children, one must ask why there are many street children in some places and few in others. One could look at the form of government. Russia, China, and Cuba during their communist eras, did not have street children. The State was powerful enough to keep them off the streets. As State power decreased, the numbers of street children rose. There are many street children in the former Eastern Bloc of communist countries, including the Ukraine, but less so in China, which has more street children since the 1980s, and there are still essentially no Cuban street children.

Whiteford (1998) makes an argument regarding the historical development of Cuba and the Dominican Republic during periods of structural adjustment programs that would help to explain why one country's population of street children rose, and the other's didn't. According to Whiteford both countries had strong central governments that provided health care for their children before structural adjustment. But they took two different approaches to resolving their debt issues. The Dominican Republic invested in central urban hospitals while Cuba continued to develop it country's primary care facilities, emphasizing preventive care, including general health education of the public. The commitment to universal equal health care correlated with healthier children and families, and fewer street children. However, it is difficult to exactly show the effect of structural adjustment policies on the number of street children. The correlation between these policies that burdened the social care systems, especially in the 1990s, and the statistics of street children are difficult to ascertain as the latter are mostly inaccurate.

One thing is for sure: when the State is weak and children are the least expensive labor, human rights can become secondary to immediate needs and profit margins. Without legislation and a means to enforce the law, there are street children in Iran, Bangladesh, India, and Pakistan for example.

Some people would consider that street children exist only in developing countries, and especially in countries that were under colonialism. This is also a misconception, as street children may be encountered also in countries that do not have a colonial past. Take for instance Thailand and Ethiopia, two countries never colonized, but which both have street children. In Ethiopia, this has been observed ever since the arrival of the first European explorers. England and European States had similar descriptions of street vagabonds for hundreds of years. There are also descriptions of street vagabonds in Beijing as early as 1900, although only Hong-Kong and Shanghai had been colonized. A French doctor, Jean-Jacques Matignon who spent 3 years taking care of beggars in the out=patient clinic of the French hospital of Nan-Tang in Beijing, wrote that beggars could be seen everywhere in the city, at each street corner, under the bridges, and at the gates of the temples (Matignon 1900). The depictions accompanied by photographs indicate that the conditions were harsher than what is observed a century later (Matignon 1900). In between, the number of street children has decreased, especially during the first decades after installation of the communist regime (1949), and increased again with the beginning of the era of economic reforms (1979) up to now, and these variations have nothing to do with external influence, but rather with domestic policies. Therefore, the influence of colonialism on the phenomenon of street children can be said to be uncertain, as this factor is intertwined with several other political, economic and socio-cultural factors.

It appears that all States in the developed world have homeless youth. Yet, the relationship between outsiders and insiders is a more likely candidate to impact the numbers of children in street situations. As tourism increases in the developing world, so do the numbers of street children, even in places like Cuba with a strong governmental commitment to children (Lutjens 2000).

In some cases there are no children in street situations because they are defined out of existence. In Serbia, there is no term for street children so they are classified into categories that do exist such as children with mental health problems or children without adequate parental care (Muskinja 2009). Thus these children are in touch with police officers, employees in State-run shelters and social workers.

In these countries, the children closest to what we are referring to as children in street situations are from marginalized ethnic groups, living in extreme poverty, and often have experienced some treatment within the institutions of the official system. Many are internally displaced from Kosovo, or refugees from Bosnia and Herzegovina and Croatia (Muskinja 2009). Others are Roma, but this group presents another definitional problem, because they are homeless, but with families.

In the developing world, countries with a relatively substantial middle class have street children. In Latin America for example, the three countries noted for their high incidence of street children are Mexico, Colombia, and Brazil (Rosemberg 2000). All of them have large middle classes and the first two are substantially involved with the drug trade. But being a country involved with the international drug trade is not a guarantee that there will be street children; take Cuba, for example.

Why Cuba? Is it because the State has become "family"? The family being united with the State means there is no economic need for street children. Single motherhood is common, historically and since the revolution, but because the State acts in the role of the errant father, there is no economic reason for children to go to the streets to work. The Cuban system is committed to children, a situation not found elsewhere in Latin America or Africa, and probably found only in certain socialist countries.

Because of the counting problem linked to the use of different definitions, as we mentioned before, it is difficult to know whether the phenomenon of children in street situations is shrinking or growing. Many rely on guesstimates when writing that the numbers have grown in the last decade and throughout all continents (Muskinja 2009). For some, this situation is linked to transitions which are accompanied by a rise of modern life (Le Roux and Smith 1998), including a street culture of petty crime, drug selling and prostitution. (We are not sure what is so modern about this). It might also be because of the rise of urbanization.

But, it should be added that other studies do not show a rate of growth among street children. In Vietnam there were steady increases until 2001, but from 2001 to 2004, numbers went down (Hong and Ohno 2005). These data might be low because they are supplied by the government, which at times wants to underestimate figures so that tourists and potential investors would feel more comfortable.[13]

[13] It also points out the difficulty of getting accurate numbers. Aptekar, in a personal conversation, remembers being at a conference where researchers were estimating thousands of street children, yet very few were visible to him, even though he had been working in the city for years.

Whatever the true numbers, when focusing on street children and to a lesser extent on homeless youth, it is very easy to ignore the more macro level social causes for their origins, which in part is a pattern of "development" that jeopardises economic and social rights condemning large sectors of the population to social exclusion.

Macro-economic trends such as international dependency, neo-liberal policies and structural adjustments imposed by the international creditors heavily affect children around the world. These plans, decided by the International Monetary Fund (IMF), the World Bank (WB), the Club of Paris (Northern creditor governments) and the Club of London (Northern private banks), are characterised by the privatisation of State enterprises and the reduction in the bureaucracy of public services, in particular healthcare, education, housing, transport, environment, and a drop in salaries, and increase in the distance between social classes, favouring the wealthy over the impoverished (George and Sabelli 1994). How this affects street children is made clear by Kilbride et al. (2000) whose work in Nairobi shows there is a direct connection between the numbers of street children and structural adjustment. And, working with Canadian homeless youth, Haldenby et al. (2007) found that the cuts in social programs and support have greatly increased the numbers of homeless youth. And, "*such structural changes are also thought to contribute to the rise of street involved youth in Canada* (p. 1232)".

Mickelson (2000) compares homeless youth in the USA with street children in Brazil and Cuba and concludes that poverty, in large part due to the globalization of economies, is the major cause of children in street situations. Despite huge differences, the three countries, like others, are increasingly affected by the globalized economy, which shape similar contours of homelessness in different countries.

The difference between the GDP of the USA and the other two countries is startling in favor of the USA, but in public health indicators, Cuba and the USA are about equal, with Brazil falling behind.

Income distribution disparities in the USA and Brazil are vast and growing wider. In the USA more children are living in poverty every year. Cuba, for the most part, has an equal distribution of wealth. Few Cuban children suffer from prolonged poverty, while 60% of children in Brazil and 23% of children in the USA do (Mickelson 2000).

In the USA, the jobs that can support a decent wage are located far from the barrios where the poor live, so in some cases the poor sleep closer to work, even if it is rough sleeping, because it is a better alternative to spending hours both going to and coming from work.

Even as Cuba is dealing with its own economic problems, there are virtually no street or working kids on the streets. It appears that it is not just global economics that contributes to the numbers of street children, but other factors as well.

According to Veale et al. (2000) in *The State of the World's Children 1996*, a document published by UNICEF, there are some 800 million people in 40 countries living with reduced incomes due to the debt crisis and structural adjustment programs, which have brought cuts to essential social service programs, which in turn has increased the numbers of street children.

Among the major fallout of this that affects the lives of the poorest segments of the population are a growing number of slums without any basic amenities; inadequate educational policies – ignoring the direct and indirect costs of schooling, lack of vocational training and an exceedingly rigid and repressive juvenile justice system with legal norms that are often not fully applied or even lacking, and are replaced by unofficial norms based on power relationships which are sometimes preferred, imposing corrective measures with limited or no legal foundation. Interests related to the maintenance of public order overrule Article 3 of the Convention for the Rights of the Child (The best interests of the child) and the required formalities (probationary procedure, separate detention of adults and juveniles, etc.).

According to the world report on Violence Against Children (Pinheiro 2006), the economically difficult situation is affecting the family. Because men are frustrated by unemployment, some tend to become violent, and the home situation deteriorates, mostly aggravated by alcohol and drugs, with children sometimes involved in trafficking. Numerous forms of child abuse are reported in the document, including child trafficking and other intolerable violations of the rights stipulated in the United Nations Convention on the Rights of the Child (UNCRC 1989), particularly with regards to the right to live a decent life, have a home and an identity, the right to protection, food, health, education, and the right to express oneself. Because of the downturn in the global economy, many States have had to reduce or strop providing a social net. This and other factors mentioned above might "produce" what we call children in street situations.

Cheng (2008) reports that in China it is macro social changes that have lead to the failure of the traditional extended family. This in turn has caused children to migrate into the public streets. The peer-group relations of the street children phenomenon are constantly interconnected with macro social transformations (Stoecklin 2000b). What happens is that societal reaction and peer sociability influence children in street situations. How the child incorporates this input depends on many psychological variables (see the previous chapter), such as their age, gender and health, their experiences and expectations of street life, which vary from escape from abuse, to an opportunity for work, to the need to survive.

The point of view that considers the macro-social phenomenon, adult's ability and desire to raise children, and the immediate social network of the child is called the "new paradigm in childhood studies", initiated almost 25 years ago by James and Prout (1990).[14] It shows that childhood is a social construction and therefore, rather than look at childhood or adolescence, (and children in street situations) as an

[14]Really this work is based on the work of the French historian Philippe Ariès (1960) whose breathtaking assertion was that childhood was a creation of the Renaissance. Before that historical period, people would not look at childhood as its own developmental category. In contrast, Archard (2004) claimed that previous societies did not lack a concept of childhood, only that it was different than what we have today.

essence, we should see multiple childhoods and varieties of adolescence depending upon local, international, national and specific cultural factors.[15]

Societal Reactions to Children in Street Situations

Societal reactions to children in street situations are based on a moral view of childhood and child rearing practices. These reactions and what behaviors the public allows and which are considered inappropriate, mold the children's public personas, and the concept of self. It is also possible to look at the information about street children and the way it is presented in narratives and in the media as a locus of study (de Moura 2002). This would be in line with the sociology of knowledge (Berger and Luckmann 1966), which is to say that the information presented about street children can be seen as more than declarative comments, but also adds a certain version of reality.

There is a relationship among street children and homeless youth and their respective societies which defines their group dynamics, at what we are calling the macro level. For example, children in street situations are often portrayed as polar opposites, one as victim the other as perpetrator. Given this variety, it is strange that social workers and scholars still refer to children in street situations as if they were a clearly outlined group.

Aptekar (1988) and de Moura (2002), refer to their mythic image. The image stays, in spite of its inconsistent reference points, because it produces the desired effect, a call for action and funding. And the two sides, the children in street situations and the larger culture, interact to maintain this image as it benefits both of them.

Ennew (2000) notes that abandoned children (we could put in children in street situations) are used to stigmatize the poor. By showing that the poor cannot take care of their children, children in street situations allow civil society to justify its view of the poor as morally inferior.

Street children as a group of children began with UNICEF (1986) claiming there were categories of street children; candidates to become street children, children on the streets but returning home at night, and finally children of the streets, those without home or adult supervision. The implication was that there was a causative linear movement from a good family home to a dysfunctional family home, to working on the street, to becoming a fully fledged street child. The belief was that their families were dysfunctional, because of economic conditions that forced rural to urban migration, because of economic hardship, and because they had too many dependents that needed to be taken care of most often by a single parent (a mother with allegedly questionable moral values as she prefers a series of men who abuse her children), and who lived in shantytowns amidst crime and squalor. Street children are thus

[15] See Balagopalan (2002) for an in-depth view of a Calcuttan street child's reaction to a vocational education program that shows how culture, including those in developing countries which have been affected by colonialism, post-colonialism and modernism, confirm childhood and adolescence as social constructs that prevail upon the biological realities of age.

placed outside of the normal flow of poor urban life in the developing world, and the street then becomes their home; the evil place where unbridled youth with their own secret codes (their own idiom) and values (crime, drugs and prostitution), confront traditional life and values. Thus, the description of street children is more than defining a social group; it includes the demise of their families and the moral values of the children. It is stigmatizing and perpetuating their exclusion and low status.

Domiciled children live within the acceptable norms of family, schools, and religious life. Children in street situations define themselves by their independence from these norms. Through a constant, subterranean, set of negotiations children in street situations press through a cycle of advances, parries, and retreats between themselves and the adult society, which becomes the text of who they are, and how others define them. This can roughly be divided into two categories; their relations with each other, and in their interactions with society.

But even their relations with each other are closely linked to fictive comparisons and thus social in nature because they actively situate themselves against some of the dominant normative family standards in order to build an in-group identity. In Brazil for instance, street children define themselves by referring to domiciled children as "children of mama and papa". Lucchini (1993) found their comparisons to the norm were a mixture of contempt and envy.

Societal reaction to life on the street fluctuates among extreme violence, indifference and assistance. There are too many examples of individual violence and institutional hostility against street children and runaway youth to list them all (Aidswatch 1989; Aptekar 1988, 1994; Cheng 2008; Dimenstein 1990; Leite and Esteves 1991; McLachlan 1986; Patel 1983, 1990; Pereira 1985; Pinheiro 2006; Randall 1988; Swart 1990; Verma and Dhingra 1993; West 2003). The UN Secretary-General's study on violence against children (Pinheiro 2006) indicates that quite often judges resort to needless incarceration of children who pose no specific danger to the public and that bail is almost never, if ever, considered an option for street children.

The fact is that the streets are not a neutral venue; they are a public space with symbolic meanings including the culture's view of what is public and private including what behavior is permissible and what is not. In most places children do not belong in the streets and adults see their presence as a hostile intrusion on their rights. On the streets, the children earn a living, they have their own domiciles, their own social groups, and they take control over their means of pleasure; all of which adults see as an affront to their rightful domain of adult roles.

The impact on the child of the public's reaction depends a lot on the nearly invisible skills of the child. Many authors have shown the importance of street children's moral sensibility, or the capacity to have and make moral judgments.[16] However, the media focuses almost exclusively on the visible and spectacular behavior, reinforcing the cycle of stigmatization and secondary deviance.

Although any intervention should, by international law, include the participation of youth in all phases of planning (something we go into in more detail in Chapter 4),

[16] See Aptekar 1988; Ennew 1994; Lucchini 1993; and Parazelli 2002.

top-down approaches are still predominant in programs. This has been observed in programmes for homeless youth and street children where it is still mainly according to adult intervention agendas that children's views are taken into consideration (Parazelli 2002; Rizzini et al. 2007).[17]

In the most extreme cases, torture and killings of street children have been perpetrated. Torture on street children was common in Guatemala and Honduras in the 1990s (Casa Alianza 1997). Police abuse and killings of street children in India have also been reported (Human Rights Watch 1996) as well as police abuse and detention of street children in Kenya: Human Rights Watch (1996) found that street children were committed for years to juvenile correctional institutions just because they had been labelled "in need of protection or discipline" in some summary proceedings without any legal representation.

Social reactions and sometimes even deprivation of liberty through judicial acts are closely linked to status offences: things that are seen as a crime only if perpetrated by a category of population (in this case by people too young to be considered adult) not allowed to do such things according to their specific status. For children in street situations, these status offences may include running away from home, or simply being "beyond parental control". According to Wernham (2004), 60% of boys detained a remand home in Lagos, Nigeria, in March and April 2003, were non-criminal cases sent for protection. This proportion was up to 80% for the girls detained in another remand home.

Rwanda rounds up street children and puts them in "re-education centres", regardless of their supposed offences (WHO 2001). In numerous other settings, street children may be sent to detention in remand institutions or adult prisons, and kept indefinitely (Peres 2004). Stoecklin (2003) once visited a prison in Guinea-Conakry where more than 200 children and adults were detained together in a compound around 80 square meters and where the heat and lack of facilities were intolerable. When asking what a randomly selected child of around 13 years old had done to be here, he was told that the child had stolen a bicycle some years ago. No one knew how many years it had been, and the boy was still waiting for his trial.

How then do we define the atrocities perpetrated on children in street situations? In Brazil, Hecht (1998) describes a street child who had committed some petty thievery being held upside down by police who simultaneously slowly dripped cleaning detergent into his nostrils.[18] Another incident in Brazil was the Candalaria massacre of 1993, where police fired on a group of 40 street children sleeping by the Candalaria Church. Before they could awaken, six were dead (two more would die later) and many were wounded (Scheper-Hughes and Hoffman 1998).

[17] A certain domination is playing out in the form of a hidden "habitus" (Bourdieu), or typical way of perceiving and defining reality. Therefore the social relationships between actors within the project are the ones that the planning process, and the dominant forces in it, produced (Mosse 2001).

[18] What is worse, is that children in street situations are now being hired by perpetrators of other violence such as police or paramilitary groups such as drug traffickers to do their work for them (Hecht 1998).

What brought about this massacre? Evidently, the day before, some street children threw stones at a police car, but this wouldn't account for it. What needs to be added to understand this?[19] According to the authors of the study some possible factors include; social shame at the failure of the country to achieve its economic goals; the children out in the public space, often in the most affluent public space, portraying the image of social failure; and the fear of an eruption of violence from the favelas.[20]

The behaviors of children in street situations that the public observes indicate to the public that children in street situations have violated the norms and rules of accepted childhood behavior. Think of all the things they do as adults would. They do not live under the roof that their culture assigns them, they bypass school, they work while "under age", and perhaps most important they enjoy the fruits of their behavior with alcohol or drugs, in full public view.

Why is it that the biggest fears of children in street situations worldwide center around the police (Aptekar and Stoecklin 1997)? Is it because they are enforcers of local rules? The problem is that children in street situations do not see the police as fair arbiters. For street boys in Bangalore, India, who "experienced the police as their major problem in their daily existence" (Nieuwenhuizen 2006, p. 79), the greatest fear was of being arrested and sent to prison, often for crimes they did not commit, or having their money taken from them, or being forced to pay bribes or fines or even being used by the police to steal or commit other illegal acts such as collecting money for the police. A similar reaction was found from the public in Port-au-Prince Haiti, where Kovats-Bernat (2006) found that the fact that much of the trouble between street children and the police who patrol the streets and local business owners, comes from the public's resentment of the fact that street children are acting as if they were adults. Again, the response is only to what they see, not to the interior motivations of their behavior.

On the other side of the spectrum of social reactions, we find assistance to children perceived as victims. In between violence and assistance, another possible social reaction is indifference, which is less common. We can consider the three possible reactions to street children – violence, indifference and assistance – as a continuum with the most frequent reactions polarized in the two extremes (Fig. 3.5).

Strangely, the two extremes are often present at the same time, which can be explained by the fact that the street child is an ambivalent character defined as both

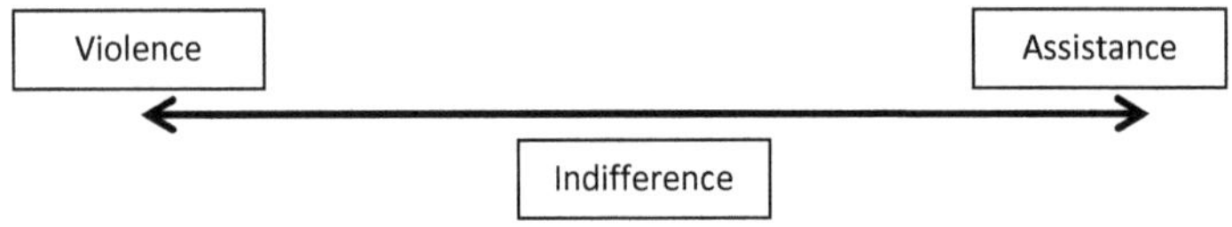

Fig. 3.5 Continuum of social reactions to children in street situations

[19] Twenty percent of the public supported the police based on being fed up with dirty aggressive street children (Scheper-Hughes and Hoffman 1998).

[20] A similar situation, the authors' point out, exists in the poor urban areas of the USA. Here too, there is fear of an eruption of violence in a public space and of police brutality.

victim and delinquent (Aptekar 1990a, c; Lucchini 1993; Pérez Lopez 2009). Even the term street children acts as an oxymoron because it is composed of two terms that do not match well together; together they challenge the social representations of childhood (Chombart de Lauwe 1983; Jodelet 1993).

When the street child is seen as a delinquent (illegal work, theft, drugs, and sexual acts), a vicious circle of deviance and repression begins. This begins from the moment that being a vagabond is considered a status offence, which in turn criminalises children in street situations in a way that provokes greater delinquency. In the beginning, the child commits petty crimes just to survive, then, as he is already branded a criminal, he takes on the role of a true delinquent and ends up specialising in this career.

The State sponsored repression through criminalization of status offenses encourages the career paths of street children and runaway youth toward further deviance. Add the economic globalization that forces males into the streets and tensions created by domestic violence, and we can see that the presence of children in street situations looms large in the public's eye. Then, it is the nature of the media to provide statistics and define categories without realizing how conducive they are to the discrimination that contributes to the widespread derogatory labels of "street child", and "homeless youth" that make such children the objects of both sentimental compassion and violent repression.

Cultural Contexts of Children in Street Situations: a View Through the Media

How do the media portray children in street situations? *Hugo*, the recently acclaimed Martin Scorsese movie based on Brian Selznick's 2007 novel, *The Invention of Hugo Cabret*, starts with a cute boy as a street child with the special skills of fixing clocks and other mechanical things. Neglected and abandoned by abusive parents, he is taken over by his uncle, an alcoholic abuser himself. When his uncle dies, Hugo moves forward on his own, save for a single omnipresent police man, himself a wounded ex-member of the orphanage who threatens Hugo and the other urchins with jail time. Why isn't *Hugo* an objective portrayal of a street child? Well, for one he is too clean, and his sleeping quarters include a bed, rather than a soft space on the ground. Just as important are his contacts and skills. Even more importantly, Hugo socialized with children of the well to do. Indeed he finds a young woman whom he befriends and over time she takes him in. Also, society recognizes his alleged high moral standing (in his relationship to the man selling mechanical toys, with whom he eventually works). His intelligence is acknowledged as he out-foxes his nemesis, the policeman. While this is the dream of any child in a street situation, the dream is only realized in, say, one hundredth of one percent of all cases, if that. The dream of the movie viewer is that all children in street situations could be like Hugo and that they would be able to succeed, but the reality is that the problems of children in street situations remain complex and difficult to deal with.

At the other extreme is the protagonist of the movie *Pixote*, whose life is filled with crime and violence, and in whom the viewer can only see a slight sliver of goodness. This allows us to think he too might be reborn into better circumstances. In real life, the street child actor playing Pixote, after his moment of glory returns to his former life and ends up dead from violence.

The Mexican movie, *Los Olvidados* (*The Forgotten Ones*), seems more real to us. The hero is forced to live by scavenging garbage in the Mexico City dump and remains there because he is still poor. He demonstrates his coping skills by befriending a blind man, who can protect him from being abused by bigger boys in exchange for offering the blind man the eyes he is missing. The emphasis in *Los Olvidados* is on coping with poverty, which seems more real than emphasizing the alleged special attributes which draw the attention of a savior in *Hugo* or result in self-defeat in *Pixote*.

Through these media portrayals, we can see that life on the streets is made-up of various constraints affecting children and their survival strategies, and their lives vary according to the context. We can ask ourselves; when, where, how and why is living on the street a problem?

To respond to this question requires that we also cast light on those who are in contact with street children, because they are part of the problem, and hopefully also part of the solution. When talking about street children and homeless youth, the people who usually analyse the situation use their own values, positions and interests, which in turn influence public opinion. For some, such children are delinquents; for others victims. Some people exaggerate statistics. This may increase the feeling of public insecurity, which, in turn, can be exploited to justify "cleaning-up" the streets. Others underestimate the problem or simply censure the topic, thus potentially ignoring a very real humanitarian problem.

In almost all cultures, childhood and adolescence are in large part defined by their powerlessness in relationship to adults. To the extent that children in street situations feel abused or neglected at home, they carry a double dose of powerlessness, because in addition to being powerless as part of their developmental stage, they believe that power has been used unfairly at home. From this belief, and their inability to negotiate fairer rules and regulations, their pain (anger, depression, self-abuse, coping via drugs) gains ground. As they continue trying to gain some power, and step by step they find no success they finally come to the realization that they are powerless to make a change.

Perhaps correctly, they feel the only way to solve the problem is by leaving the scene. Thus they run away and the public reacts. But the public's reaction needs an explanation. One narrative is that these children are inadequately socialized and let loose to run wild and create havoc. This script is conducive to seeing children in street situations as delinquents rather than victims. Even when they are seen as victims of single-parent homes, of abusive stepparents, or poor child rearing practices, the narrative locates responsibility within the abusive family rather than at the level of larger socio-economic structural processes which impoverish and marginalize whole sectors of society.

A study regarding the trends of intervention since 1989, when the UNCRC was adopted, confirms that the narrative of the child victim is less concerned with structural socio-economic violence than with the individual violence exerted in the immediate surroundings of the child (Hanson 2012).

Historical Contexts of Children in Street Situations

Children in street situations can suffer from multiple and complex problems. Take the case of Bangladeshi, Afghani and Burmese children living in street situations in Karachi, Pakistan (Ono 2008). In addition to living in street situations, they are also unwelcome migrants. There are an estimated 1.2 million children living and working on the streets in Karachi. About 18% of the total are immigrants.

There is almost no research about them and most of the information we have comes from NGOs who are assessing and monitoring their programs. There are essentially no studies of nor programs for female children in street situations. And, finally, many of these immigrants are not Muslim.

The single most important variable that is left out of explaining the origins (and narratives) about children in street situations is the cultural and historical context. These multinational children living in street situations in Karachi, Pakistan cannot be understood without taking into account their multifaceted context.

America was founded in part by homeless youth who as early as the 1600s were running away from home to travel to the new world (Libertoff 1980). By the time the colonies were more affluent and building a modern State in the 18th and first half of the 19th century, many homeless youth were indentured into service, placed in orphanages run by churches or charitable organizations, and made to go to almshouses. They were treated no differently than adult vagrants, and records suggest that in many almshouses these youths were severely malnourished. By the mid-to-late 19th century, public attention was brought to bear on the horrific conditions of many of these institutions. These efforts led to the creation of juvenile courts, the criminalization of running away, and to youth and adult homelessness being addressed separately.

Teeter (1995) shows that the study of historical antecedents of American homeless youth is important in understanding modern adolescence, particularly extending the culturally acceptable age for leaving home from 14 to 18. The first American urban slums developed in the 1830s and 1840s. This was the time of the "street arabs", so-called because of their comparison to nomadic tribes. Increasingly portrayed as waifs, they were known for their multitudes, their disregard for authority, and their petty crimes. Many of them were abandoned, others ran away from home, and some made the choice to live more freely and in many cases a better life than staying in the slums. They earned money legitimately and illegitimately. They were of both genders, including female gangs of youth ("The Forty Little Thieves" and "Lady Locusts" in New York).

A decade before the civil war, New York had, according to the author, about 30,000 homeless youth. In 1846 Boston, there were some 5,000 homeless youth. The public feared the alleged criminality of homeless youth was taking over the city. American society responded by initiating programs to take children off of the streets and out of the sweatshops.

In response to the alleged problems of misconduct of homeless youth, American society built what became the modern high school and increased the ages of compulsory education. This was not a motivated by altruism; it was based on fear.

Another societal reaction to homeless youth at this time was a religious revival, much of which took place in urban slums. The pitch was based on moral threats; if youth did not follow a religious path, they would end up in jail or die. These urban religious efforts were, according to Teeter (1995), the prototype for today's church-affiliated Sunday Schools.

During the 1850s, charitable and benevolent organizations began to offer more secular responses to homeless youth. These programs were based on the alleged character defects of homeless youth; they did not take into consideration larger social issues such as economic conditions. Children were put in foster homes or on rural farms. From this time until the eve of the great depression, some 150,000 "orphan trains" went west to resettle these children.[21] At each stop the children were paraded in front of the community for families to choose among them. Those who weren't chosen went to child-run communities, which were self-governing laboratories for modern citizenship in a democratic society. These communities were seen as good investments in youth and explain the founding of Boys Town in 1917. Likewise, the YMCA (Young Man's Christian Association) provided homes and communities for homeless youth. City-sponsored clubs for boys were begun throughout the country, and later brought together under the national umbrella of Boys' Clubs of America in 1906. The scouting movement, begun in 1910, was an effort to channel youthful instincts into constructive citizenry. Parks and playgrounds were created to provide safe places for play.

Just before the 20th century, Anthony Comstock began a campaign to limit reading material for children and youth (Teeter 1995). At about the same time, *Huckleberry Finn* was published (in 1884). The two views of homeless youth, Huck Finn as a care-free, adventurous, homeless youth, and Comstock's fears of other homeless youth becoming like Huck, illustrated the battle between the moralists and the secularists.

As these programs failed, America began to take another approach; the advent of the modern American high school. At the beginning of the 20th century, there were about 7,000 high schools in the US, and fewer than 10% of American youth completed high school. Teachers were as rare as the students, often one teacher per high school. It was not until the depression ended that high schools were abundant and not until the 1950s did they become essential. Thus from the turn of the 20th century, coinciding with the apex of homeless youth, the American secondary school grew from a small part of American life to the major institution for adolescents. As the American high school grew, the numbers of homeless children declined.

A similar historical analysis was conducted in Britain (Carlen 1996). One comparison in this study is the historic correlation between the lack of affordable housing and homeless youth in the UK. Prior to the 20th century, homeless youth in the UK carried the image of the wandering mendicant.

Aptekar (1988, 1989a, 1990a, 1992) demonstrated this with Colombian street children. He begins on April 9, 1948, the day the dictatorial government of Ospina Perez was overthrown and the populist president elect Elieazar Gaitán was

[21] In the depression of the 1930s, some two million Americans were homeless (Smollar 1999).

assassinated. Gaitán was the first man of the masses to have won the votes of the people as well as the support of the political system, thus instilling a renaissance of possibility in the populace.

Before Gaitán, access to political life, as well as inclusion in high society, depended on one's family name; civic life was dictated by family connections; different families not only belonged to different social classes and to different political parties, but the very identity of those parties was inexorably intermingled with certain family names. With Gaitan's election, the country became more egalitarian and meritocratic, which increased many people's opportunities to participate in civic, social, and political life. This put a great deal of strain on the heretofore unquestioned power of the dominant families.

Street children had been part of the Colombian landscape since the late 1800s. They were called *chinos de las calles*, (*chino* is an affectionate word for child in Quechua, the language of the Incas, and *calle* is a public street). Sometimes they were called *puluelos* (little rascals or scamps).

The origin of the word *gamin* dates to 1874. At that time, the boys working in the Zipaquira salt mine walked out because of the inhumane working conditions. The viceroy, Manuel de Guirar, ordered the State to round up the boys and place them in custody. But the authorities did not blame their parents for improper childrearing. It was a labor issue, not a problem of parental abuse or neglect.

It wasn't until Gaitan's victory that street children were labeled "abandoned". Thus their families were judged to be at fault and moral values were applied. Streets are outside of family control. The public nature of the streets makes people in them anonymous. They are no longer known members of a family.[22]

Gaitan's election threatened the hegemony of the traditional family. In great part the new concepts of "losing the children to the street" and "abandoned and neglected children" were a warning from those recently elected to the defeated upper social class regarding the turmoil that would result from opening up society to different social and racial groups, as well as from a different set of rules that would change participation in civic life. Vying over the eventual extent of this change, those who held power and those who sought it found, in the presence of the street children, a symbol over which claims for each side's position could be made. Thus street children inherited a particular social class and cultural struggle that would determine not only how their childhood would be defined, but would also set the boundaries of appropriate child rearing, which included basic moral values (Aptekar 1988).

A similar situation exists in Venezuela where street children are also greatly influenced by the Spanish culture (Marquez 1999). Historically, upper class Venezuelan men of Spanish descent have headed powerful extended families and fathered children with their mistresses. Because these men did not recognize their mistresses and their children as legitimate, these children of mixed ethnicity were left without documentation and thus without citizenship. Being unable to

---

[22] A constant theme of Indian authorities is that they have limited control over the use of space by the poor on the streets, and that street children without family contacts are a major social concern (Huchzermeyer and Karam 2006).

marry legally, the male offspring of these relationships grew to adolescents and fathered children, some of whom became street children.

The street children found themselves in a war against the socially conservative traditional Spanish higher socio-economic class who, because of where the children came from, the fact that they lived on the streets and the multiple examples of their unacceptable behavior, used the media, government agencies, and the juvenile justice system to define them pejoratively.

The same societal factors and family changes contributed to the dynamic of street children in Haiti (Kovats-Bernat 2006). The Francophone elite over-harvested the forests, over-grazed the land, and over-mined for minerals, all for export. While they prospered, many rural families without the natural resources were forced to look for work in urban areas. Traditional extended families became dismantled and foster care among relatives became scarce.

In the urban environment, many families were so poor that there simply was not enough money to feed everyone. They coped by having only the young children remain at home, while the older male children were forced out to find work and bring back money. In some cases, there were situations of abuse or neglect, but many children forced into the streets maintained loving relationships at home. The public reaction, in this case from the French (similar to the Spanish), demeaned the traditional Haitian family for not taking care of its children. They classified them as unhealthy caretakers, which thus allowed Haiti to sanction street children under law (Kovats-Bernat 2006).

In Kenya, Kilbride et al. (2000) showed that the origins of street children could be found in the unfortunate intersection of the Western-oriented market economy and indigenous cultures. Traditional Kenyan cultures (of which there are many, but referring here to Bantu cultures) contained large extended and joint families who lived closely together. Their marriages extended beyond a single man and woman to include the families of the bride and groom. Their children grew up in peer groups of similar ages, creating life-long ties among them.

As the post-colonial market economy gained strength, a series of changes ensued that led to devaluing many relationships that had held the culture together. One was the decline in the number of elder men who had been seen as sages and political conciliators. Adult men had to move to the city for employment. In the absence of men, the older male children went to work in the fields earlier, matured earlier and went to town sooner to find work to support their families, while the girls went to school less and peer-related childhood became less viable.[23]

In colonial India, certain Indian individuals were chosen by the British because of their Western values to be social-cultural interpreters, to work essentially as colonizers to instill Western values in the lower class Indian children (Balagopalan

[23] Children in street situations from Northern Somalia stand out because they remained relatively mentally healthy in spite of being considered to be of the highest mental health risk (Rousseau et al. 1998). According to the authors it was the lack of pull from the international marketplace. Thus these children still grew up in age-related peer groups and participated in the intergenerational social structure, whereas elders were leaders whom youth respected and learned from.

2002).[24] This continues today so that poor children, including street children, have modern cultural values. Street children are not a traditional subculture.

Among the Portuguese-speaking Brazilian elite, government sanctions ranged from incarcerating to murdering street children. By 1990, more street children had been killed in Brazil than the number of people who died in the civil war in Lebanon (Leite and Esteves 1991).[25] This appeared to be the apogee of this epoch of harmful societal reactions to street children.

As in Colombia, Venezuela, Haiti, Kenya, Brazil and India, the media and government, controlled by the established power brokers, castigated street children instead of owning up to how their role in the world economy, increasing their economic power and the national debt, would only increase the factors that lead to the existence of street children.

The importance of social reactions in shaping peer-group dynamics is very clear in the case of Chinese street children where political factors play a major role. In the 1990s especially, street children were not only shaped by the traditional values and expectations regarding all children, but specifically by the authorities who fought to keep street children in their homes in a period of huge economic transition (Stoecklin 2000a). As a result, street children received very repressive sanctions.

Another societal intervention into the lives of Chinese street children came as a result of the massive rural–urban migration, increased urbanization and the fines that had to be paid for children born outside of the "one-child policy". Most of the children interviewed by Stoecklin (2000a) were born "out-of-plan" and had to come to the city to work or beg under adult supervision in order for their families to escape from the penalties and measures that they would been subjected to if they stayed in their hometowns. A smaller number of the interviewed children had to work to compensate for the fines the family had to pay. The fines affected the poor because wealthier families could afford the fines or resort to paying corrupt officials.

When one considers the numeric importance of the total number of births outside of the limits of the family planning policy: officially recognized statistics show that in the 1980s, every year this was some 40% of births (Stoecklin 2000a). We can see the enormity of the problems in China. For example, a part of these "unplanned" births remain "unregistered" and thus do not "officially" exist: these children are called "*hei haizi*" ("black children"). The label "*hei haizi*" applies to children who are born outside of the limits set by China's family planning policy, and thus referred to as "out of plan", and who are also not registered in the Civil Registers held by the Ministry of Public Security. The results of research in China (Stoecklin 2000a; Cheng 2008) highlight a particularly interesting topic, namely the impact of the *hei hazei* (unregistered, out-of-plan children) and the fact that street life is not just a matter of socialization, but can also be politically induced.

---

[24] This is essentially an example of the filtration theory of cultural assimilation.

[25] Scheper-Hughes and Hoffman (1998) report 5,000 street children were killed in Brazil during the 3 year period of 1988–1990. For a world view of how street children are treated by their communities see Boyden and Holden (1991).

Because there are no retirement schemes for the vast majority of China's rural population, relying on offspring for securing one's old age remains a common strategy. In this context, the patrilineal and patrilocal social structures and the introduction of a strict policy on birth limitation serve to reinforce the preference for boys. The behaviors and strategies of children in the streets are thus quite constrained by these macrosocial elements.

The Internationalization of Childhood

In 21st century western settings and more and more in all places around the world, childhood is giving sway to international social contexts. The older paradigms of James et al. (1998) and James and Prout (1990) argued that childhood is a universal biological phenomenon, but differs according to the social significance and interactions attached to it. Nowadays one realizes that what is becoming more important to children in street situations is the internationalization of adolescence.

As a result of feeling of tenuousness about home and feeling the tendrils of international materialism, Hanson and Vandaele (2003) found that more and more parents have come to see the street as dangerous and to keep their children away from it. The streets are so dangerous that regulation of them and surveillance over them is necessary. In many western settings, there is a debate about the legitimacy of video surveillance for public security.

Into this social mix come street children and homeless youth who are attracting a lot more attention as they are living in that threatening place, the streets. The more autonomous they become, the more governments threaten to impose another kind of social regulation whereby the authority of adults is not only challenged but overthrown.

Ironically, the wandering around of street and homeless children is seen as indicating a lack of self-control, whereas it is a survival strategy. Actually, the symptom (wandering around) should not be seen as the cause (lack of self-control) but as an adaptation to the real problem, which is that the means to lead a domiciled life in a stable family are not accessible to everyone. Blaming the poor for disturbing the public order doesn't address the root causes of street life.[26]

The more the family is consumed by the evil "out there" in the streets, in the public place, and in any event not at home, the more children in street situations become the property of contemporary criminology, public moralizing and current debates over pedagogic practice. This view assumes that evil, corruption and baseness are primary elements in the constitution of the "child". It derives from the perspective of the Leviathan (Thomas Hobbes) as a collective force that has to impose restraints on individuals. People must renounce the use of individual powers and

[26] See Pupavac (2006) who questions if societies are expected to take different development paths, and the effects of this on considering a global child development path.

restrain their instincts, in exchange for which they are protected by a "social contract", conferring powers to specialised institutions; that is, to the State (Leviathan). Childhood is therefore to be shaped by the exercise of restraints on natural dispositions. In the Freudian perspective, which has pervaded a great deal of today's common sense, drives and instincts are a common explanation for aberrant behaviour. Sexual intercourse by street children appears therefore as indicative of uncontrolled drives. These conceptions of childhood are informing the dominant social reaction towards children in street situations.[27]

Take for example countries where punishment of children is considered a duty of parents. Serbian children are considered bad social beings; they would need to be punished in order to become good (Trebjesanin 2001). In Serbian patriarchal culture, punishment has become synonymous with upbringing. Society fosters a protectionist attitude rather than investing sufficient efforts in the development of institutions and services which provide support for parenting and children's education and health. Children are 'protected' and 'empowered' for as long as their needs, views and conduct do not interfere with the established order in the family, but also with that in educational and social welfare institutions. The needs and problems of children are subject to interpretation by adults (Zegarac 2007). Paternalism is reflected in restrictions on children's rights to participation, privacy and free expression of their views rather than in the protection and promotion of the rights of the child (Vuckovic-Sahovic 2000).

At the end of 20th century, post-colonial NGOs changed from direct care to advocacy of children's rights (Klees et al. 2000). The "Children's Movement" had something to do with this, as did the UN Convention on the Rights of the Child (1989). The "Children's Movement" gained strength in part by going public. In the past, television media showed graphic portraits of violence toward street children along with imagery and stories showing children as law breakers while depicting store keepers and paramilitary personnel as defenders of the law. Because of the "Children's Movement", the image of street children changed and the press found it could sell copy by showing the intelligence of the children as they organized and spoke for their cause. They could do this because in a newly flourishing democracy lower classes are less disenfranchised and upper classes (of small populations) lose their hegemony.

This pattern of change in political dynamics and family structure directly translating into effects on street children, are similar to the case of homeless youth. Over different historical epochs, values changed. So did the attitudes toward homeless youth. At the beginning of the American Republic when expansion was necessary,

[27] This is Freud's psychoanalytical hypothesis of the evil nature of man where primal libidinal drives (instinctive energies), and the pleasure principle are incompatible with collective life, and therefore need to be curbed. In this perspective, successful development into adulthood derives from proper management of this repression. Street and homeless youngsters probably trigger the unconscious fear of an evil that would reside within children, and parents increasingly identify the world outside the home as one from which their children, must be shielded and in relation to which they must devise strategies to reduce risk. The children are perceived as being vulnerable to physical harm such as traffic accidents and strangers as a source of attack or abduction.

runaway youth were conquering heroes who left home to seek a fortune. During the great depression, when endurance and ingenuity were valued, leaving home to find a job was condoned. One can imagine that during these times it was poverty more than abuse that was the impetus for leaving home. In this way the situation was much like the conditions confronting male street children today.

From the end of WW1 until the end of WW2, runaway youth, in the context of the world wars, were seen as psychologically deviant because they were assumed to be escaping from fighting. During the 1960s and early 1970s, youth running away from home were seen as part of the peace movement or counter culture, and to some extent were given a reprieve, until rampant drug use went public and society became alarmed.

When the Diagnostic and Statistical Manual (American Psychiatric Association 1968, 2nd ed.) of the American Psychiatric Association was published, it labeled runaway youth as having a mental disorder characterized by; fleeing from threatening situations, timidity, feelings of inadequacy, and a lacking of friends, thus making the runaway's dysfunctional psyche the central focus of societal reactions.

Since then, public policy and public attitudinal change have broadened to include the pathology of the runaway, the pitiful family circumstances, and delinquent behavior. This coincided with rising figures for child abuse in the 1980s (maybe because of more abuse or maybe because of more reporting or reporters).

The view of their personal unfavorable characteristics grew to include depression, suicidal behavior, low self-esteem, and a closer look at family dynamics, which were also considered dysfunctional, (intergenerational troubles with the law, including drug abuse, domestic violence, etc.). Even their school problems were included; confrontations with teachers and peers, truancy, and poor grades (Roberts 2000).

There are several social science theories that can be used to understand these reactions to children in street situations. Cognitive dissonance theory (Festinger 1957) suggests that society's attitude about what children should be doing in public and what they see children in street situations doing in public are not in synch. The dissonance between the beliefs that children belong at home under caring adults, and the behaviors of children in street situations in public is uncomfortable; it produces a psychological tension which the person wants to reduce. The two ways to reduce the tension are either to think of children in street situations as having been abandoned or abused and therefore still children, but children who have a reason for acting this way, or to think that children in street situations have no excuse; they are acting delinquently, and thus they are in need of action to get them back in line with what is appropriate children's behavior. Take this news item: It has become widespread in many African countries to hear that street children are carrying syringes filled with contaminated HIV positive blood and are threatening anyone who refuses to give them money with lethal injections. Not one case alleged behaviour has ever been authenticated, yet the public's perception is that it is a common occurrence. Notice that neither response allows the public to accept the children in street situations as early entrants into adulthood, so it is impossible to resolve the cognitive dissonance without resorting to blaming the children's parents and highlighting the children's delinquency, drug abuse, promiscuous sexuality, etc.

Rational choice theory suggests that each action is the result of a previous action which the actor considered to be personally beneficial. Because all the information to make an optimal rational choice is not available to the actor at all times, people act to meet their immediate needs, thinking that this is the rational choice. In fact, what appears more hedonistic in the short run, may be the rational choice in the long run. Sen (1999) makes an argument about the "information bias" and shows that the selection of information that is necessary to make a rational choice is always problematic because in the end, a rational choice depends on the selection of all relevant information which is hardly ever possible.

Under rational choice theory children in street situations are on the streets because they have made a rational decision that it is better than staying at home, either because it was abusive or neglectful, or because as boys they were expected to leave and earn money to help the family. This decision might not be the optimum decision in the long run, but the best one available at the time, given the lack of complete information.

The public can assume that children in street situations are not making a long-term rational choice and thus need immediate help. The same can be said of their parents who are not making a rational choice to be abusive or neglectful, in which case they also need help. Even if the public can accept that the children are acting rationally, it still does not provide an option to grant them adult respect. There are always strings attached to this way of thinking.

Social constructivism theory explains that reality is formed by the interaction of the children and their environments. This helps to explain children in street situations as being abandoning and abandoned, having abusive or neglectful families and families that are rearing them to do their best with what life has to offer, and of a supporting or ostracizing society. Children in street situations under this theory must be considered in the context of multiple realities, and the way to help them is to focus on the quality of the multiple relationships of the child and his or her diverse social world. However, the wider and more complex the children's stimuli, the more difficult it is to help them, because too many components have to be changed. Again, there is no mention of accepting them as early entrants into adulthood.

The sociological perspective looks at what society demands of the child. James et al. (1998) propose a critical exploration of the various ways in which the sociological tradition has conceptualized childhood. First is the functionalist approach to explain that uniform and predictable standards of action from participating members of society are the only way to maintain stability and integration. The first participants in the social order are children and they must be socialized in ways that are functional for the social system.

The critique made by James et al. (1998) to this functionalist approach is that children are seen as passive receptacles of society. There is no consideration for children's specific skills, which continue to be simply measured against adult skills.

Socialization is seen as the process through which children learn to conform to social norms. The social order depends on the efficacy of socialization, which involves the successful transmission of culture from one generation to the next.

Street children break this cycle of virtuous behaviour by disobeying older people, making decisions on their own and leading independent lives, since these norms are more functional with regard to street conditions.

The analysis of socialization made by social scientists within mainland China may be taken as a reflection of the normative definition of children. In mainland China, socialization is reduced to cognitive abilities and conformity, or in other words achievement and virtue. Socialization allows the passage from *sheng wu ren* (or *ziran ren*, natural being) to *she hui ren* (social being). They insist on the importance of society for the individual. Socialization is intended to perpetuate the succession of generations, and to guarantee continuity and stability through the transmission of norms (Wang 1989, p. 31). The political interpretation of socialization is clearly normative and calls for conformity. This definition of socialization in prescriptive terms is justified by the opposition between nature (animals = low value) and culture (social being = high value). Basically, in the mainland Chinese view, socialization seems to be the development of virtue.

The functionalist paradigm accommodates quite well with the traditional and instrumental approach to children, whereby actors are seen mainly as an outcome of social reproduction. Street children are thus seen as non-functional or deviant and, as it happens, moral judgements often pervade the analysis, especially when the researchers are not really in a position of axiological neutrality (Weber 1968). In China, sociology is a field that has been heavily affected by political control for decades. It was even banned from 1953 to 1978 (Ming 1989). In this context, there is still a relatively low differentiation among political discourse, public attitudes, and sociological analysis.

But the case of China is not as individual as it seems. Actually, there is no scientific perspective that would be totally free from some kind of normative framework. To begin with, the choice of the topic and the funding of research on that topic are to some extent dependent on political forces. By extending the cross-cultural comparisons to China, we broaden the scope of our understanding of children living in the margins, as this case allows highlighting the barriers to scientific analysis itself. The challenge is to arrive at a perspective that is less dependent on political forces, including the normative framing of NGOs. The task is not easy, as access to street children is quite often mediated by these institutions and hence their own priorities. Contributing to a more complete theoretical perspective should start with procedures and tools that are more child-friendly, allowing them to reflect on their own experiences with as little interference of normative frameworks as possible.

A "New Paradigm" in Childhood Studies?

What we learn from the developed and developing worlds is that children in street situations do not exist in a vacuum. Who they are depends upon cultural factors and political processes. Worldwide, children in street situations have come to represent to the civil politic the moral decay of the current generation. People worry about what is wrong with their communities and fear what the future might bring to their own families.[28]

The "new paradigm" in the sociology of childhood (James and Prout 1990) can be qualified as social constructionism, a combination of structuralism and interactionism. The structuralists emphasise power and domination. They show that children constitute a dominated social category. The interactionist's perspective highlights the continuous negotiation between child and adult in the process of socialisation. Since the rise of the "new paradigm" in childhood studies, the social construction of childhood and the necessity to observe their agency have been underlined (James and Prout 1990; Archard 2004; Qvortrup et al. 1994; Corsaro 1997; Sirota 2006).

The difference between visible and invisible skills is very important to understand and intervene in relevant ways with street children and homeless youth. The difference between ability and competence is that the latter is more than just technical skills, as it comprises the capacity to evaluate and to compare events, persons and things (Lucchini 1998, p. 363). Another way to understand the distinction between ability and competence is to consider the difference between *poiesis* and *praxis*. *Poiesis* qualifies the action that produces an object that is external to the person, whereas *praxis* is a reflection over what is produced. People generally to focus on immediate visible outcomes (*poiesis*) and forget inner and longer term changes (*praxis*). Action cannot be reduced to only concrete activities. It involves symbolic and reflexive dimensions such as the image of self, the motivations, the values one has, as well as the actor's appraisal of his relationships (Stoecklin 2013).

The tendency to reduce actions to a concrete visible outcome (*poiesis)* is especially detrimental to people who do not have access to the conditions necessary to produce objects that are socially considered valuable. Therefore there is an invisible violence in expecting street and homeless youth to behave (to perform) like others, while ignoring the obstacles they encounter to display visible and valued actions. The ignorance of their competence to reflect critically denies the moral dimension of their action (*praxis*) on the grounds that whatever they do will not meet the expected standards. The standards they cannot meet are conceived as being normal, while what they do is not.

The visibility of children in streets situations contributes to conflating their ability and their competence, thus reducing their moral value to what can be seen. This reaches its climax in modern cities where public places are used by the vast majority as merely intermediary spaces in between home and the workplace. Thus, the children in street situations who are hanging out in this space are perceived as deviants.

As there is a growing limitation on access to public places situated in the city centre, children in street situations are forced into increased mobility, and even greater devaluation (see Rizzini et al. 2007 for the situations in Rio de Janeriro).

Children in street situations do not carry a single identity because the sources of their evaluation are multiple. While this might be true for anyone in society, the

[28] As we move to Chapter 5, which discusses programs, we will see how taking into account culture is necessary in helping them.

consequences depend on the social status of the individual, as well as on the social visibility attached to this status. The visibility of a status is positively correlated with three elements: the social control on the roles attached to one's status, the marginality of the group one is affiliated to, and the low degree of diversification of one's socio-cultural environment (Lucchini 1993, pp. 208–209).

Children in street situations have a high degree of visibility, and a corresponding low degree of diversified social identity. As they are hanging around in a place instead of just circulating from one place to another, their visible immobility tends to favor a stereotyped social identify as people who are "doing nothing". Their visibility then leads to prejudice about their moral value. They are perceived as "thinking nothing good" and most probably "preparing something bad". Therefore, behaving in a fugitive way, induced by a low and visible status, reinforces the impression that these children have something to hide. This is why children in street situations display their presence in the streets with some claim for pride. This is how they can defy those in power who label them as deviants without actually knowing them. At the same time, we see that the low social status and high visibility of street children are factors contributing to their reflexivity and critical in determining the way they are treated. The adverse situation they are facing obliges them to develop competencies that remain largely invisible because they are at the symbolic level (thinking, reflecting on things, assessing situations, etc.).

Of course, the influence of peers is rather important. Many studies show that in their decisions, street children affiliate to models of behavior most frequently transmitted by peers. Behavior imitation, mostly aggressive and violent, is a way to impose one's authority on younger children and/or on newcomers. Thus, the idea that they have chosen to be on the streets often comes from the position they have gained within the group. Not surprisingly then, they also consider it to be in their own best interest to stay in the streets, a "choice" that may be, in fact, the only alternative to a violent familial or institutional environment (Muskinja 2009).

Children living in the streets are invisible to the social welfare system in their countries: they lack personal documents, mostly birth certificates, and become unknown to social welfare, educational, justice and health systems (UNICEF 1986). Muskinja (2009) writes of female children in street situations in Belgrade, who have a high visibility on the street but are called "invisible" because they are acknowledged as competent. Yet they have invisible competencies: for example, the capacity to negotiate with much older men. The relationship between the visibility of children in street situations and their invisible competencies (because these are symbolic competencies) is a rather new concept. Only a few studies and some intervention programs make a systematic evaluation of street children's competencies. If we want to evaluate the status-related competencies of a particular child in a street situation, we have to identify the sources of evaluation or the symbolic references of this child. This evaluation depends: (1) on the values, beliefs, prejudices, of the larger culture of the group(s) in which the child lives; (2) on the goals and objectives of the larger culture, on the importance or the (practical) functional value of children in street situations, on the context and the event in connection to which the evaluation takes place, and (3) on the level of realization of the goals and aspirations of the child (Lucchini 1993).

When children are placed in the category of "street child or homeless youth", they are already considered to have nothing but weak or negative capacities. If, on the other hand, we put more emphasis on considering the way these children make sense of and use of their street environment, then we talk of "children in street situations" and we are in a different state of mind. The capabilities of children in street situations depend simultaneously on their personal characteristics and the social organization they live in. In fact, children in street situations show impressive capacities for association, and quite important symbolic competencies: empathy, negotiations among peers and with the larger society, such as police and social welfare workers, and a critical mind that can evaluate and react quickly to many situations.

These same skills, ironically enough, are the very competencies needed in a modern world. Meanwhile, the dominant intervention is still very repressive or paternalistic. For instance in Serbia: "*The perception of the child as vulnerable, passive, dependent on the physical, emotional and financial assistance of adults is inconsistent with the real circumstances in which some of the children in Serbia live. The life and work of street involved children poses an ethical challenge to experts, scholars and the broader public, giving rise to ambivalent opinions and responses ranging from tolerance and minimization to moral panic, public attacks on accountable persons, calls for protection, forced removals from the street and repressive measures against parents and children themselves*" (Zegarac 2007, p. 139).

A less paternalist intervention is the rights-based approach based on the UNCRC which includes the opportunity for children in street situations to be heard and therefore participate in the decisions about how they will be treated. This might be the only way their invisible competencies can be recognized and valued.

It has been shown that for all children there is a general blindness to their competencies. There are powerful social and economic forces limiting children's voice, and most young people feel that decisions are taken elsewhere (Matthews 2003). This is even more the case with street children and homeless youth. Thus favouring their genuine participation is a challenge. With Stoecklin's (2013) "actor's system" (see Chapter 4), attempts are now being made to have child participation based on the children's subjective reality.

What the new paradigm is telling us is that the way in which street children and homeless youth come to their identities, and develop their agency, is always related to the diverse and multiple conceptions of childhood. And these conceptions are still dependent on power relationships, thus reinforcing structuralism as an important perspective.

In other words, a cross-cultural comparison of categories such as "street children" or "homeless youth" should look at how these categories have been socially constructed. In this theory there is no universal street child or homeless youth. Thus, studying street children only within their peer-group interactions, as if one could study other children only in schoolyards, playgrounds, or clubs, would have the same shortcomings as any micro-level approach ignoring macro-level influences (economy, politics, etc.).

At the same time, studying peer-group dynamics is helpful in understanding how street children's social actions are structured. Concentrating on street children's language and codes is actually a good starting point to reveal the larger influence of societal of major structural factors (poverty, power distribution, etc.).

The diversity of situations is reflected in the literature about street children but also about homeless youth (Zeneidi-Henry 2002). But what are diverse are not childhoods but the experiences different children make of similar conditions.

Conclusion

We divided the social interactions of children in street situations into two categories: How they relate to each other and their relations with the public. Among themselves they have intimate dyads, small work-related groups, larger social groupings and they have places that are conducive to each of these. These places include their private hangouts, the places they sleep and to gatherings of more than one group of children in street situations.

The dyads often begin with an affectionate same-sex relationship with another child. Through dyads the children are incorporated into the group. In their groups they have a complex set of rules for reciprocity.

We showed that gender is an important distinction in intra and intergroup behavior. Although females are often portrayed as engaging in sex for money while the boys are portrayed as bullies and "johns", we presented other research which shows that they relate to each other in less stereotypical ways. Their use of drugs is better understood not as a personal characteristic, but as a social behavior.

We described how street children and homeless youth looked and acted differently than gang members. Groups of children in street situations are not organized around a common ethnicity as they often are with gangs. While crime often defines the gang, crime is usually opportunistic among groups of children on the streets. Gangs are delinquent and deviant; children in street situations are deviant but not very delinquent.

Societal reactions to children in street situations are based on a moral view of what the majority believe is proper behavior for children and what are acceptable child rearing practices. What behaviors the public allows and which are considered inappropriate, mold the children's public personas and self-concepts.

We showed that societal reactions to children in street situations fluctuate among extreme violence, indifference and assistance, and in the most extreme cases, torture and killings. The biggest fears of children in street situations world-wide center around the police.

Across cultures and history, street children and homeless youth are among the most marginalized by society. When the public associates them with violence, they react with hostility. Because the numbers of street children in some societies is large, they can manipulate public opinion, which they often (and perhaps surprisingly) do by behaving in a way that encourages society to view them pejoratively, such as taking drugs in full public view. This makes them stronger as a subculture.

We showed that because of the proportional scarcity of homeless youth in comparison to street children, and being more abused and from a culture with few adult role models for them, homeless youth have little ability to roam the streets or earn money legitimately. They rely more on the State or engage in extra-legal behavior.

Groups of children in street situations are found in differing degrees in different cultures, making it hard to understand their relationship to the State. We did find that a State's commitment to universal equal health care correlates with healthier children and families, and fewer children in street situations.

The passage of the UN Convention on the Rights of the Child (1989), and later the "Children's Movement", have had considerable impact on children in street situations, some good and some not so good. We presented the new paradigm of children studies, which is based on accepting the UNCRC and its corresponding claim to recognizing children's agency in forming their own lives.

As we have mentioned, the public distinguishes between two types of behaviours; instrumental abilities and symbolic competencies. Instrumental abilities are visible, concrete and evident in multiple activities in the street; shoe-shining, buying and selling, stealing, begging, etc. Symbolic competencies are invisible, and include the capacity for association (social skills), the ability to evaluate the environment (critical mind) and the capacity to influence the reactions of others (creation of opportunities).

The public's attitude toward children in street situations focuses on activities that are directly visible while passing over the invisible skills that are needed to survive (and which are quite similar to adult behaviours). In order to stop both condemning children in street situations as delinquents and/or accepting them in the powerless role as victims, society needs to be encouraged to pay more attention to their symbolic than visible competencies. The problems that come from behaviours that appear shocking to the public are likely to be responded to by the visible behaviour alone, and not the symbolic competencies such as negotiation, solidarity, and the critical mind.

References

Aidswatch (1989). Death squads kill one child every two days in Brazil. *American Medical Association Council on Scientific Affairs, 7*, 1.

American Psychiatric Association. (1968). *Diagnostic and statistical manual of mental disorders* (2nd ed.). Washington, DC: American Psychiatric Association.

Aptekar, L. (1988). *Street children of Cali*. Durham: Duke University Press.

Aptekar, L. (1989a). Picaresque tragedies: The 'Abandoned' children in Colombia. *Phenomenology and Pedagogy, 7*, 79–92.

Aptekar, L. (1990a). Family structure and adolescence: The case of the Colombian street children. *Journal of Adolescent Research, 5*(1), 67–81.

Aptekar, L. (1990b). Colombian street children: Gamines and Chupagruesos. *Adolescence, 24*(96), 783–794.

Aptekar, L. (1990c). How ethnic differences within a culture influence child rearing: The case of the Colombian street children. *Journal of Comparative Family Studies, 21*(1), 67–86.

Aptekar, L. (1992). Are Colombian street children neglected? the contributions of ethnographic and ethno-historical approaches to the study of children. *Anthropology & Education Quarterly, 22*(4), 326–349.

Aptekar, L. (1994). *Environmental disasters in global perspective*. New York: G. K. Hall/Macmillan.

Aptekar, L. (2004). The changing developmental dynamics of children in particularly difficult circumstances: Examples of street and war traumatized children. In U. Gielen & J. Roopnarine (Eds.), *Childhood and adolescence in cross-cultural perspective and applications* (pp. 377–410). Westport: Praeger Press.

Aptekar, L. (2010). *In the lions mouth: Hope and heartbreak in humanitarian assistance*. Bloomington: Xlibris.

Aptekar, L., & Abebe, B. (1997). Conflict in the neighborhood: Street children and the public space. *Childhood, 4*(4), 477–490.

Aptekar, L., & Ciano, L. (1999). Street children in Nairobi, Kenya: Gender differences and mental health. In M. Raffaelli & R. Larson (Eds.), *Homeless and working youth around the world: Exploring developmental issues: New directions for child and adolescent development*, Number 85 (pp. 35–46). San Francisco: Jossey Bass.

Aptekar, L., & Stoecklin, D. (1997). Growing up in particularly difficult circumstances: A cross-cultural perspective. In J. Berry, P. Dasen, & T. S. Saraswathi (Eds.), *Handbook of cross-cultural psychology* (Basic processes and human development 2nd ed., Vol. 2, pp. 377–412). Boston: Allyn & Bacon.

Archard, D. (2004). *Children, rights and childhood* (2nd ed.). London: Routledge.

Ariès, P. (1960). *L'enfant et la vie familiale sous l'ancien régime*. Paris: Plon.

Balagopalan, S. (2002). Constructing indigenous childhoods: Colonialism, vocational education and the working child. *Childhood, 9*, 20–34.

Barrett, D. (Ed.). (2011). *Children of the drug war: Perspectives on the impact of drug policies on young people*. New York: International Debate Education Association (iDebate Press).

Becker, H. (1963). *Outsiders: Studies in the sociology of deviance*. New York: The Free Press.

Berger, P. L., & Luckmann, T. (1966). *The social construction of reality: A treatise in the sociology of knowledge*. New-York: Anchor Books.

Boyden, J., Holden, P. (1991). *Children of the cities*. London ; Atlantic Highlands, N.J.: Zed Books.

Carlen, P. (1996). *Jigsaw: A political criminology of youth homelessness*. Bristol: Open University Press.

Casa Alianza/Covenant House Latin America. (1997). Report on the torture of street children in Guatemala and Honduras, 1990–1997. San José, Costa Rica: *Casa Alianza*.

Cheng, F. C. (2008). *Negotiating exclusion: An ethnographic study of the street children in Shanghai, China*. Unpublished doctoral dissertation. Hong-Kong: University of Hong-Kong.

Chombart de Lauwe, M.-J. (1983). La représentation des catégories sociales dominées. *Rôle social, intériorisation, dans: Bulletin de Psychologie, XXXVII*(366), 877–886.

Corsaro, W. (1997). *The sociology of childhood*. Thousand Oaks: Pine Forge Press.

Davies, M. (2008). A childish culture: shared understandings, agency and intervention: An anthropological study of street children in northeast Kenya. *Childhood, 15*(3), 309–330.

de Moura, S. (2002). The social construction of street children: Configuration and implications. *British Journal of Social Work, 32*, 353–367.

Dimenstein, G. (1990). *A guerra dos meninos: Assassinatos de menores no Brazil* [The war of the children: Assassinations of minors in Brazil]. Sao Paulo: Brasilense.

Diversi, F., Filho, N., & Morelli, M. (1999). Daily reality on the streets of Campinas, Brazil. In M. Raffaelli & R. Larson (Eds.), *Homeless and working youth around the world: Exploring developmental issues* (New directions for child and adolescent development, Number 85, pp. 19–34). San Francisco: Jossey-Bass.

Ennew, J. (1994). *Street and working children – A guide to planning* (Developmental Manual #4). London: Save the children.

Ennew, J. (2000). Why the convention is not about street children. In D. Fottrell (Ed.), *Revising children's rights: 10 Years of the UN Convention on Rights of the Child* (pp. 169–182). Boston: Klauser Law Institute.

Festinger, L. (1957). *A theory of cognitive dissonance*. Stanford: Stanford University Press.

George, S., & Sabelli, F. (1994). *Crédits sans frontières. La religion séculaire de la Banque mondial*. Paris: La Découverte.

Glazer, C. (2000). *Bo-Tsotsi: The youth gangs of Soweto, 1935–1976*. London: James Currey.

Haldenby, A., Berman, H., & Forchuk, C. (2007). Homelessness and health in adolescents. *Qualitative Health Research, 17*(9), 1232–1244.

Hanson, K. (2012). Schools of thought in children's rights. In M. Liebel et al. (Eds.), *Children's rights from below. Cross-cultural perspectives* (pp. 63–79). Basingstoke: Palgrave Macmillan.

Hanson, K., & Vandaele, A. (2003). Working children and international labour law: A critical analysis. *The International Journal of Children's Rights, 11*, 84.

Hecht, T. (1998). *At home in the street: Street children of northeast Brazil*. Cambridge: Cambridge University Press.

Heinonen, P. (2011). *Youth gangs & street children: Culture, nurture and masculinity in Ethiopia*. New York: Berghahn Press.

Hong, D., & Ohno, K. (2005, July). *Street children in Vietnam: Interactions of old and new causes in a growing economy* (Discussion Paper, No. 6). Hanoi: Vietnam Development Forum.

Huchzermeyer, M., & Karam, A. (2006). *Informal settlements: A perpetual challenge?* Cape Town: University of Cape Town Press.

Human Rights Watch. (1996). *Police abuse and killings of street children in India*. New York/London/Brussels: Human Rights Watch.

Hutson, S., & Liddiard, M. (1994). *Youth homelessness. The construction of a social issue*. London: Macmillan.

James, A., & Prout, A. (1990). A new paradigm for the sociology of childhood? Provenance, promise and problems. In A. James & A. Prout (Eds.), *Constructing and reconstructing childhood. Contemporary issues on the sociological study of childhood* (pp. 7–34). London: The Falmer Press.

James, A., Jenks, C., & Prout, A. (1998). *Theorizing childhood*. Oxford: Polity Press.

Jodelet, D. (1993, April). Les représentations sociales. Regard sur la connaissance ordinaire. *Sciences Humaines, 27*, 22–24.

Johnson, K., & Tyler, M. (2006). Trading sex: Voluntary or coerced? the experiences of homeless youth. *Journal of Sex Research, 43*(3), 208–216.

Kevin, A., Yoder, L., Whitbeck, D., & Hoyt, R. (2003, June). Gang involvement and membership among homeless and runaway youth. *Youth & Society, 34*(4), 441–467.

Kilbride, P., Suda, C., & Njeru, E. (2000). *Street children in Kenya: Voices of children in search of childhood*. London: Bergen and Garvey.

Klees, S., Rizzini, I., & Dewees, A. (2000). A new paradigm for social change: Social movements and the transformation of policy for street and working children in Brazil. In R. Mickelson (Ed.), *Children on the streets of the Americas* (pp. 79–98). NY: Routledge.

Kovats-Bernat, J. (2006). *Sleeping rough in Port-au-Prince: An ethnography of street children and violence in Haiti*. Gainesville: University of Florida Press.

Le Roux, J., & Smith, C. (1998). Causes and characteristics of the street children phenomenon: A global perspective. *Adolescence, 33*(321), 683–688.

Leite, L., & Esteves, M. (1991). *Escola Tia Ciata*: A school for street children in Rio de Janeiro. *Environment and Urbanization, 3*, 130–139.

Libertoff, K. (1980). The runaway child in America: A social history. *Journal of Family Issues, 1*, 151–164.

Lucchini, R. (1993). *Enfant de la rue. Identité, sociabilité, drogue*. Genève/Paris: Droz.

Lucchini, R. (1994). *The street children in Montevideo and Rio de Janeiro: Elements for a definition*. Fribourg: Institute for Economic and Social Sciences, University of Fribourg.

Lucchini, R. (1998). Enfant de la rue : réalité complexe et discours réducteurs. *Déviance et Société, 22*(4).

Lucchini, R. (2007). "Street children": Deconstruction of a category. In I. Rizzini, U. Mandel Butler, & D. Stoecklin (Eds.), *Life on the streets. Children and adolescents on the streets: Inevitable trajectories?* (pp. 49–75). Sion: Institut International des Droits de l'enfant.

Lusk, M. (1992). Street children in Rio de Janeiro. *International Social Work, 35*, 293–305.

Lutjens, S. (2000). Schooling and clean streets in Socialist Cuba: Children and the Special period. In R. Mickelson (Ed.), *Children on the streets of the Americas* (pp. 55–65). New York: Routledge.

Magazine, R. (2003). Action, personhood and the gift economy among so-called street children in Mexico City. *Social Anthropology, 11*(3), 303–318.

Marquez, P. (1999). *The street is my home: Youth and violence in Caracas*. Stanford: Stanford University Press.

Martin, J. (2011). *La rue des précaires. Soins psychiques et précarités*. Toulouse: Editions Erès.

Matignon, J.-J. (1900). *Superstition, crime et misère en Chine*. Paris: Masson & Cie Editeurs.

Matthews, H. (2003). Children and regeneration: Setting an agenda for community participation and integration. *Children & Society, 17*(4), 264–276.

McLachlan, F. (1986). Street children in prison. In N. Pines (Ed.), *Street children perspectives* (Paper No 40, pp. 3–6). Johannesburg: Institute for the Study of Man in Africa.

Mickelson, R. (Ed.). (2000). *Children on the streets of the Americas*. New York: Routledge.

Ming, Y. (1989). Sociology in China: Its past, present, and future. *Chinese Sociology and Anthropology, 22*(1), 3–29.

Mosse, D. (2001). People's knowledge, participation and patronage: Operations and representations in rural development. In B. Cooke & U. Kothari (Eds.), *Participation: The new tyranny?* London: Zed Books.

Muraya, J. (1993). *Street children: A study of street girls in Nairobi, Kenya*. Swansea: Center for Development Studies, University College of Swansea.

Muskinja, M. (2009). *Best interests and participation of children in street situations. How to bridge theory and practice?* Master thesis. Sion: IUKB.

Naterer, A., & Godina, V. (2011). Bomzhji and their subculture: An anthropolitical study of street children subculture in Makeevka, Eastern Ukraine. *Childhood, 18*(1), 20–38.

Nieuwenhuizen, P. (2006). *Street children in Bangalore, India: Their dreams and future*. Antwerp: Het Spinhuis Publishers.

Ono, M. (2008). *Migrant children in the streets of Karachi with special focus on Bengali Children*. Master thesis in children's rights (unpublished). Sion: IUKB.

Paradise, M., & Cauce, A. (2002). Home street home: The interpersonal dimensions of adolescent homelessness. *The Society for the Psychological Study of Social Issues, 2*(1), 223–238.

Parazelli, M. (2002). *La rue attractive. Parcours et pratiques identitaires des jeunes de la rue*. Sainte-Foy: Presses de l'Université du Québec.

Patel, S. (1983). *An overview of street children in India*. New York: Covenant House.

Patel, S. (1990). Street children, hotel boys and children of pavement dwellers and construction workers in Bombay – How they meet their daily needs. *Environment and Urbanization, 2*, 9–26.

Pereira, P. (1985). *Retrato do Brasil. A situaçâo da infancia Brasileira* [Profile of Brazil: The situation of Brazilian children]. Sao Paulo: Editora Politica.

Peres, M. F. T. (2004). *Firearm-related violence in Brazil – Country report*. São Paulo: Centre for the Study of Violence, University of São Paulo.

Pérez Lopez, R. (2009). *Vivre et survivre à Mexico. Enfants et jeunes de la rue*. Paris: Karthala.

Pinheiro, P. S. (2006). *World report on violence against children. United Nations Secretary-General's study on violence against children*. Geneva: United Nations Publishing Services.

Pupavac, V. (2006). *Global children's rights, sustainable development and punishing childhoods*. Unpublished manuscript.

Qvortrup, J., Bardy, M., Sgritta, G., & Wintersberger, H. (1994). *Childhood matters*. Aldershot: Ashgate Publishing.

Randall, G. (1988). *No way home: Homeless young people in central London*. London: Centrepoint Soho.

Rizzini, I., Mandel-Butler, U., & Stoecklin, D. (Eds.). (2007). *Life on the streets. Children and adolescents on the streets: Inevitable trajectories?* Sion: Institut International des Droits de l'enfant.

Roberts, A. R. (2000). An overview of crisis theory and crisis intervention. In A. R. Roberts (Ed.), *Crisis intervention handbook: Assessment, treatment and research* (pp. 3–30). New York: Oxford University Press.

Rosemberg, F. (2000). From discourse to reality: A profile of the lives and estimates of the number of street children and adolescents in Brazil. In R. Mickelson (Ed.), *Children on the streets of the Americas* (pp. 118–135). New York: Routledge.
Rousseau, C., Said, T., Gagne, M., & Bibeau, G. (1998). Resilience in unaccompanied minors from the North of Somalia. *Psychoanalytical Review, 85*, 6125–637.
Schaffner, L. (1999). *Teenage runaways: Broken hearts and "bad attitudes"*. New York: Haworth Press.
Scheper-Hughes, N., & Hoffman, D. (1998). Brazilian apartheid: Street kids and the struggle for urban space. In N. Scheper-Hughes & C. Sargent (Eds.), *Small wars: The cultural politics of childhood* (pp. 352–388). Berkley: University of California Press.
Sen, A. (1999). *L'économie est une science morale*. Paris: La Découverte.
Sharf, W., Powell, M., & Thomas, E. (1986). Stroller-street children of Cape Town. In S. Burman & P. Reynolds (Eds.), *Growing up in a divided society: The context of childhood in South Africa* (pp. 262–287). Johannesburg: Raven.
Sirota, R. (2006). *Eléments pour une sociologie de l'enfance*. Rennes: Presses Universitaires de Rennes.
Smollar, J. (1999). Homeless youth in the United States: Description and development issues. In M. Raffaelli & R. Larson (Eds.), *Homeless and Working Youth Around the World: Exploring Developmental Issues: New Directions for Child and Adolescent Development, Number 85* (pp. 47–58). San Francisco: Jossey-Bass.
Stoecklin, D. (2000a). *Enfants des rues en Chine* [Street children in China]. Paris: Karthala.
Stoecklin, D. (2000b). *A baseline survey of the street children of Chittagong City in Bangladesh*. Dhaka: Aparayeyo-Bandladesh. Terre des homes.
Stoecklin, D. (2003). Rapport de mission. *Terre des hommes et Sabou-Guinée. Projet Enfants en situations de rue. Guinée-Conakry, Avril 2003*. Terre des hommes (Internal unpublished report).
Stoecklin, D. (2013, November). Theories of action in the field of child participation. In search of explicit frameworks. *Childhood*. Issue 4, pp. 443–457.
Stoecklin, D., & Chuard, N. (2003). *Les enfants en situation de rue à Antananarivo, Madagascar*. Terre des hommes (unpublished report).
Suda, C. (1993). The impact of changing family structures on Nairobi children. *African Study Monographs, 14*, 109–121.
Sullivan, H. S. (1953). *Interpersonal theory of psychiatry*. New York: Norton.
Sullivan, M. (2006). Are "gang" studies dangerous? Youth, violence, local context, and the problems of reification. In J. Short & L. Hughes (Eds.), *Studying Youth Gangs* (pp. 15–36). Lanham: Alta Mira Press.
Swart, J. (1990). *Malunde: The street children of Hillbrow*. Witwatersrand: Johannesburg.
Tao Zhiming. (1995). *Liulang ertong yu shehui huanjing* [Street children and social conditions] (p. 9). Unpublished Paper.
Teeter, R. (1995). Pre-school responses to the 19th-century youth crisis. *The Free Library*. Retrieved May 01, 2013 from, http://www.thefreelibrary.com/Pre-school+responses+to+the+19th-century+youth+crisis.-a017150109
Trebjesanin, Z. (2001). *Predstava o detetu u srpskoj kulturi* [The image of the child in Serbian culture]. Belgrade: Child Rights Centre.
UNCRC. (1989). *United nations convention on the rights of the child*. New York: United Nations.
UNICEF. (1986). *Children in especially difficult circumstances. United Nations Children's Fund*. New York: UNICEF.
Van Leeuwen, J., Boyle, S., Salomonsen, S., Baker, J., Hoffman, A., & Hopfeer, C. (2006). Lesbian, gay, and bisexual homeless youth: An eight-city public health perspective. *Child Welfare, 85*(2), 151–170.
Veale, A., Taylor, M., & Linehan, C. (2000). Psychological perspectives of 'abandoned and abandoning' street children. In C. Panter-Brick & M. Smith (Eds.), *Abandoned children* (pp. 131–145). Cambridge: Cambridge University Press.
Verma, S., & Dhingra, G. (1993). Who do they belong to? A profile of street children in Chandigarh, India. *People's Action, 8*(1), 22–25.
Vuckovic-Sahovic, N. (2000). *The rights of the child and international law*. Belgrade: Yugoslav Child Rights Centre.

Wang, B. (1989). Ren de shehuihua [Socialization of man], *Ren Yu Shehui [Man and Society].* Shanghai shehui kexueyuan chubanshe, [Publishing house of the Shanghai Academy of Social Sciences], pp. 27–42.

Weber, M. (1968). *Economy and society*. New York: Bedminster Press.

Wernham, M. (2004). *An outside chance: Street children and juvenile justice – An international perspective*. London: Consortium for Street Children.

West, A. (2003). At the margins: Street children in Asia and the Pacific. *Poverty and Social Development Papers*, *8*. Asian Development Bank.

Whiteford, L. (1998). Children's health as accumulated capital: Structural adjustment in the Dominican Republic and Cuba. In N. Scheper-Hughes & C. Sargent (Eds.), *Small wars: The cultural politics of childhood* (pp. 186–291). Berkley: University of California Press.

WHO (World Health Organization). (2001). *Small arms and global health*. Geneva: World Health Organization.

Yablonsky, L. (1979). The delinquent gang as a near-group. In D. Kelly (Ed.), *Deviant behavior: Readings in the sociology of deviance*. New York: St. Martin's Press.

Young, L., & Barrett, H. (2001). Issues of access and identity: Adapting research methods with Kampala street children. *Childhood, 8*(3), 383–395.

Zegarac, N. (2007). *Children speak out: Trafficking risk and resilience in southeast Europe: Serbia report*. Belgrade: Save the Children.

Zeneidi-Henry, D. (2002). *Les SDF et la ville. Géographie du savoir-vivre*. Paris: Editions Bréal.

Chapter 4
Research with Children in Street Situations

Problems in Determining the Population

Before we can begin research with street children and homeless youth we need to be clear we are using the same definitions so that we have faith in the validity of the numbers that are being reported. There are many problems with this, including the fact that politics take over the scientific model. For political reasons, international organizations inflate numbers to compete for funding. The inflation of numbers also comes from children in street situations who inflate their woes, also to take advantage of limited resources. They too want to eat and stay sheltered.[1] Since most people rarely engage children in street situations beyond brief, uncomfortable interactions, the mere use of the words "street child" acts like an advertising slogan to catch the public's attention. From these few prickly encounters and from information received from the sensational stories and images found in the media, most people believe that there is a street children problem of epidemic proportions. At times, high numbers are used to increase the community's feeling of insecurity which can justify street "cleansing" operations, just like at time the numbers are under-reported, to show a brighter picture of the community (see some estimates in Table 4.1).

In July 1994, the *Kenyan Daily Nation* reported that there were half a million youth living on Kenyan streets, 300,000 of them in Nairobi ("*We Will Care for Nairobi's Children*"). However, according to an article appearing in the same newspaper 2 weeks later, the number of street children in Nairobi was 30,000 ("*City Street Children Now 30,000*"). Yet, the Undugu Society, the largest and most experienced group working with street children in Kenya estimated 5–10,000 street children in Nairobi, a figure far below that of public opinion.)

[1] Hecht (1998) notes that the national movement of street children, which thrived as a political interest group in Brazil in the 1990s had, in fact, very few street children involved.

L. Aptekar and D. Stoecklin, *Street Children and Homeless Youth: A Cross-Cultural Perspective*, DOI 10.1007/978-94-007-7356-1_4,

Table 4.1 Numbers of street children

Continent	Country	# of Street Children	Data Source
Africa	Sudan	70,000	Kudrati et al. (2008)
Asia	Bangladesh	400,000	US-DOS (2005)
Asia	Bangladesh	8,020	Koehlmoos et al. (2009)
Asia	China	300,000	Zhang and Yang (2002)
Asia	China	150,000	CSC (2011)
Asia	India	11,000,000	Mathur et al. (2009)
Asia	Iran	200,000	Ahmadkhaniha et al. (2007)
Asia	Nepal	5,000	Gurung (2004)
Asia	Nepal	40,000	Thapa et al. (2009)
Asia	Pakistan	70,000	Iqbal (2008)
Asia	Phillipines	50,000	Lamberte (2002)
Asia	Philippines	1,500,000	Njord et al. (2010)
Asia	Thailand	30,000	Faulk (2010)
Asia	Vietnam	23,000	CSC (2011)
Asia	Vietnam	21,016	Hong and Ohno (2005)
Europe	Georgia	2,500	CSC (2011)
Europe	Romania	5,000	CSC (2011)
Europe	Russia	3,000,000	Kissin et al. (2007)
Europe	Ukraine	50,000	Kerfoot et al. (2007)
Latin America	Bolivia	72,000	C. C. Huang et al. (2004)

Using focus groups, Aptekar and Ciano (1999) tried to ascertain the public's estimate of the numbers of street children in Nairobi. The responses ranged from 1,000 to 100,000, and when asked to estimate the number of street youth in Kenya, answers ranged from 5,000 to 1,500,000.

The use of high numbers, in spite of knowing that the estimates are high, provides service agencies, from local NGOs to international humanitarian agencies, a chance to claim a bigger piece of the pie. Street Kids International in their applications for funding (Sauve 2003) uses the UN's estimates of 100 million street youth in the world, even though it includes many who are not homeless. UNICEF estimated that the crowded and busy streets of Latin American cities are home to 40 million children and that there are 100 million worldwide (Taçon 1981). This was a successful strategy for fund raising and scaring the public (Ennew 1994). Despite the obvious over estimation, the figure of 100 million street children is still the benchmark for use in raising funds and for writers who want to catch the eye of readers (de Benitez 2011). Writing for the Consortium of Street Children, Ennew and Milne (1989) worked by a simple demographic method to estimate about 23 million homeless children worldwide.

The following examples show just how inaccurate the estimates are. In Brazilian studies, the estimates of the number of street and working children on the streets of Brazil have varied from 17 million (Barker and Knaul 1991) to between 20 and 30 million (de Moura 2002).

Yet, Hecht (1998) points out, quoting the UNICEF magazine *Ideas Forum,* which gave a figure of more than 30 million children living on the streets of Brazil, that there were only 29.5 million Brazilians between the ages of 5 and 19. He argues that at the time of his study there were "*fewer than 39,000 children sleeping in the streets of Brazil* (p. 22)", or just over a tenth of one percent of the 30 million that were then being estimated by the international organizations.

Fujimora (2005), an anthropologist who studied street children in Russia, says that the Russian Children's Fund estimates 2.5 million children living in the streets, of which 250,000 are in Moscow. The author shows that the real numbers are much smaller. Russian children who are abandoned are not allowed on the streets. They are put into state run orphanages and counted as disabled children.[2] Of the 15,000 children who leave state orphanages each year, 6,000, a far smaller numbers than a quarter million, will become homeless street children.[3]

Another scientific problem with collecting accurate numbers is shown by Tanon and Sow (2010) who gathered data on children from Mauritania who illegally went to France. The problem was that the people collecting data were not clear about who their subjects were. They mixed criteria for enumeration, and they had difficulty tracking the population because it was so mobile.

The same problems exist in the developed world. For example, one study estimated from 5% to 7.7% of American children are homeless each year (Robertson and Toro 1999). The USA has an approximate population of 300 million. Children under 18 are about 40% or 120 million. Five percent of 120 million is 6 million and 7.7% is 9.24 million.

In another study the estimation was that one American child in eight (about 12.5%) run away from home before they are 18 years of age, and nearly a half of them do not return to the same domicile from which they fled (Whitbeck and Hoyt 1999). Paradise and Cauce (2002) used a national sample of 6,500 youth between ages 12 and 17 to show that 1 in 20 youth (5%) are homeless (defined as using public housing but not sleeping rough) during a 12 month period.[4]

In a well-respected study, Lutjens (2000) found about 1 million homeless youth in the USA, or about a third of one percent. In another respected study, Cauce et al. (2000) found that each year among American youth between one and one and a third million spend some time being homeless or in shelters (adolescents are about half the total homeless population). Other studies corroborate this lower figure. Williams et al. (2001) quote a US Department of Housing and Urban Development's study in 1994, which calculated between 300,000 and 1.6 million youth are homeless each

[2] They are grouped by disability and age. The conditions in these institutions are far below standard care for nutrition, cleanliness, and over-crowding. They all combine to cause extreme stress.

[3] One thousand five hundred of them will commit suicide. One reason for the suicides is that while the Russian people love children, orphaned children are symbols of suffering and victimization and thus a cognitive dissonance is set up, and suicide is one way of escaping the pain caused by it (Fujimora 2005).

[4] The ages were from 10 to 24 and the vast majority were male (Alteena et al. 2010). Hyde, (2005) studied young people in Los Angeles from 18 to 23 years of age. The sample was split evenly between men and women. Repeated studies in Denver, Colorado between 1998 and 2005, showed a 55% increase in the number of homeless youth (D'Alanno 2005). Yet, there is no way of knowing if this change was an actual increase, a political distortion, or a research artifact.

year. Approximately the same numbers were found by the National Coalition for the Homeless in 1990 (Stonge 2000). Also, as reported by Schaffner (1999), between a million and a million and a half adolescents in America run away from home each year which is about 2% of all American adolescents.

One reason for the disparities among estimates of homeless youth is the difference in state laws, which have different definitions of runaways.[5] Sometimes the numbers include only those who have been away for a certain minimum period of time, or exclude youth who are living on the streets. The wide differences in these estimates challenge the validity of all the research in which they are used.

An additional difficulty comes from the fact that children in street situations are not a constant percentage of the population. The numbers go up or down depending on many factors. For homeless youth, the degree to which compulsory schools laws are enforced affects the numbers. Another factor is the demand for child labor (Schrader and Veale 1999; Veale 1996). The less that child labor laws are enforced, the greater the number of children in street situations. Tougher the policies against child abuse or, a greater number of alternatives to living with abusive parents, can positively change (reduce) the number of runaway youth on the streets.

Numbers of street children increase whenever there is violence; it does not matter if the violence comes from the State toward one ethnic group within its domain or comes from inter-State violence (Uvin 1998). Violence increased the numbers of street children in South Africa during apartheid (Swart 1990), and in the wars in Sudan (Veale 1996), Kenya (Aptekar and Ciano 1999), Ethiopia, (Schrader and Veale 1999), and Angola (Moberly 1999).

In Rwanda, there was a precipitous increase in the number of street children post-genocide. According to Veale and Dona (2003), one reason for this was changing family dynamics. After the genocide there was a spike in female-headed families, both from men dying in fighting and from men being in detention on charges of genocide. There was also an increase in the numbers of orphans, separated children and child-headed households to 40,000 (World Vision 1998).[6]

The differences in numbers and demographics in Rwanda are dramatic. In the year 2000, 90% of street children in Rwanda came to the streets after the genocide (Veale and Dona 2003). Conflict rather than poverty or child abuse was the main cause of children going to the street.[7]

They found that 70% of the survivors were women. They had no money, no housing, and no medical care. At the same time there were over a million men who were in prison or being charged with genocide. The majority of the nearly seven million

---

[5] Running away is against the law in all states in the USA (and in most countries in the developed world). Thus these adolescents will become law breakers; albeit of a particular offense because they have not reached the age of majority (between 16 and 21 years of age depending on state statute). These are called status offenses and include such acts as being out late at night, drinking alcohol, having sex, being truant from school and of course, running away.

[6] This also placed an enormous strain on traditional foster care systems.

[7] While there were street children in Rwanda as early as the 1980s, their numbers were few and their origins could be accounted for by work-related rural to urban migration. In this they were typical of other African street children.

children under 18 who lived during the war were exposed to a brutality that defies description either as witnesses, victims or in some cases as participants. The same pattern of civil unrest and displacement was the main causal factor for the origin of street children in Sudan (Veale 1996). There was an increase in the number of child-headed households while and at the same time numerous programs for unaccompanied children opened (Veale and Dona 2003).

Within 3 years the availability of services declined abruptly in Rwanda and an estimated 120,000 children were outside their family of origin in extended families or substitute family care. It was at this point and under these circumstances that the authors arrived to study the increased numbers of street children (Veale and Dona 2003). Traditionally, if a parent died, the responsibility for the child went to the father's family as part of the patriarchal nature of Rwandan society.

We are including details of the research protocol because of its quality. They began by sampling 110 key informants in four sites around the country to establish a working definition of street children. The definition that emerged was a child without any adult to take care of him or her. If the child was working in the informal sector, kept himself clean and had a relationship to parents, he was not considered a street child.

After establishing the local definition of street children, the authors mapped, during various times, the places where street children congregated. They looked at what they were doing at work and play. Their research team included street educators, social work students, and older street youth. They were able to interview nearly 300 children in four locations around the country that fit their definition of street children. The interview was both structured and open ended. It took about a half hour to complete, which is within the attention span of the children.

They sampled children based on their mapping of high concentrations of street children, including the usual areas of bus stations, market areas, and public recreational spaces. Interviews were carried out during different parts of the day to insure valid time sampling. Of the nearly 300 children who were interviewed, 91% were males and 9% were females (with the percentage of girls on the street decreasing during the day).

They checked on reliability by comparing their final sample to their original observational mapping. They also included focus group discussions with street girls (they were highly fearful of sexual assault in the streets at night). They checked for validity by triangulating their methods, using the interviews, observations and focus groups as data points.[8]

The findings disclosed that those without local families or guardians were significantly more likely to be sleeping on the streets, significantly fewer were

[8] The mean age of the 290 children sampled was 14.2 years. The older children were on the streets longer than the younger children. And the older children were significantly more likely to have experienced the death of their mother. Nearly 90% first came to the streets after the genocide of 1994. They found no significant differences with regard to the reason for going to the street based on whether their father or mother were alive. What was significantly different was their mental health when viewed pre-genocide and post-genocide.

attending school, and children without local guardians had more nightmares. When the authors used the chi square test (verifying with multiple responses) to compare the characteristics of children who slept mainly at home with homeless children, the homeless children fared less well on all measures. A multivariate logistical regression analysis determined that the children who had mothers as guardians were significantly less likely to be homeless. The other significant variable was family discord. Sixty percent of the street children said they had bad memories, four in ten had nightmares, nearly two-thirds suffered from headaches and 44% were anxious "often" or "sometimes."

In summary, there are more Rwandan street children sleeping on the streets and they are older than those street children of other African countries. Nearly a third of Rwandan street children are orphans. Their uniqueness is seen when contrasted to studies of street children in other parts of the world. Fewer than 1 in 10 Nepalese street children were orphaned (Panter-Brick et al. 1996). And a study in Honduras conducted by Wright et al. (1993), showed that fewer than 5% were orphaned. Neither of these studies was conducted in war zones. There was a similar degree of orphans found in Veale's study of different places in Ethiopia that experienced war (Veale et al. 1993). "*Perhaps the most significant social impact of genocide has been on family structures. Thousands of children were catapulted out of their families of origin into alternative guardianship care. Street children sampled here reported a complex variety of guardianship arrangements. Research examining the care of reunified and fostered children in Rwandan communities has found that children grapple with complex negotiations around issues of identity, grief and loss, and the child's position in the family*" (p. 264).

Many of the problems are associated with the loss of fathers and male relatives in a patriarchal society. Thus, street children lost their inheritance, and being male they were not comfortable in being dependent on a new family with new male non-related men who, by tradition, should have no authority over them. When the boys have only their mothers as heads of households (and no paternal uncles), they feel compelled to become men by earning an income. As a result of the death and imprisonment of men, the remaining families are destitute. The economic hardships follow the effects of the war.

A further war-related cause of street children has to do with housing. Not only were houses destroyed during the war, but as the result of displacement and resettlement, the remaining houses were often taken over to be used for the relocation of 650,000 internally displaced. The result was that 3 years after the genocide, when the study was carried out, Veale and Dona (2003) found, "*rather than poverty, urbanization, or modernity, it was conflict, death and displacement that constituted the roots of street life involvement in Rwanda. While poverty and conflict are integrally mixed, it is argued here that it is the effects of civil conflict, and the human, material, social, and cultural losses that stem from conflict, that is fundamental to the experience of Rwandan street children*" (p. 266).

In most non-conflict situations street children have families, while the vast majority of street children in post-conflict areas do not. These children are part of the new face of street children who are on the streets as a result of being war orphans and whose demographics and problems are considerably different.

In Angola, more than 60% of street children had run away from families because of the post-war changes in family dynamics. They were commonly the oldest in the family and the ones given the responsibility of caring for younger siblings when the parents were gone. As they gained strength and maturity from this, they no longer were willing to accept authority, particularly if it was from a non-family member living with their mother, or if it was abusive (Moberly 1999).

Another variable that affects the numbers of street children is the global economy. In Brazil, for example, like other countries in the global economy who are being restructured by the World Bank or International Monetary Fund, there is a widening inequality gap between rich and poor and a reduction of social safety nets for the poor, increasing the numbers of street children (Mickelson 2000).

Redefining the Population

Another research problem is coming up with a clear definition of the population to be studied. The most commonly used definition of street children separates them into two categories, children of the streets (who live in the streets without family and which amounts to about 2% of the total) and children on the streets who are working children who go home at night to give what they earn to their families.[9] As we will see, this is problematic.

The scientific issues related to the numbers problem often is the result of overlapping categories which include "street children", "children in the street", "homeless children", "abandoned children", "children at risk", "minors in conflict with the law", "children in especially difficult situations", etc. Take for example, Egypt's report to the Committee on the Rights of the Child (1998) which offered to put street children into a compilation of categories, which included children placed with foster families, foundlings, illegitimate children, homeless, and stray children. Should we assume that only the homeless (1.8% of the total) and stray children (less than 1%) are street children, or should all of the categories be combined?[10]

The same overlapping of categories is used to classify street children under "child labour" so working children with homes and homeless working children are put together. This also multiplies the problem because children in street situations constitute only a small fraction of working children (Bhalotra and Tzannatos 2003).

Lucchini (2007) developed a diagram (see below) to show the problems of this two-dimensional definition of children **on** the street and children **of** the street (Fig. 4.1).

---

[9] This off and on distinction started in 1985 when Peter Taçon of UNICEF coined the phrase (Taçon 1985).

[10] See also Koller and Hutz (1996) on how differences in definitions cause confusion in results.

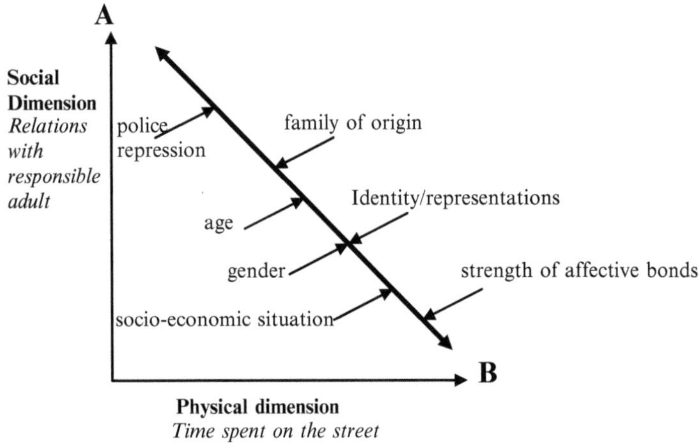

Fig. 4.1 The two-dimensional definition of the 'street child' (Lucchini 2007, p. 50)

In this figure, children in street situations are defined by the two dimensions: time spent on the street and relations with parents or other responsible adults. Axis A defines the intensity of the child's contacts with responsible adults and axis B measures the time spent on the street. "Children **on** the street" would be located high on axis A and low on axis B: they regularly return home and they spend less time on the street. The situation for "children **of** the street" is the reverse: they stay mostly on the street and have few contacts with family or other responsible adults.

Between A and B (diagonal arrow), there are a number of intermediary situations that raise important issues regarding this approach to defining children in street situations. The child who moves on the axis from A to B progressively actualizes her/his status as 'street child' (child of the street). But the reverse is also true: the child who is going from B to A would not be a real "street child" anymore but a "child on the street". Then, one may ask: when does a child become or cease to be a street child? The criterion of duration of stay on the street is insufficient to answer this question. This raises interesting questions like what amount of time spent on the street is required to be considered a homeless youth?

Numerous other factors influence the position of a specific child in the continuum between A and B, including factors we considered earlier such as age and gender. There are also factors directly linked to the family, such as family composition and organization, the strength of family ties, the economic situation of the family and the degree to which the family is rooted in the city (bringing up questions of migration).

The movement from A to B also highlights problems with the **on** or **off** criteria used by the funding agencies. For example, the notion of the 'responsible adult' is less of an **on** or **off** divide than a graded dimension. The role of 'responsible adult' might be divided among various people who do not necessarily live in the same place. This role can also be temporary as when the child circulates from one domestic unit to another, going back home daily and yet without necessarily maintaining a relationship with a responsible adult. The two-dimensional model is not adequate in these cases.

It is also problematic that UNICEF defines children at risk in the context of the relationship between a child and the child's family, even though "contact with the family" is not clear. The same applies to homeless youth, only in this case the definition is based on what those homeless youth have left behind. Do we mean the frequency or the quality of the contact? A child may have numerous contacts but of poor quality, and these contacts with the family may even be negative or abusive as is often the case with homeless youth.

If the regularity of the "contact with the family" is a criterion to define a normal childhood, children who spend more time on the streets would be seen as deviant simply on the basis of an objective measure. This ignores the subjective meaning the child attaches to the quality of the contact with the family. The family responses that are given to the child are subjectively perceived by the child who may consider that, at some point, the street offers better responses to his or her needs.[11] Many 'street children' suffer from a lack of affective and material responses at home, but find these conditions in the peer-group in the street.

The same can be said of factors directly connected to the street: the image that the child has of the street, the contacts the child has had with persons who already have experience of the street, the presence of the child within a group or network of other children, the initiation rituals by peers to be accepted on the street and in the deviant underworld, the profitability of activities, police repression and the violence between children. These dimensions are difficult to discern, yet invaluable in understanding the child.

There is a similar analysis of factors connected to urban spaces: the significance of the distance which the child would have to cover from home to the street in which she or he practices her income generating activities, and the nature of the urban space which the child has to cross to reach this place. This last issue has to do with the survival opportunities that the child encounters in moving within or towards the city centre.

Also, the simple on and of the streets does not deal with the macroscopic variables referring to the social, political and economic situation of the country, such as the fact that war and structural readjustment increase the numbers of street children.

The criticism of this dichotomous model also does not take into account that street children are not affected with the same intensity by similar events or situations. This is why children with similar life conditions at home do not all take to the street. Otherwise the cities of the world would literally be invaded by children.

Because of the dichotomous model of definition, we are left with the problem of defining the population we are studying. What we need is a systematic technique of analyzing data gathered with children so we can conduct research on a clearly defined population.

---

[11] Thus, Cosgrove's criticism (1990) that street children are defined with reference to where they hang out, not by common characteristics of a collective group. And Rizzini et al. (2007) questioned whether what was being called a street child corresponded to either a clearly delimited social category or a perfectly homogeneous psycho-sociological unity.

The Child-Street System

The Child-Street System (Lucchini 2007) stems from the observation made throughout the years by Riccardo Lucchini in Brazil (Lucchini 1993), Montevideo and Mexico (Lucchini 1994, 1996). This framework captures the diversity of relationships that children may have with their social environment. For each child, there are eight dimensions which are either strong or weak. All of them make up the child's subjective experience of street life in a systematic way. Also, as time changes, the dimensions change because they are interdependent; any change in one category affects the child's overall experience.

The value of this framework has been confirmed through observations of children in the streets of Shanghai (Stoecklin 2000), and has been adapted by Stoecklin (2007) as a tool for intervention or consultation with various INGOs, local associations and networks from 1998 to 2007 in 15 countries: Afghanistan, Albania, Bangladesh, Brazil, Burundi, China, Egypt, Guinea, Honduras, Madagascar, Niger, Morocco, Pakistan, Senegal, and Vietnam.

It has also been used as an intervention to foster the participation of children in their own needs assessment. The children can participate in the definition of their realities and their accounts would constitute solutions on a more individual, or at least a profile-like, basis.

While working on this model and its application, Lucchini (2007) and Stoecklin (2007) came to the conclusion that instead of a typology of "street children", it would be better to elaborate a typology of "street situations", which included the subjective relationship a child may develop within a given setting, as every child's situation on the street is specific (Fig. 4.2).

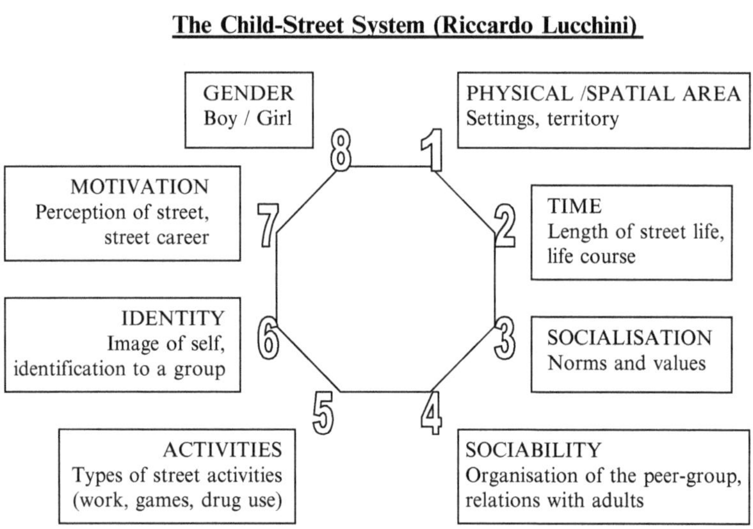

Fig. 4.2 The child-street system (Lucchini 2007)

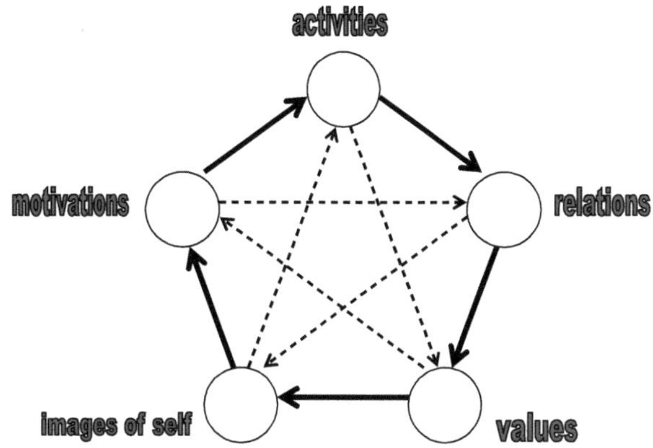

Fig. 4.3 "The actor's system" (Stoecklin 2009a)

Stoecklin (2007) stressed the child's or youth's subjective relationship with a particular environment, showing that children in street situations are those for whom the street has become a major part of the cognitive and emotional dimensions of their lives. This new approach is a definition which obliges the researcher to understand the meaning attached by specific children to street life; the emphasis is on the interactions the child builds with other people. Thus the child is considered a social actor, which is in line with children's rights. This means that we should not be so concerned about the number of children found in the street, but more with the quality of their lives on and off the street. Therefore the important question is that of the interaction between individuals and social groups, and the preferred approach is to use the expression "children in street situations", since the question is not two dimensional, instead it takes into account many situations and the degrees of involvement in which the child may find him/herself.

Lucchini's "Child-Street System" proved to be useful to identify specific profiles of children in street situations (the reader may go back to the example of Bangladesh in Chapter 2). However, the implementation of this tool proved to face several obstacles, among which are the limited resources dedicated to staff training and the corresponding difficulty for the staff to deal with a tool that requires time for cross-checking. In an attempt to simplify this tool, Stoecklin (2009a) came up with another model called the "actor's system", which proved to be applicable not only with children in street situations, but also with other children (and therefore heads towards non-discriminatory research protocols). This models allows us to consider the social actions of any actor (in street situations or not) as a general system made up of five dimensions: activities, relations, values, images of self, and motivations. The model is called the "actor's system", as action is not reduced to "activities" but encompasses all the above-mentioned components (Fig. 4.3).

The five dimensions are what Blumer (1969) calls "sensitizing concepts" (p. 148) and are open to be defined by the respondents, suggesting only directions to look at and therefore acting as lenses through which the actors may read and give meaning to reality. The model considers that former activities may influence new ones by

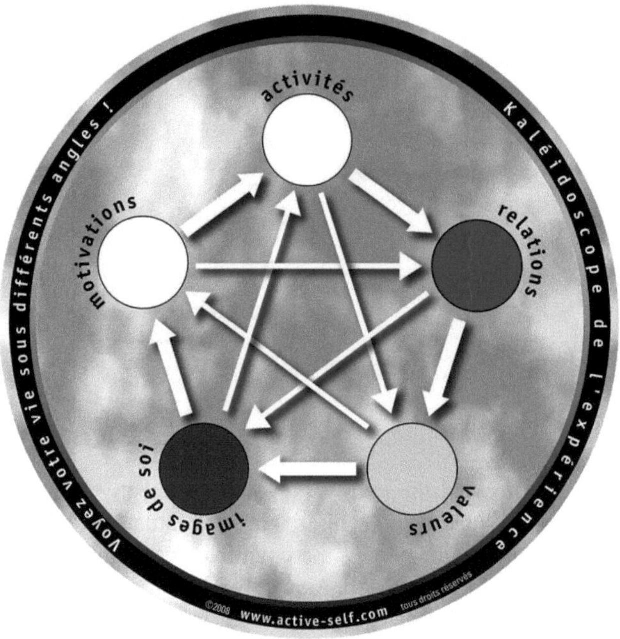

Fig. 4.4 The kaleidoscope of experience (Stoecklin 2009b)

producing changes in relations, values, images of self and motivations. With this cyclical aspect, Stoecklin's model tries to capture and reflect the cumulative nature of experience (Dewey 1910). Out of this model, Stoecklin (2009b) has produced a concrete tool called the "kaleidoscope of experience" (Fig. 4.4).

The kaleidoscope of experience is a concrete tool which one can use to speak about one's experience by turning the colours (red, yellow and blue) and place them alternatively on the five dimensions, following different techniques (which we don't detail here for lack of space). This tool has had several applications (Stoecklin 2013), and it has also been used with 80 children and young people in street situations, aged 10–18 years, of the working child clubs of Biratnagar Municipality, in the Eastern Region of Nepal (Tronchet-Pradhan 2011). The application of this tool in Nepal was described as very valuable to understanding the way children and young people conceptualize some of their rights, and notably ideas of non-discrimination and social justice (Tronchet-Pradhan 2011, p. 27). One major outcome of this application is that street children realize the various aspects of their decisions and reflect upon them. It also helps to avoid the side-effect of social desirability which is the tendency to answer in a way thought to be socially acceptable and desirable (McBurney 1994). It is anchored in the new paradigm in childhood studies, understanding children as social actors having agency, i.e. some degree of power over the construction of their everyday lives.

Several applications in the field of child participation have been made and allowed children's heightened participation in situation analysis (Stoecklin 2013). On this basis, attempts to use this tool in fieldwork with children in street situations are currently made but it is too early so far to assess the outcomes.

Random Sampling: The Aptekar Method

As we have mentioned, finding reliable demographics and defining children in street situations has been practically difficult for scientific and political reasons. To begin to solve some of the scientific problems, it will be necessary to establish a valid procedure for choosing a random sample. Almost all research with street children continues to use convenience samples, which rely on opportunistic sampling. This method does not lead to randomization, and makes inference very questionable. The numbers of street children and their characteristics remain, as we have seen above, not much better than guess-work. The same can be said about many significant demographics such as gender ratios, income and ethnicity of families, etc.

Aptekar and Ciano (1999) developed in Kenya a random sampling technique based on peripatetic groups. They began by defining the sleeping places (which in Kenya are called *choums*) to define households. Households are the central concept in census data but are lacking in most estimates of street children (Fig. 4.5).

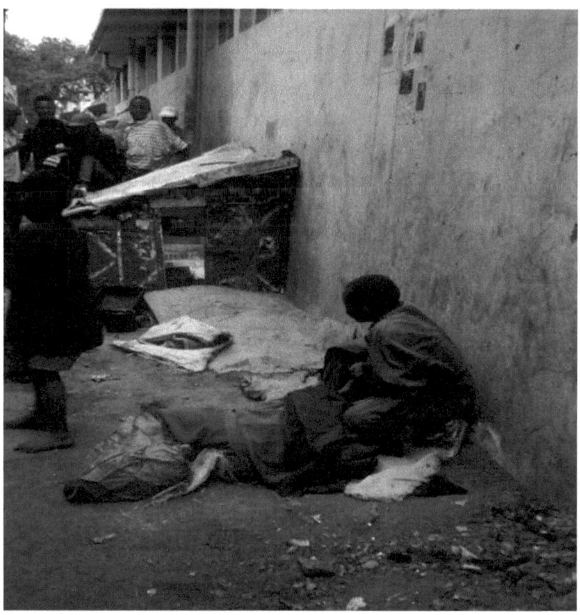

Fig. 4.5 A street household

They then placed the *choums* on the map of the city. This map was divided into equal grids, which were then labelled with high or low concentrations of households. They then selected a stratified random sample of the high and low areas of households for collecting census data.

Local people who were known by the street children were chosen to walk these random areas each night for 2 weeks collecting data on the numbers of street children in each *choum* in the randomly selected areas for three successive nights, and then at weekly intervals for 3 weeks.

Because street children are not good reporters of demographic information, such as ages and family circumstances, they worked in pairs. While one member of the team asked the child's age, the other made an independent estimate of the child's age. Similar procedures were used for comparing the children's stated tribal affiliation with physical characteristics and language skills. The degree of discrepancy noted gave them some idea about the validity of information the child was supplying, and by using this procedure three times they had some notion of reliability. Because they were working with a relatively small sample and were checking on them daily and nightly, they were able to understand the degree to which they moved from *choum* to home and the gender ratio.[12]

The census data was then used to estimate the population, which would determine how large samples had to be for statistical comparisons. For example, they ascertained the differing degrees of street experience, from those who had just arrived on the streets to those who had been around a while, and compared this with various measures of mental health. Because they had a random sample, they were able to use inferential statistics to test if the length of time on the streets diminished mental health (not necessarily).

Participants in the study were sampled from five programs that served street and working children. The children had different degrees of street experience, ranging from living without supervision from parents or assistance from helping agencies to working on the streets but returning home to families at the end of each working day. Boys were randomly selected from client lists, but it was impossible to get an equal number of randomly selected street girls because so few street girls were available, so they chose them non-randomly (as they were made known to them by agencies, researchers, and so on), which tempers the robustness of their conclusions.

The 61 street children (42 male, 19 female) in the study ranged in age from 8 to 17 (*Mean* = 12.70 years, Standard Deviation = 2.17). Each child was administered three psychological tests. The Bender-Gestalt (BG) was used to assess neurological functioning. The Draw a Person (DAP) test was used to measure the child's overall emotional well-being and to give an idea of the degree of abuse or neglect they might have experienced. Finally, the Raven's Progressive Matrices test was used for

[12] By checking in on the *choums* at various times they were able not only to collect demographic data, but also to assess the stability of who lived where. There were times when they would see a couple of boys in one place for a few nights and then see them in another place. This movement was not only within Nairobi, boys often left Nairobi for the coast or Western provinces and then returned.

intellectual assessment. These tests were chosen because they had been successfully used before in cross-cultural contexts, including in Kenya with children of similar ages, as well as with street children in other cultures (Aptekar 1988). The tests were translated into Kiswahili and then back-translated into English to verify the accuracy of the translation. All but four children were given the tests in Kiswahili. The tests were scored by Kenyans and Americans who did not have an interest in the outcomes of the study or knowledge about the hypotheses. For more information on the testing, see Aptekar and Ciano (1999).

In order to avoid ethnographic bias, they matched the children's answers to different data collectors. They suggest that data collectors should come from different academic disciplines, ethnic groups, genders, social statuses, ages, and so forth. In future research, they suggest exploring the ways in which street children respond differently to different people asking the same question, as this may well represent a significant bias.

Random Sampling: The Sao Paulo Counting Method

Other sampling techniques are also valid. Rosemberg (2000) defined a process of counting street children (the Sao Paulo count) that began with compiling a list of places where street children congregated. They then divided the city into sectors where street kids were found and organized walking routes so all of the children were counted. They put trained teams of counters along the routes in cars and on foot to count (without double counting) and record the information using only a few variables, such as gender and age. Their conclusion was that the numbers of street children were considerably lower than what had been reported in the press, and from organizations (such as UNICEF) that help street children. They also found that in spite of the fact that there were more children sleeping rough than there were beds for them in shelters, the shelters were running at only a 65% occupancy rate.

The children in their count were overwhelmingly male, yet in districts where girls could earn an income, for instance near nightclubs, there were more girls. The ages seen were between 10 and 15 years of age and rarely did they encounter young children. There were almost no observations of the children using drugs, being involved in delinquent acts, or prostituting themselves. What the team did observe was the children working most of the time (and not begging much at all), and being together in groups for work and sleep.

In summing up what was learned from the Sao Paulo count, Rosemberg (2000) noted that only a very small percentage of the poor children were street children and inflating the numbers of street children had the effect of over-funding for this group and less funding for poor children. Street children are predominately male and the genders do different kind of work. Criminality is only a minor element of what their activities; they are usually working. And they found that many street children have loving families, whom they care for by being on the street, thus countering the idea that all street children are the victims of neglect and abuse.

Random Sampling: The Count-Recount Method

This method is based on a sampling approach used with wild animals or highly mobile populations (Gurgel et al. 2004). The data was collected in Aracaju, a town of nearly half a million in northeast Brazil where estimates of street children ranged from 2 to 300, to several thousands. They began with lists of street children from several different sources. Then the lists were scanned for recurring names. They had 20 data samplers walking the streets that were already identified as having street children on them. They asked the children to give their names and other demographic information. The results depended upon the honesty of the responses, which we will see can be problematic. The authors concluded that all but one child in their sample were male, that the majority were attending school and providing financial help to their families, and they returned home at night (note the expanded category). The top age was 19 as that is the age for official entry into adulthood in Brazil.

Palusci et al. (2010) used the capture-recapture method to estimate the total number of child maltreatment deaths in Michigan, USA. This methodology was originally developed to estimate the size of wild animal populations by estimating total population size based on proportions of animals that were captured, tagged, released and recaptured in two or more random samples. The method has been adapted for human populations and used to estimate the number of individuals affected by a number of different-problems such as for better estimates of fetal alcohol syndrome, physical abuse cases, and of course as stated above, difficult-to-count populations such as street children (Gurgel et al. 2004).

Validity, Trust and Manipulation

Street children, and to some extent homeless youth, cope for better or worse, by eliciting pity and avoiding disdain. The more successful learn and apply the skills they need to receive the responses that will profit them. The less successful cannot help but present themselves in ways that bring disdain or fear.

Children in street situations know they must be adept at creating images which will be profitable to them because their livelihoods depend on it. Lying about their ages, family backgrounds, reasons for being on the street, and their current circumstances is part of their well-rehearsed scripts. Aptekar and Ciano (1999) by using multiple data collectors with different demographic characteristics (gender, age, expatriate vs. local, etc.) found one boy who told them he was in the state reform school because he was beaten by his father, while later the same day, he told a female investigator that he was abandoned by his family and had no other place to go. Another boy was 8 years old when he was admitted to a program that served lunch to children eight and younger, then later the same day he was admitted for dinner at another program for children over 12 (Fig. 4.6).

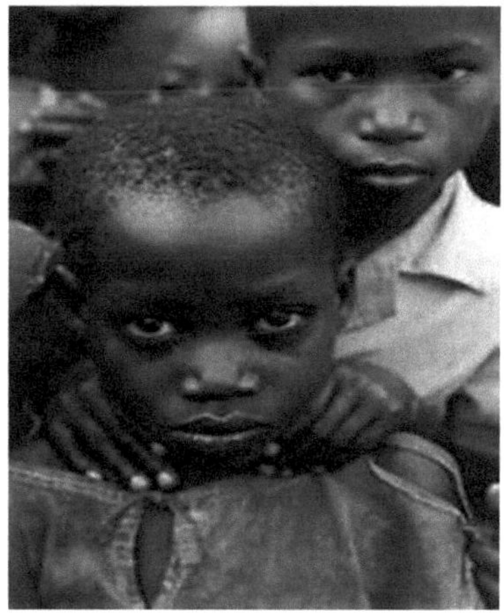

Fig. 4.6 Difficult to determine age

Conticini (2008), who worked in Bangladesh and Ethiopia, noted that the issue of getting to know street children and being trusted by them is vital to getting valid data. But how is this done? Should we accept what they say as valid? Honest no, valid yes. Even though what they say is made up to manage the impression they are giving, it does not mean it is invalid because it is both meaningful and important to understanding them.

Hecht (1998) found that in north east Brazil, when street children spoke about their mothers, they also made up information. He took this to mean that the topic held something of importance, namely the children's troubled relations to their mothers. So it seems that sometimes important information may not be true, but it can still hold validity.

Hecht found that these kids wanted to tell their stories. They did not fear the tape recorder, in fact they wanted to record their stories (or the stories they wanted the listener to hear). To one another, they boasted about their drug use, they told of imaginary do-gooders among them, they admonished others boys to get off the streets, they repented to the imaginary jailor or social worker, and they spoke of their religious conversions when playing up to imaginary clergy. What was unique was that at group times during radio workshops, the boys would speak openly and positively about their mothers, but in private sessions they would express their sense of being rejected by them.

In India, Nieuwenhuys (1994) found that the children were interested in talking to her and took some pride when she wrote down their information. She felt that the questions she asked were taken seriously by the street children and they tried to go as deep as they could in answering her. In her study of child labor in Zimbabwe, Reynolds (1991) found that her child informants took careful notes that were detailed and valid.

Davies (2008) conducted a participant observation study of street children in a regional town in north western Kenya. Because of the size of the town, Davies was able to identify the majority of the street children in his geographical area. He collected data without using questionnaires or surveys. He did not use formal interviews until the end of project, by which time he had a close relationship with the interviewees. Also the questions he asked in the interviews were for specific reasons, based on questions he found during his participant observations of the street children. Some of this had to do with clarifying demographic information such as the children's living conditions and whether or not they had parents.

He collected data nearly every day from morning to night, including a special emphasis on getting data at night which meant on a few occasions of staying overnight with them. He found certain places, such as the center of town, were not conducive to collecting data. It was too busy and he became too much of an object of curiosity. Data collection was more successful in the more intimate places where the children rested or were otherwise out of public view.

Heinonen (2011) decided not to look for answers to specific questions by using questionnaires. She believes that only by getting very close, indeed involved with her subjects, can she find the social meaning behind their behaviors. She became very familiar with social, work and leisure activities at home and in the street. But, she did this only after eschewing what she called the "*reality behind the contemporary social constructions of childhood within their social environment* (p. 7)". She explains what she finds from the point of view of the actors in the local environment she studies. She understands that street children and their families have their own narratives for their common customs and norms. She works to find their common culture, embedded in Ethiopian history and society.

She discusses the many problems beginning with choosing a field site so she could find street children and their families. Unlike in other places where there are concentrations of street children, she found that there wasn't a stable place nor any one location in the city where they could be found. She points to the uniqueness of Addis Ababa where social classes in one neighborhood can be quite heterogeneous. The street children and their families live in socially diverse communities, in all parts of the city. She shows how they roam nearly every part of Addis Ababa.

Nor, as she points out, do the street children and their families form a homogenous group. They have different backgrounds, different ethnic origins, speak different languages, and have varied types of households they come from.

As a result she had to work in nearly all parts of the city. Because of this she was able to find that urbanization has not created social tension. It has in fact encouraged various forms of integration. She points out that inter-marriage across ethnic, and even religious lines, is common, and it was not a cause of street children. She was able to ascertain that in some families the street children's mothers had taken men from different ethnic groups so that the siblings in these families did not share many cultural variables we commonly associate with our studies of street children. The common bond was poverty and overcrowded living conditions, which in turn proved important in how the poor socialize their children.

Another aspect of her work is that she went into her long years of ethnographic study free from preconceived hypotheses. She allowed herself time to wait until the middle of her study to identify the themes, because it wasn't until then that she was sure what the important material was. Briefly stated here (and more thoroughly elsewhere) she found three blocks upon which to build the culture of street children. The first block is *yilunta* (shame, honor and family pride), which she relates to the male hegemony in the wider Ethiopian context. It is this that accounts for how Ethiopian children are socialized and how gang members operate.

Her second central building block is reciprocity. What the children said is that this mattered most to them. Thirdly, she talks about the need for the researcher to confront one's own issues when working with street children. These include such sensitive topics as sex, drugs, violence, and theft. Throughout her work, she doesn't flinch from these methodological problems. Instead she discusses how she worked with them, which is invaluable to other researchers. The same can be said of how the children and their families react to her and how she reacts to them.

Also, she talks about the delights of the work. Her participant observations were composed of easy talk about interesting things. What she calls a continuous form of chitchat. As she moves between questions and answers sitting in a variety of places with parents and their street children, she captures their voices though first person narratives and by contextualizing people and ideas in a way that, coupled with ethnographic method, results in descriptive writing that brings to life not only context but characters.

Heinonen (2011) cites the Amharic word *yilunta* to explain the value that the street children she studied in Addis Ababa place on this concept. *Yilunta* means shame and honour, which plays out in a gender sensitive manner. "*Traditional masculine traits of assertiveness, power, independence and rationality were more important than traditional feminine traits such as docility, irrationality, submissiveness, and dependence* (p. 30)". *Yilunta* is the informal code of the general population. It is through this concept that she is able to bring forth a unifying theme that connects street children with larger cultural values. This connection marks her work as indispensable to the study of street children and to childhood studies. *Yilunta* essentially expresses the gender-based status of people as citizens in a culture where women are subordinate to men, which is deeply embedded into Ethiopian social values and mores. This is so important, she tells us, to being Ethiopian that it transcends ethnicity and religion. *Yilunta* makes it legitimate for men to dominate women and the values which are generally associated with masculinity – rationality, independence, assertiveness, and physical strength – receive higher status than characteristics associated with females – docility, submissiveness, irrationality, dependence and physical weakness. The other aspect of *Yilunta* is that parents must dominate children. According to Heinonen, these are the basic values which define Ethiopian culture and which people use to define themselves as members of a family and a community. It is not as if people are forced to follow these rules, but by history and culture they hold powerful sway and they are the basis upon which people feel honor or shame.

Because she defines street boys in relationship to *Yilunta*, masculinity and pride are central to their identity as they are to the general population of boys. Since power and wealth are associated with masculinity, street gangs cannot be proud without looking to other masculine traits. In fact, they feel shameful of who they are. For boys and men, *yilunta,* in association with their concern with status, means not losing face, protecting and honoring the family including financially helping relatives if necessary. Sensitivity to and concern about the opinion of others and a strong sense of propriety in dealing with friends and family alike are key to having Y*ilunta.* She tells us that among the youth she worked with, the expression they used to justify their disapproval of an unpopular comrade was that he had no *yilunta,* meaning that he had no scruples or shame. For upper-class-and upper-middle–class males, *yilunta* meant being conscious of and taking pride in the knowledge of one's class position. This precluded certain types of work and other social activities, which ranged from housework, accepting lower-status jobs like portaging, or marrying beneath one's status.

Warnings About Data Collection

Most readers of this book will be aware of the general cross-cultural research problems (such as translations and back–translations, the importance of local norms, etc.), but the mistake of overlooking the obvious can be dramatic.[13] For example, in Kaliti, an Ethiopian camp for the displaced, a group of researchers that Aptekar and Heinonen (Aptekar 2010 and Aptekar and Heinonen 2003) belonged to began a research project by taking a random sample of the people in the camp, then used tests developed in the U.S. and northern Europe on Post-Traumatic Stress Disorder (PTSD), but which were chosen for their appropriateness to the topic of study and their widespread international use. They subsequently worked on translations and back-translations, establishing local norms, training local data collectors, and otherwise working on the issues of taking tests from one culture and administering them in another. They did ignore the fact that many of the children did not have adequate age documentation, even though all the standardised tests were normed on age.

In their attempt to get the best data collectors, they chose the brightest and most competent university students. Several problems emerged. First, these students came from privileged backgrounds and were not familiar with the living conditions of the adolescents in the refugee camp. Because of this and other social class differences, the researchers sat together in one tent to collect the data, ate lunch together, and left together at the end of the day. Because the data collectors sat together in one place, the adolescents found that they could not talk about their personal problems without their peers overhearing them. This skewed the data to make them appear less troubled than they were.

Second, because the adolescent subjects were very poor and were being paid for participating, they vied for the option to participate. Some children on the list took the psychological testing that was the basis of the study more than once under

[13] Klein et al. (2006) in studying European gangs (and some from the USA) found that there were several advantages to using the cultural comparative approach. Some of these were using the same data collection methods, common sample procedures, and having and resolving conflicts among research teams to arrive at a consensus cross-cultural view point.

different names, since many preferred to sell their right rather than to sit for the several hours it took to administer the test. Since the data collectors were new to the camp and did not venture out to learn more about their subjects, they were not aware that some of them bought the names of others.

In addition, when the children were answering the questions on the tests, there was no check on how accurately they were responding. Many subjects rushed through their tests so as to complete them and get paid. They were more interested in getting the money than in telling some person they did not know details of their awful war experiences in full hearing of their peers. The tendency was to finish fast and inflate psychological difficulties, because they thought that their fictitious circumstances would bring them more aid. Since the data collectors were being paid per test administered, they too had their reasons to get through the protocols quickly, rather than take the time to have accurate responses.

Many of these research problems could have been avoided by having the data collectors and the people in charge of the study work more closely with their subjects. Like most studies by expatriates, the people with the knowledge of research methodology remain in their offices, preferring to hire out non-experienced data collectors instead of getting involved in the day to day work of the study. The lesson is: "mind the store, no one else will."

Methods to Avoid in Collecting Data

We have known for three decades that questionnaires are not answered honestly by children in street situations. Yet we persist. The same can be said of formal interviews, which are similar in format to the questionnaire. Davies (2008), who used formal interviews in Kenya, suggested that if you use questionnaires or interviews do not do so until the end of the research, when the children are known to the researcher who then can customize each interview to each child. He suggests using the formal interview as a validity measure that triangulates the information about the same child.

Young and Barrett (2001) report that time was a key factor in their work in Uganda which attempted to overcome the two problems inherent in research with street children, namely access to the children and the identity of the researcher as perceived by the street children.

In their case, they did not want to meet the children on the street (access) because they would be seen as rich tourists and thus receive a predictable pitch (identity). So they began working at an NGO where they were seen as donors. By staying longer and getting more involved, their identity and access improved because the children had to construct a new meaning about them.[14]

[14] It has also been recommended to follow kids as they leave day care programs or the parks to the streets where they hang out (Aptekar 1988; Kilbride et al. 2000). In Kenya, Aptekar and Ciano (1999) report on the advantage of having an older street child at their side. In any event, the public nature of the street conversations might keep them limited to acceptable and gender-sensitive topics

Their approach to the research was not related to psychosocial processes *per se*. They were looking at the street children's geographical space. Young and Barrett (2001) believe that street children have a particular relationship to their environment based primarily on the public presence and their devalued status as minors, their impoverished appearance, and their alleged delinquency. The aim of their study was to bring to light how street children (in this case in Kampala, Uganda) managed their spatial environs in order to survive.

The value of their work with regard to methodology is their direct communication about the difficulties in doing research with street children and the ways they explored to find solutions. The problems center on getting access to the children in order to build trust, and with how to manage what the children do and say given the demographic characteristics of the researcher. Over 9 months the authors collected ethnographic notes, orally derived information and drawings from the children. They make the case that these diverse methods helped them overcome the inherent bias in doing research with street children.

Young and Barrett (2001) did not provide any long-term incentives to the children for their participation. They claim that for the children just being in the research process was fun for them. The authors discussed with the children the purposes of the study, and they believe their consent was given without pressure. They were informed they could stop at any time, and the authors say that some did.

They add a dimension to the difficulty by stating quite clearly what is often left out in research with street children, that the children can be dangerous: high on drugs, involved in illegal activities, dirty and suspicious. Because they are weary of being arrested or detained, they are not likely to offer any accurate information about themselves. Race, gender, age, social class and language of the researchers influence how the children respond. The researchers describe themselves as female, white English speakers. The children are also adept at controlling their researchers; being researched is nothing new for street children, not only in the case of the street children in Kampala, but all over the world.

What we want to highlight here is that the situation of being known or unknown to the children is not as straight forward as it may seem. One could argue that the more the children knew and trusted the researcher the more biased the data might become, because having more of a stake in the relationship, a child might be more inclined to manage what is being said. And, there are, of course, many type of closeness that might develop, so the issue of bias can get even more complicated with having a more personal relationship.

What Young and Barrett (2001) do to meet these challenges is to include the children in adopting research methodologies, and, as mentioned above, to use more than one method to collect data. They discuss how each method they used helped to alleviate the bias inherent in researching street children. To overcome the children's past history with researchers and tourists, they volunteered at an NGO drop-in

(Kovats-Bernat (2006). While Kovats-Bernat is unable to talk freely with street girls, particularly about sex, Mtonga (2012) was able to do so. Presumably, the issue is not one of gender, but that Kovats-Bernat is an expatriate while Mtonga is a Zambian interviewing Zambian children.

center where they could work with bilingual volunteers and the children. Since the volunteers were Ugandans whom the children knew, the authors reasoned the children would become more relaxed with them. The authors mention that at first, the children asked them for money and to be taken to America to attend school, which the authors attributed to experiences with other program donors at the drop-in center in the past.

Young and Barrett (2001) also participated in the NGO's street outreach work, which allowed them to be seen by the children on the streets. They mention taking some kids to the local clinic, which we believe is instrumental in forming alliances with the children. Then they offered the opportunity to the children of being researchers like themselves. They believe that over time (9 months) this broke down many of the barriers which are often associated with trusted lack of trust.

The authors quote studies which show that interviews and questionnaires are not very reliable tools for research with street children. They felt that a lot of the problems with these methods were related to the fact that the researchers set the questions. So they used more child-centered oral methods. For example, they had the children simulate a radio program about street children. The children prepared for their radio program by brainstorming with the researchers and among themselves. They were able to have the children accept the use of a tape recorder. The children enjoyed listening to themselves and enjoyed controlling the tape recorder.

In addition, the authors enlisted the help of the children by asking them to control the logistics of the data collection, such as choosing the times and places to collect data. It became apparent that the children preferred to participate in their own spaces, rather than in some place provided by the NGO. They also had certain times when they wanted to collect data which were centered on the children's work schedule. All of this meant the children were involved, thus minimizing the potential bias of the adult researchers.

Finally, they had the children tell their stories through drawing which they felt was particularly helpful in getting the type of spatial information they wanted to learn regarding how children negotiated the urban streets. This brought into the sample children who were not literate, and who spoke different languages and dialects. The use of mental maps and photo diaries were the most helpful visual methods. By drawing the maps, the children were able to show what areas of the city were important, which ones to stay away from, etc. It also allowed the researchers to get an idea of the spaces that they could not enter. The authors believe that both the maps and the pictorial images drawings allowed them to avoid influencing the children's' stories.

Pictorial images were gathered by children using disposable cameras to capture their activities over a 24 hour period. The authors believe that this method has the advantage of getting actual images of places they would not go, like where illegal activities took place. The photos provoked interesting discussions with the children.

Kovats-Bernat (2006) conducted in-depth interviews and life history conversations with children while his guide told him whom he should talk to and where he should go. He cites Hecht as the source of what he refers to as this participatory approach, meaning being involved with the children, teaching them to find their voices, possibly using the researchers' connections to help them present their information to people who, because of his (and Hecht's) prestige as expatriates, might be valuable.

Another good approach is the triangulation of data, that is, taking three different methods, each with its own problems in validity, but which taken together counter the adverse affects of each one; for example, locally normed tests, interviews, and projective techniques.

Since most street children's ages are not properly documented and the children are often malnourished and thus small for their ages, it is difficult to determine their correct ages. This makes it difficult to do psychological testing that is age-based (see Kovats-Bernat (2006) for Haiti, Aptekar (1988) for Colombia, Aptekar and Ciano (1999) for Kenya, and Le Roux and Smith (1998) for a global perspective). In some cases, standardized tests have been locally normed, which helps. Also a case can be made for estimating children's ages by having independent local observers.

Methods to Use in Collecting Data

The best methods for research with children in street situations include projective techniques such as open-ended sentence completions, human drawings, drawings of mental maps and photographic diaries (Young and Barrett 2001). Also good are observations and performance related information. Finally we suggest a new method, the mental status exam.

Even if the street children are not literate, they can build their own life stories by cutting out photos from magazines. These photographs can be used as projective techniques; children can explain what they see in relationships between people, or to tell the wishes the adolescents in the photos might have for their future. While this does not give standardized data, it does help toward getting a triangulated source to see how reliable the collected data is.

Other projective techniques include answering incomplete sentences, such as, "*my father was …*", or, "*the best thing that ever happened to me was…*" or, "*if I could choose I would …*". This is similar to the three wishes test, which asks the child if he or she had three wishes, what would they be? The researcher can make these up and use them for conversational starters. Or, the answers of any of these questions can be sorted into common themes for nominal data for descriptive statistics.

Many performance related tasks can be used as forced choice (Q sorts). Say for example, asking children to rate their preferences or their fears on a five point Likert scale. This will result in ordinal values, which can be used for some rudimentary inferential statistics such as chi-squares.

A much overlooked and an extremely important method of collecting mental health data is the mental status exam (MSE), which essentially is the psychological equivalent of a physician's physical exam thus providing a look into the child's mental health at the moment. Essentially, it is an observable structured interview.

For example, mental status includes an assessment of the child's appearance. Are there any tics or tremors? What is the degree of hygiene? Are cuts, wounds, and injuries taken care of? Fine motor coordination can be assessed by asking the child to draw. Large motor coordination can be assessed by watching the child walk to see if the cadence is even and coordinated.

There are three kinds of memory: immediate, short term and long term. Asking the child to remember the names of three objects, say ball, pants, and bird, and then asking for those names 15 min later, tests immediate memory, which is affected by one's ability to concentrate and by the level of anxiety. By asking about last night and yesterday, the child's short term memory can be assessed. The child's level of consciousness from hyper-vigilant to non-responsive can be noted.

We can assess thought processes. Are they logical? Are there delusions? Does the child exhibit depressive thinking, or have manic thoughts? Are there obsessive thoughts or compulsive behaviors? Are there perceptual hallucinations such as seeing things that aren't there or hearing voices, or in the case of alcohol withdrawal feeling bugs crawling over one's skin?

Is the child's speech tone appropriate? Is the flow of speech slow or forced? Is the volume appropriate? What is the child's level of vocabulary? Does the child have a problem finding words, using words appropriately or in recalling the names of well-known objects?

There is more to mental status assessment, but suffice it to say that it can be taught to data collectors and can yield information on how well or the degree of difficulty the child is having in functioning, if there are mental health issues that need treatment, and a variety of important intellectual and cognitive measures.

The use of observations can also yield information about the validity and reliability of the children's histories. For example, if a child says that he goes home to give money to his family every day, but in fact you see him sleeping rough, there is a validity problem, and if he tells different stories about himself each day, you have a problem of data reliability.

Ennew (1994) suggests participating with the children in their lives and recording notes each day to document the observations. The observer can look for themes, and measure the number of recurring words or phrases. Another option is structured observation, in which the observations are done at pre-set time intervals (including in this case hopefully at night), or recording the number of events within a certain time limit. This data can be tabulated into frequencies, and compared to expected frequencies with the chi-square test.

When it comes to the presentation of results, there is often a problem of over-generalizing. Many authors, either in refereed journal articles or in evaluative studies of programs, over-generalized their findings by moving from a small non-random sample to a title that suggests a much larger population. For example, the study's sample is 50 street children in Johannesburg, but the title becomes "South African Street Children".

Sometimes, the publisher asks for a concise title. Stoecklin (2000) was not able to maintain the title "*Enfants en situations de rue en Chine. Une exploration sociologique*" (*Children in Street Situations in China. A Sociological Exploration*) as it was considered too long. The title eventually became "*Enfants des rues en Chine*" (*Street Children in China*) which both doesn't account for the important paradigmatic change that we expose here (focus on the situations) and tends to over-generalize his findings about 40 children in Shanghai. Although he considers his study as only an exploration, the market-oriented publication logic took over the cautious and scientific considerations of the PhD student he was at that moment.

Readers tend to believe the numbers printed in scholarly articles, no matter how much the author discounts the validity of these numbers. Once an article is published it is common that others in the field will cite the numbers in future research. In this way, faulty numbers, once published, become research facts prominent in the field, even if the original author provides disclaimers that down-play their validity. We saw this problem in the case of estimates of numbers of street children.

Children's Rights Bring Changes to the Research Paradigm

Children in street situations, based on their status as children, were historically used as objects to be studied. This is no longer the case. Once the UN Convention on the Rights of the Child became international law in 1989, research with children in street situations took a turn. The children were no longer seen simply as being objects of study, but as social actors with agency. Their ability to change their circumstances was stressed, emphasised. This included their relationships to the researchers and to the research. The researchers must now involve, inform, and consult with children in any area of research that involves them. This approach parallels new social science methodologies that see research and subjects as co-producers and co-researchers.

It also complies with Article 12 of UN Convention on the Rights of the Child which says that children have the right to express their opinions about matters that concern them and that they have the right to be heard as well as-Article 13 which declares that children are entitled to freedom of expression and have the right to seek, receive and impart information and ideas of all kinds.

Therefore, it is no longer legitimate or even legal to say that children are too little or too young to understand or to have a say in decisions concerning themselves. Thus a new term, "ethical symmetry": meaning the equal ethical treatment of children and adults in any investigation (Christensen and Prout 2002). They believe that rather than a single consent form, there needs to be a continual arbitration of ethical issues between adults and children.

This also means that children and youth are told (in terms they can understand) the nature and goals of the study, and that they have the right to withdraw from it at any time without suffering from any adverse consequences. More inclusive modes of communication can be used to adapt participative processes to the cognitive capacities of children.

Thus, full participation means ethically that the child and youth subjects should be involved in the whole research process and design; including the interpretation of data, the dissemination of results, and the consideration of the potential benefits of the project. This is not an easy law to follow or agree with.

Efforts towards more participatory modes of research, including the respect of children's rights in the research procedure itself, require that the tools used during research are made child-friendly. This is the case, as was mentioned before, with Stoecklin's simplification of the "Child-Street System" (Lucchini 1993), through the "kaleidoscope of experience" Stoecklin (2013). If the child is considered a social actor, rather than an object, then the research tools and procedures should be consistent with this. They should allow active participation of the child to give meaning to and to interpret his own experience instead of leaving this to the researcher's expertise.

Research tools and social theories are closely linked together and reflect each other. If we want the research tools to be consistent with the new paradigm in childhood studies, seeing children as social actors, then these tools should also incorporate a specific theory of action. Stoecklin (2013) goes in this direction with his theory of the "actor's system".

Participatory Action Research (PAR)

Much used since the 1990s, Participatory Action Research is a method in which the researcher participates with the subjects to generate what needs to be researched, how it is to be carried out, and how the results will be presented. The theory is that this empowers the subjects (in our case, street children and runaway youth) and helps them learn how to improve themselves. PAR also provides the researcher an understanding of the children's social experiences and social competencies by identifying the commonalties and differences among children, and by understanding the way they engage with and respond to the research itself (Christensen and James 2000).

Nieuwenhuizen (2006) used the PAR approach in Bangalore, India. Over a period of two weeks, the research team met with groups of street boys in several different locations in Bangalore. They had group discussions and in-depth interviews. The point was for the researchers to get more information from them about what they saw as their problems. They were asked in group discussions what were the worst problems they were currently facing.

Using this information, the research team built a simulated game called "*Voyage of Discovery*". In the game, four to eight children sit together and try to tackle a problem they have identified in the group discussions. They begin by making drawings of what they like and do not like in their current lives. Each boy explains his drawings to the group and pastes them onto a board in order from the largest to the smallest like and dislike. Then they are asked to identify the causes of these likes and dislikes. Then boys act out causes and effects and tie them to other problems and solutions in their lives. They discuss how they might carry out these solutions and in the next step they get more specific about actions that could help which they then put into practice in real life. Afterwards, they are asked how it went and if they feel they made any progress.

Given this information, Nieuwenhuizen (2006) decided to prepare a slide show for presentation to an outside group, but first she checked with the boys to see if her interpretations were in line with their thoughts. The new edited slide presentation was used in focus groups with adults who were in various roles with the street boys.

Ataöv and Haider (2006) used PAR in a study of 400 street children between the ages of 9 and 18 in Turkey. They too wanted to have street children understand their lives in a systematic way, categorize their problems and test out solutions. They collected data in a similar fashion that Nieuwenhuizen (2006) used in her study. Then they asked the children to evaluate the results and repeated the process again. Eventually they arrived at a point where the children could draw maps of their experiences and social networks, and interview their peers.

In Uganda, Young and Barrett (2001) used microphones as stage prompts for children to tell their stories as a radio announcer might do. Street Children International (Sauve 2003) had their workers tell the kids fictional stories about street children based on their experience of working with street youth. The children then used these stories to talk about themselves. Note that this is the reverse of the usual story telling method, which begins with the street youth telling their stories to the adults.

Veale and Dona (2003) asked Rwandan non-street children to describe the characteristics of Rwandan street children. The authors then used this information to define their subject population. They used older street children and street educators to observe places (observational mapping) where the defined street children were, and to understand their activities at different times of the day. Then nearly 300 identified street children were interviewed to obtain demographic information, including their psychological well-being. The researchers also used structured interview format with open and closed questions, which was developed, pretested and administered in Kinyarwandan to Rwandans.

In all of these studies, the children and youth took an active role in the research which allowed them to challenge the negative public perceptions of them, and to gain knowledge of themselves. This process is best when it systematically collects information with the children in the hope of improving the ability of the beneficiaries to take charge of their problems. Making strategic choices involves understanding the local situation to the greatest possible extent. And to achieve this bottom-up transfer of information, we must begin by strengthening the ability of both the children and the staff to translate their immediate concerns into more general problems. Each activity should therefore be given sufficient space, and should include the qualitative language of significant facts, a variety of explanatory hypotheses, and lessons learned. The participation of all levels in defining the strategy of intervention calls for a bottom-up consultation process (Participatory Action-Research - PAR).

Research taking quality of life into consideration, paying attention to the way in which the children themselves consider their lives on the streets, has definitely eliminated certain prejudices and improved the quality of intervention. In many countries, those who think a strong hand is the best way to deal with such problems now have to face the opposition shown by NGOs and various public movements, as well as, which is quite new, the academic world. Networking organisations have been set up, thanks to participation of some researchers. Part of the information which flows between those involved is made up of analyses of situations and capacity-building carried out in collaboration with social science experts. Their input helps in understanding the relationship between the development of personal capabilities and the nature of the institutional environment.

The Absence of Longitudinal Studies

The absence of longitudinal data reveals the largest gap in the research agenda on children in street situations. One of the most important reasons to conduct a longitudinal study of street children is to determine their ability to have productive intimate relationships and to survive economically as adults.[15] But all we have is a few small semi-longitudinal studies. Hecht (1998) revisited his sample of street boys 3 and 5 years after his original stay. Of the 23 boys he originally studied, 9 were murdered, and another died in an accident, all of the survivors were homeless (Fig. 4.7).

Heinonen (2011) contemplates that the street children in her study showed they "*joined the ranks of jobless destitute men and women found all over Addis Ababa* (Heinonen 2011, p 148)." Aptekar (1988) in a wistful contemplation speaks of some Colombian street children moving into small scale entrepreneurial pursuits, typical of the urban poor.

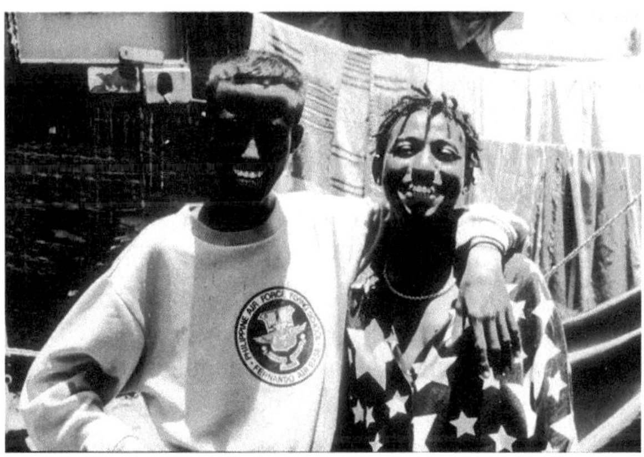

Fig. 4.7 Street boys revisited years later

[15] There is, for example, no study about love relationships of children in street situations. Although bonding and intimate relationships are not reducible to sexual intercourse; the focus on the latter, especially sexual abuse, in the media but also in academic research, is also a part of to the social construction of the street child's stereotype.

In Ethiopia, Aptekar (2010) found, several years after he studied street children raised in a camp for the displaced, that some joined the army to fight against Eritrea. One became schizophrenic, another felt he had a religious awakening, but to his knowledge, none became criminals.

Research Problems Associated with the Researcher

Aptekar (1992) believes that no one who collects data with children in street situations has such a unique relationship to the children to be able to completely eliminate the distortion of information that the children are likely to produce.

To understand the difficulty of knowing the validity of what the kids are saying, Aptekar (1992) suggests reading Berland's (1982) ethnography of the Qalander. The Qalander annually roam a 2,000 mile circle where they perform magic tricks, train animals for shows, and where children as young as five are taught to tell lewd sexual jokes for money. Because nomadic entertainers make their living this way, they are particularly adept at manipulating their audiences, either by begging or devising schemes to get work. The Qalander easily fool their marks. Like the sedentary groups who are prey to the Qalander, data collectors who are accustomed to a sedentary life are rarely exempt from the skills of children in street situations.

In fact, even if the ethnographer could develop a relationship of trust or friendship, it might easily lead to increased distortion because the researcher is more invested in the relationship which leads to ethnographic bias, and which makes street children more adept at manipulating information to get what they want. How the ethnographer comes to terms with this and how they help to align what they learn with objective and subjective reality should be part of the ethnography. This is the best way for ethnographers to assure the reader that they have not overly romanticized the children, which tends to create a bias toward resilience, or overly dramatized the children, depicting them as worse off than they are (Aptekar 1992).

Research can and does have a serious "*real world effect*" on the children we study. It might be life and death (witness the death squads in Brazil), or it might mean imprisonment and loss of freedom (witness the incarceration rates for dark skinned homeless youth in the U.S.). Yet, self awareness of the researcher is not easy given that as part of the scientific discipline researchers are asked to participate, but with distance, and asked to belong, but to remain objective. If they write about how they have been changed by the research experience, then the text will be described as sentimental, as a self-indulgent embellishment. If researchers explain how they have altered the text, because of their past experiences, then their conclusions will be dismissed as subjective. On the other hand, if researchers give only the cool presentation of the detached narrator, they open themselves to criticisms of a narrative without the convincing depth that comes from personal experience as well as one that forces the reader to accept what is written on faith alone.

Stoecklin (2000) experienced how much his interviews with street children in Shanghai attracted the attention of passers-by. As a white European speaking in

Chinese with children who were usually roughly pushed out of the way, he was highly visible. In order to protect his informants, Stoecklin chose to conduct his interviews mostly at night, "*when all the cats are grey*". But even then, he often had to stop his interviews, as there were too many people assembling, and it only took a few seconds until he and the interviewed child would literally be surrounded by dozens of people. He had to stop interviewing not only as the changing conditions would modify what the child was able to tell the researcher, but also and primarily in order to avoid police intervention and most likely trouble for the child, and maybe also himself (remember that in the 1990s, Stoecklin would not be allowed to do research on that topic in China).

The fact is that all research and writing involve abstractions of actual experience. The process of abstracting includes deciding on which phenomena are worthy of putting into words, how much each event will be emphasized in the document, and how the researcher sees the subject's experiences. These are combined to form ideas, concepts, and hypotheses. In short, the whole document, its form and content, is a matter of choice. What makes research valuable as well as valid is that this process is clearly defined. The goal should not be the elimination of the effects of the researcher, but a clear and concise description of their work.

While engaged in an ethnographic study of Colombian street children, Aptekar (1988) found that as surprising as it might seem he did not think about his own childhood and how it might have influenced the study of these children. In part he attributes this embarrassment to professionalism, which he equated with being objective. He had learned as part of his professional way of doing things to exclude what might well be the heart of the ethnographer's life blood, the personal values that connect them to their subjects. In this case, he assumed he was to sever the connection between his own childhood and the children he was studying.[16] This is obviously a factor facing all academic researchers who are working with children and youth.

This makes it difficult to ascertain just what these children are truly like, not only for researches but also for the public. The greater the confusion about them, the wilder the accusations about them become, either exaggerating or underestimating their behaviors. In fact, making an appraisal of them is even more difficult because children in street situations participate in contributing to the formation of the myths about them.

The importance of what the writer writes should not be underestimated. Aptekar's (1988) ethnography about street children in Colombia took a decided tack (as does most of his more current work). He pointed out that at that time according to the Colombian populace and to the international organizations that served the children, street children were considered "abandoned". However, he described many of the children as growing up in an orderly fashion and usually coming from matrifocal homes that stressed an earlier independence from their parents than was common in the socially dominant patrifocal society in which they lived.

---

[16] Aptekar wants to thank Phillip Fucella, University of California at Berkeley, for his rich editorial comments on counter transference.

Marquez (1999) in her study of Venezuelan street children, showed the relationships among street children, family structure, social class and political history. In both of the countries of her study there were two types of family structure: the Spanish patrifocal and the African matrifocal. These two family structures represented not only different family and cultural traditions, but also different sources of power in the society.

The dominant social class was composed of patriarchal families of Spanish descent. The family began with marriage in the Catholic Church and was sanctioned by kinship ties. The man took charge of the family's economic affairs. When children came he was also in charge of directing the childrearing. His wife and children were considered his assets. The conjugal relationship was important in defining the family (and hence the man) publicly, and placing itself (himself) within the strata of the civic order, hence the over-weighted value Colombians and Venezuelans placed on the *apellido*, the father's family name. In this family structure, men teach their boys to be men.

In many ways this is the opposite in the matrifocal family, where the unions were consummated without legal, church, or even kinship sanctions. The nucleus of the family was the mother and her children of both gender, but particularly the girl. Even the man in the matrifocal family who fathers a child was not necessarily considered a part of the family. In fact, the father was given the status of family member only if the mother decided to give it to him. In the matrifocal family, the woman's role as mother, instead of wife, was of primary if not sole importance. On the other hand, in the patrifocal family, the woman was both mother and wife.

These differences were represented in the roles of the mother-child dyad which was extremely important because this dyad often mirrored the roles the children had as adult men and women, both separately and in relationship with each other. In as much as the matrifocal family puts less emphasis on the conjugal unit, they reared children to expect that the relationship between husband and wife was less necessary and less important. This threatened the integrity of the patrifocal family where the conjugal relationship was the basis of the family's ties and the backbone which instilled and maintained authority and obedience within the families.

By examining the methods of child rearing in the matrifocal family, it is easy to reject the allegations that the street children were neglected or abandoned. Matrifocal families in Venezuela (Marquez 1999) and Colombia (Aptekar 1992) and Kenya (and in much of the world and unlike patrifocal families) raise their children in a deliberate and helpful manner that includes training boys for an early independence and self-assurance, attributes needed to gain a functional place in the existing subculture of urban poverty (Aptekar 1990).

Aptekar (1988) claimed that the majority of street children had adequate mental health, while the prevailing point of view was that they had mental disorders. He described the children as being free of drugs and crime, while they were commonly portrayed as addicted and delinquent.

How much of his description, which was the opposite of what almost everyone else saw, was filtered through his childhood? It is unfortunate that he did not try to answer this as it would have made for a more valid study. What he did in writing a traditional ethnography was to present notes in the form of a lawyerly argument so that the conclusions seemed obvious. He left out the internal dialogue; in fact he did not even allow himself to have one. This deprived the reader of being able to make a judgment about how much of the relationship between him and his informants existed before either of them got to the point of actually talking to each other.[17]

To the extent that Hecht (1998) and Kovats-Bernat (2006) and others with more negative appraisals about the children are right, and those whose findings are more positive are wrong, those with a positive view hold a terrible burden. The thinking goes something like this: How could these people say that children in street situations lead anything but an awful existence? How can they see children like Roberto and Antonio as resilient rather than as sad and pitiful, or even as delinquent? Is it that shedding a positive light offers hope to the researcher's personal problems? If they can live in abhorrent conditions and survive, we can too. Disturbing questions and provocative imagery are inherent, but are they helpful to researchers in this field? We can only recommend that researchers tell a little bit more about their own motivations in a specific section that must deal with the research ethics (about the ethical aspects in research with children see Morrow 2008, and more specifically with street children see Bemak 1996).

Suggestions for Research with Expatriate Researchers

As a subset of the problems of collecting data, we present below some suggestions to address problems peculiar to the expatriate researcher as well as teams of researchers that include expatriates and local researchers.

1. Expatriate researchers should have an extended stay in the host country, so that they can, at least to some extent, learn the language and work as full participants.
2. Work collaboratively with host country researchers in the collection and the analysis of the data.
3. Know the basic values and belief systems of children in street situations, which can best be achieved by working collaboratively.
4. Be prepared to explain what is similar and different from the expatriate culture to the culture of children in street situations. These are good discussion points for inter-cultural communication.
5. Understand and adapt to cultural variations of the population.
6. Use all subgroups of the street children or homeless youth population and see that they are sampled proportionately to allow for the statistical validation of the study.

[17] Swart (1990) in South Africa and Ennew (1994) in her international review mention a similar phenomenon; the problems of having middle class people who have inherited middle class prejudices about children in street situations collecting data. Note that the middle class people are often not expatriates but people from the local culture who come from a different social class.

7. Compare what their subjects lives are like, the quality of their living places, and the style or type of work they are doing to their social peers, thus being able to show if children in street situations are worse off or better off than their counterparts. Again, work collaboratively to discuss this in a cross-cultural context.
8. Make every effort, in spite of the difficulty to distinguish street children from working children and homeless youth from domiciled youth.
9. Get informed consent directly from the youth and children, even if they cannot legally give consent.
10. Know the possible problems associated with doing research with children in street situations. These include, but are not limited to: running the risk of being labeled an expatriate pedophile, of incurring physical danger, of being used by indigenous groups for purposes of funding, and of making things worse for the children rather than better. This information can be obtained more easily when working with collaborators from the home culture.

Ethical Considerations: To Give or Not to Give?

Researchers are also advised to read important ethical considerations that are necessary when conducting research with children (Alderson and Morrow 2011), as well as the standards set by the Inter-Agency Working Group on Children's Participation (2007).

Relationships between researchers and subjects always take place within social relations and cultural contexts. For example, as we suggest above, what is the effect of the intergenerational differences between adult researchers and children and youth? In the specific milieu of homelessness there are specific problems. The most uncomfortable of which is the question: to give or not to give?

Certainly, one ethical question you will face is to be or not to be involved; and if you choose to be involved, to face the logistical nightmare of how much to be involved, and when and how to stop. Children in street situations are in need and usually poor. Researchers are middle class and comfortable, although they don't see themselves that way. Most are not prepared for an honest response when children in street situations ask; "*What's in it for us?*" or when they say; "*Many people have been here before to do research, but we never get anything*".

How much are researchers willing to share the pie? Should they give them money, or reimburse them in any way; do they take them to the doctor? If they do, do they think this "contaminates" their study, compromising their professional integrity? Do researchers give them money for their time, or do you think this too will be compromising? Researchers might think that the children are the beneficiaries of their work; but sometimes the researchers themselves are the primary beneficiaries. However, research involving personal interactions between people belonging to different worlds is as complex as the ethical dilemmas might be. Who benefits from what? A research may also have long term effects. In a short-term appraisal, we could say that Stoecklin's research in China (2000) was to get a PhD. The 40 children he observed at the railway station in Shanghai hardly got more than his occasional help and smiles. But Stoecklin moved on, and today he is engaged in teaching children's rights in China that may have a much larger impact on children's lives in China. Considered in the long-run, his research was only the starting point of his involvement in China. This however hardly depends on his sole intention, but rather on complex inter-institutional arrangements and politics. No researcher has the control over the different agendas around street children issues (the research funding agencies, the public policies, the media, the NGOs, the children themselves) that make up a specific research environment. Therefore we can see that the issue of the "real beneficiaries" has an important temporal dimension and many possible stakeholders. A black-and-white divide between beneficiaries and non-beneficiaries is therefore too simplistic. Hecht (1998) provides a more nuanced assessment. He speaks of the problems of being indifferent to the street children. It takes an emotional toll to ignore the reality of their lives. But he doesn't hide from the differences in wealth between him and the street children, and he honestly admits that while he has the upper hand in material terms, he cannot work without the street children, so ultimately they have the upper hand.

From Kaliti, a camp for displaced people outside of Addis Ababa, Aptekar (2010) writes:

"Each day when I arrive another person is either gravely ill, or has just passed on. Those who are sick lie in bed without medicine or food, and wait until they get better or die. Solomon, is barely of age. After serving in the war he came back to Addis Ababa to discover he lost his family. He lived on the streets until he moved into this refugee camp thinking he would get some compensation for military service. He did but not for long. Up until he got sick, he earned money in the streets.

When I arrive to see him, he is lying in bed too sick to raise himself to greet me, and too sick to clean himself from vomiting up his food and medicine. I know there are only a few ways for him to get help. One is to borrow money from his family or a friend. He has no family. Whatever his friends lend him comes directly out of their mouths; they are already barely eating enough to survive. The second is to borrow against his future grain rations, which he has already done. The lender knows that if he does this again he will not be able to pay off the debt, because he is dying. Third, I could give him money. Short of success on one of these options Solomon will go the way of other young street youth who are HIV positive."

My being white and foreign means the people think I am rich. I cannot argue with this. The question is what is my responsibility given this status? If I give to Solomon now, when do I stop giving? Certainly others will also ask for help. What will be my rationale for giving in one case and not in another?

Here is what some researchers have to offer. Kovats-Bernat (2006) notes that while Haitian street children will resort to some of the most abhorrent brutalities imaginable, like lashing out with razor blades or throwing rocks, when they feel sad, they cry - uncontrollably. And when they crawl into sewage culverts only to be found days later dead, he asks himself how can he keep from offering help? He helps the children with their physical needs, dressing their wounds, giving clothes and food to them, as well as other humanitarian gestures.

Heinonen (2011) in her study of street children in Addis Ababa sees one young man in front of a pharmacy quite upset. His dilemma is that his best friend has been hurt and while he has a prescription for him, he doesn't have enough money to fill it. She offers to pay for it, and tells him to put what money he has back into his pocket. Later that day she sees the boy and his comrade, they thank her for her help and from that moment on, they are friendly and welcoming. By giving, she learns that street children are not from another species.

Aptekar (2010) describes stopping at a traffic light in Addis Ababa where a blind youngster with opaque infected eyes open to public view habitually begged. While trying to ignore being seen by the eyes that could not see, Aptekar realizes why so many people doing research with children in street situations find it very difficult to give. It is too hard to accept the difference between them and us (Aptekar 2004).

He has heard and read that, "*Giving to them would ruin the research project by making it biased*", or "*it wouldn't be fair to the others*", or, "*it would reinforce the stereotype of white-skinned people giving to black-skinned people*", or "*they would just spend the money on inhalants or other drugs*". A lot of problems can be resolved by focusing on work with numbers instead of interacting with the individuals one comes to know. Is this why most researchers spend most of their time in the office making administrative decisions and calculating data?[18]

Malinowski (1926) at a time when Western anthropologists were confronting their own wealth in relation to indigenous peoples was the first one to address Hecht's dilemma. He realized the reasons for giving ranged on a continuum from selfless altruism to giving only in order to receive something in return. The exchange of gifts maintains social obligations. Hecht knows he wasn't really giving altruistically, but out of self-interest to keep the children obliged to him.

While it is hard to give because it is impossible to be altruistic, it is also hard to stop. If we decide to give, children in street situations will have to accept that we the professionals and well-wishers are helpless in meeting all of their demands. And, we have to realize that the only way we can help any of them is to have them accept that not everyone is going to be helped. This can become a programmatic or personal night mare.

Once one gives, there is the nearly impossible heartbreaking burden of deciding whom to give to and when to stop. This is why there are so many rules for not giving. How could Aptekar stop giving to Solomon? Should he wean him of the money that buys his food that keeps his drugs down that keeps him alive? Maybe yes, if it means accepting Solomon's demise and using what he would have received to help the next person who might be more productive. Can you be the mother that doesn't feed one of her two child because he or she is the weaker of the two?

About the only way through this morass is to follow the philosophy of Sister Mary, from the Italian Comboni order, a group that specializes in working with

[18] On the other hand, Hutz and Koller (1999) show that giving to children can lead to unreliable data; the result of street children fighting to be interviewed more than once in order to get more than one payment.

"outcasts". She provided a feeding program for the indigent for several years. Aptekar (2010) recalls seeing a young woman with a 10-month old girl waiting to see the Sister. The little girl had been burned on her face. A soiled white piece of cotton cloth was wrapped around her head, as if she had a toothache. As the woman reached out to say hello to Sister Mary, he could see that the fingers of her hands were stubs, a product of her leprosy. Sister Mary welcomed the girl in her arms and complained to the girl's mother that the child had a runny nose.

Here is the logistical lesson. Sister Mary developed her own *modus operandi*, one that was filled with caveats, judgements, exceptions, and broken rules. In short a system devised, probably as subconsciously as consciously, to keep her going. She had continued giving by finding a way to ignore the incurable obvious and embrace the barest of possibilities. The ethical champion is not the purist, but the one that stays around the longest.

Conclusion

We demonstrated that research focused on street children and homeless youth has several problems beginning with being clear about defining who is being studied. Without a clear definition, it is difficult to form an accurate picture of their numbers and characteristics.

Most research data on street children and homeless youth comes from evaluative studies with non-random samples. In order to go beyond basic descriptive statistics, we need a random sample. We showed three different ways to do this. The Aptekar model is based on what is used for peripatetic groups. This begins with a clear definition of households, mapping high and low concentrations and taking a random sample of the map sectors. Potential problems include the time of day the data is collected, who the data collector is, the difficulty of using standardized tests, and the importance of translation and back-translation.

Another model, the Sao Paolo Count, begins with compiling a list of places where street children congregate. Then the city is divided into sectors where the subjects are found and walking routes are organized so that everyone can be counted. Potential problems include double-counting and the limited number of variables, such as gender and age, which can be counted.

The count-recount method is based on a sampling method used with wild animals which are tagged, released and recaptured in two or more random samples. Lists of subjects from several different sources are scanned for recurring names. Multiple data collectors walk the streets that are identified as having populations. They ask the children to give their names and other demographic information. They repeat the process. The results depend on the honesty of the responses.

We mentioned some good and not so good data collection methods. Because children in street situations have developed skills in saying what they think the researchers want to hear, they often provide invalid data, for example regarding their ages, family backgrounds, and reasons for being on the street. We showed the advantages of multiple data collectors with different demographic characteristics (gender, age, expatriate vs. local, etc.).

We provided some solutions to these problems, and gave a series of suggestions. Researchers should know the basic values and belief systems of children in street situations. They should be able to proportionately sample subgroups, and compare data to show if children in street situations are worse off or better off than their domiciled counterparts. Researchers know that these children are likely to be experienced subjects. The best methods for research with children in street situations include projective techniques such as open-ended sentence completion, human drawings, drawings of mental maps, photographic diaries, and performance related information. The mental status exam is introduced as a guided observational tool. It is important to triangulate methods, avoid questionnaires or other paper and pencil tests that ask direct questions.

At a more paradigmatic level, we showed the limits of the classical and Cartesian bi-dimensional definition (children of the street/children on the street) and how systemic tools better help understand the actor's relationship to the street, like in the Child-Street System (Lucchini 2007) and in the Actor's system and Kaleidoscope of experience (Stoecklin 2009a, b).

Because of the adoption of The UN Convention on the Rights of the Child, researchers are asked to involve, inform, and consult with children in any area of research. As a result there are many Participatory Action Research (PAR) projects where children take over many research functions previously carried out only by adults.

We lamented the lack of longitudinal studies, thus making it difficult to know how the street children and homeless youth eventually function as adults. There are research problems associated with the researcher's collection and understanding of the data. Data should be put into the context of local culture and history. There are also ethical considerations, including the question of giving money.

References

Ahmadkhaniha, H., Shariat, V., et al. (2007). The frequency of sexual abuse and depression in a sample of street children of one of deprived districts of Tehran. *The Journal of Child Sexual Abuse, 16*(4), 23–35.

Alderson, P., & Morrow, V. (2011). *The ethics of research with children and young people: A practical handbook.* London: Sage.

Alteena, A., Brilleslijper-Kater, S., & Wolff, J. (2010). Effective interventions for homeless youth: A systematic review. *American Journal of Preventive Medicine, 38*(6), 637–645.

Aptekar, L. (1988). *Street children of Cali.* Durham: Duke University Press.

Aptekar, L. (1990). Colombian street children: Gamines and Chupagruesos. *Adolescence, 24*(96), 783–794.

Aptekar, L. (1992). Are Colombian street children neglected? the contributions of ethnographic and ethnohistorical approaches to the study of children? *Anthropology & Education Quarterly, 22*(4), 326–349.

Aptekar, L. (2004). The changing developmental dynamics of children in particularly difficult circumstances: Examples of street and war traumatized children. In U. Gielen & J. Roopnarine

(Eds.), *Childhood and adolescence in cross-cultural perspective and applications* (pp. 377–410). Westport: Praeger Press.

Aptekar, L. (2010). *In the lions mouth: Hope and heartbreak in humanitarian assistance.* Bloomington: Xlibris.

Aptekar, L., & Ciano, L. (1999). Street children in Nairobi, Kenya: Gender differences and mental health. In M. Raffaelli & R. Larson (Eds.), *Homeless and working youth around the world: Exploring developmental issues: New directions for child and adolescent development*, Number 85 (pp. 35–46). San Francisco: Jossey Bass.

Aptekar, L., & Heinonen, P. (2003, Spring). Methodological implications of contextual diversity in research on street children. *Children, Youth and Environments, 13*(1). Retrieved from: http://colorado.edu/journals/cye

Ataöv, A., & Haider, J. (2006). From participation to empowerment: Critical reflections on a participatory action research project with street children in Turkey. *Children, Youth and Environments 16*(2), 127–152.

Barker, G., & Knaul, F. (1991). Exploited entrepreneurs; Street and working children in developing countries (Working Paper No1). New York: Childhope.

Bemak, F. (1996). Street researchers. A new paradigm redefining future research with street children. *Childhood, 3*, 147–156.

Bhalotra, S., & Tzannatos, Z. (2003). *Child labor: What have we learnt?* (Social Protection Discussion Papers 27872). Washington, DC: The World Bank.

Blumer, H. (1969). *Symbolic interactionism: Perspective and method.* Englewood Cliffs: Prentice Hall.

Berland, J. (1982). *No five fingers are alike*. Cambridge: Harvard University Press.

Cauce, A., Paradise, M., Ginzler, A., Embry, L., Morgan, C., Lohr, Y., & Theofelis, J. (2000). The characteristics and mental health of homeless adolescents: Age and gender differences. *Journal of Emotional and Behavioral Disorders, 8*(4), 230–239.

Christensen, P., & James, A. (Eds.). (2000). *Research with children: Perspectives and practices* (1st ed.). London: Falmer Press.

Christensen, P., & Prout, A. (2002). Working with ethical symmetry in social research with children. *Childhood: A Global Journal of Child Research, 9*(4), 477–497.

Conticini, A. (2008). Surfing in the air: A grounded theory of the dynamics of street life and its policy implications. *Journal of International Development, 20*(4), 413–436.

CSC (Consortium for Street Children). (2011). *Street children statistics*. Retrieved on-line at: http://www.streetchildren.org.uk/

D'Alanno, T. A. (2005). *Homelessness in the Denver metropolitan area: A base line point in time study*. Denver: Metropolitan Denver Homeless Initiative.

Davies, M. (2008). A childish culture? shared understandings, agency and intervention: An anthropological study of street children in northeast Kenya. *Childhood, 15*(3), 309–330.

de Benitez, S. (2011). *State of the world's children: Research* (Street children series 2). London: Consortium of Street Children.

Dewey, J. (1910). *How we think*. Washington, DC: Heath & Co Publishers.

de Moura, S. (2002). The social construction of street children: Configuration and implications. *British Journal of Social Work, 32*, 353–367.

Ennew, J., & Milne, B. (1989). *The next generation: The lives of third world children*. London: Zed Books.

Ennew, J. (1994). *Street and working children – A guide to planning* (Developmental Manual #4). London: Save the children.

Faulk, M. (2010). *Exploring the perceptions of youth street migration Ii Pattaya, Chiang Mai, and Bangkok*. Thesis for MSW degree, San Diego State University, San Diego.

Fujimora, C. (2005). *Russia's Abandoned Children: An Intimate Understanding*. Westport: Praeger.

Gurgel, R., et al. (2004). Capture-recapture to estimate the number of street children in a city in Brazil. *Archives of Disease in Childhood, 89*, 222–224.

Gurung, H. (2004). *Study of policies and programmes addressing the right of street children to education research report*. Pokhara: Child Welfare Scheme UK.
Hecht, T. (1998). *At home in the street: Street children of northeast Brazil*. Cambridge: Cambridge University Press.
Heinonen, P. (2011). *Youth gangs & street children: Culture, nurture and masculinity in Ethiopia*. New York: Berghahn Press.
Hong, D., & Ohno, K. (2005, July). *Street children in Vietnam: Interactions of old and new causes in a growing economy* (Discussion Paper, No. 6). Hanoi: Vietnam Development Forum.
Huang, C.-C., et al. (2004). A comparative analysis of abandoned street children and formerly abandoned street children in La Paz, Bolivia. *In Archives of Diseases in Childhood, 89*, 821–826.
Hutz, C., & Koller, S. (1999). Methodological issues in the study of street children. In W. Damon (Series Ed.) & M. Raffaelli, & R. Larson (Vol. Eds.), *Homeless and working street youth around the world: exploring developmental issues* (New directions in child development, Vol. 85, pp. 59–70). San Francisco: Jossey Bass.
Hyde, J. (2005). From home to street: Understanding young people's transitions into homelessness. *Journal of Adolescence, 28*, 171–183.
Iqbal, S. (2008). Street children: An overlooked issue in Pakistan. *Child Abuse Review, 17*(1), 201–209. Online: Wiley InterScience (www.interscience.wiley.com). doi:10.1002/car.1026
Kerfoot, M., Koshyl, V., Roganov, O., Mikhailichenko, K., Gorbova, I., & Pottage, D. (2007). The health and well-being of neglected, abused and exploited children: The Kyiv Street Children Project. *Child Abuse & Neglect, 31*, 27–37.
Kilbride, P., Suda, C., & Njeru, E. (2000). *Street children in Kenya: Voices of children in search of childhood*. London: Bergen and Garvey.
Kissin, D., Zapata, L., Yorick, R., et al. (2007). HIV seroprevalence in street youth, St Petersburg, Russia. *AIDS, 21*(17), 2333–2340.
Klein, M., Weerman, F., & Thornberry, T. (2006). Street gang violence in Europe. *European Journal of Criminology, 3*(4), 413–437.
Koehlmoos, T., Uddin, J., Ashraf, A., et al. (2009). Homeless in Dhaka: Violence, sexual harassment, and drug-abuse. *Journal of Health, Population, and Nutrition, 27*(4), 452–461.
Koller, S., & Hutz, C. (1996). Meninos e meninas em situacao de rua: Dinamica, diversidade e definicao (Boys and girls on the streets: Dynamics, diversity, and definition). In: *Compiled Papers of ANPEPP* (Brazilian National Association for Research and Graduate Studies in Psychology), 1(12), 11–34.
Kovats-Bernat, J. (2006). *Sleeping rough in Port-au-Prince: An ethnography of street children and violence in Haiti*. Gainesville: University of Florida Press.
Kudrati, M., Plummer, M. L., & Yousi, N. (2008). Children of the Sug: A study of the daily lives of street children in Khar-toum, Sudan, with intervention recommendations. *Child Abuse& Neglect, 32*(4), 439–448.
Lamberte, E. (2002). *Ours to protect and nurture, the case of children needing special attention*. PhD thesis, De la Salle University, Manila, Philippines.
Le Roux, J., & Smith, C. (1998). Causes and characteristics of the street children phenomenon: A global perspective. *Adolescence, 33*(321), 683–688.
Leite, L., & Esteves, M. (1991). Escola Tia Ciata: A school for street children in Rio de Janeiro. *Environment and Urbanization, 3*, 130–139.
Libertoff, K. (1980). The runaway child in America: A social history. *Journal of Family Issues, 1*, 151–164.
Lucchini, R. (1993). *Enfant de la rue. Identité, sociabilité, drogue*. Genève/Paris: Droz.
Lucchini, R. (1994). *The street children in Montevideo and Rio de Janeiro: Elements for a definition*. Fribourg: Institute for Economic and Social Sciences, University of Fribourg.
Lucchini, R. (1996). *Sociologie de la survie. L'enfant dans la rue*. Paris: PUF.
Lucchini, R. (2007). "Street children": Deconstruction of a category. In I. Rizzini, U. Mandel Butler, & D. Stoecklin (Eds.), *Life on the streets. Children and adolescents on the streets: Inevitable trajectories?* (pp. 49–75). Sion: Institut International des Droits de l'enfant.

Lutjens, S. (2000). Schooling and clean streets in Socialist Cuba: Children and the Special period. In R. Mickelson (Ed.), *Children on the streets of the Americas* (pp. 55–65). New York: Routledge.

Malinowski, B. (1926). *Crime and custom in Savage Society*. New York: Harcourt, Brace & Co.

Marquez, P. (1999). *The street is my home: Youth and violence in Caracas*. Stanford: Stanford University Press.

Mathur, M., Rathore, P., & Mathur, M. (2009). Incidence, type and intensity of abuse in street children in India. *Child Abuse and Neglect, 33*(12), 907–913.

McBurney D. (1994). *Research Methods*. Pacific Grove, California: Brooks/Cole.

Mickelson, R. (Ed.). (2000). *Children on the streets of the Americas*. New York: Routledge.

Moberly, C. (1999). The "voluntary separation" of children in Angola: Recommendations for preventive strategies. In *Prevention of street migration: Resource pack*. Cork: Consortium for Street Children/University College Cork.

Morrow, V. (2008). Ethical dilemmas in research with children and young people about their social environments. *Children's Geographies, 6*(1), 49–61.

Mtonga, J. (2012). *On and off the streets: Reasons why street children escape institutional care and their survival on the streets*. Unpublished Master's Degree. Trondheim: Norwegian Centre for Child Research (NOSEB).

Nieuwenhuizen, P. (2006). *Street children in Bangalore, India: Their dreams and future*. Antwerp: Het Spinhuis Publishers.

Nieuwenhuys, O. (1994). *Children's life worlds: Gender, welfare and labor in the developing world*. London/New York: Routledge.

Njord, L., et al. (2010). Drug use among street children and non-street children in the Philippines. *Asia-Pacific Journal of Public Health, 22*(2), 203–211. Honolulu: Asia-Pacific Academic Consortium for Public Health/Sage Publications.

Palusci, V., Wirtz, S., & Covington, T. (2010). Using capture-recapture methods to better ascertain the incidence of fatal child maltreatment. In: *Child Abuse and Neglect, 34*(6), 396–402. Amsterdam: Elsevier, B. V.

Panter-Brick, C., Todd, A., & Baker, R. (1996). Growth status of homeless Nepali's boys: Do they differ from rural and urban controls? *Social Science & Medicine, 43*(4), 441–451.

Paradise, M., & Cauce, A. (2002). Home street home: The interpersonal dimensions of adolescent homelessness. *The Society for the Psychological Study of Social Issues, 2*(1), 223–238.

Rizzini, I., Mandel-Butler, U., & Stoecklin, D. (Eds.). (2007). *Life on the streets. Children and adolescents on the streets: Inevitable trajectories?* Sion: Institut International des Droits de l'enfant.

Reynolds, P. (1991). *Dance civet cat. Child Labour in the Zambezi Valley*. London: ZED (with Ohio University Press and Baobab Publications).

Robertson, M., & Toro, P. (1999). Homeless youth: Research, intervention, and policy. In L. Fosburg & D. Dennis (Eds.), *Practical lessons: The 1998 national symposium on homelessness research* (pp. 3-1–3-32). Washington, DC: U.S. Department of Housing and Urban Development and U.S. Department of Health and Human Services.

Rosemberg, F. (2000). From discourse to reality: A profile of the lives and estimates of the number of street children and adolescents in Brazil. In R. Mickelson (Ed.), *Children on the streets of the Americas* (pp. 118–135). New York: Routledge.

Sauve, S. (2003). Changing paradigms for working with street youth: The experience of Street kids international. *Children, Youth, and Environments*, 13(1). Retrieved August 25, http://cye.colorado.edu

Schaffner, L. (1999). *Teenage runaways: Broken hearts and "bad attitudes"*. New York: Haworth Press.

Schrader, A., & Veale, A. (1999). *Prevention of street migration. Resource pack*. London: Consortium for Street Children.

Stoecklin, D. (2000). *Enfants des rues en Chine* [Street children in China]. Paris: Karthala.

Stoecklin, D. (2007). Children in street situations: A rights-based approach. In I. Rizzini, U. M. Butler, & D. Stoecklin (Eds.), *Life on the streets. Children and adolescents on the streets: Inevitable trajectories?* (pp. 77–97). Sion: Institut International des Droits de l'enfant.

Stoecklin, D. (2009a). L'enfant acteur et l'approche participative. In J. Zermatten & D. Stoecklin (Eds.), *Le droit des enfants de participer. Norme juridique et réalité pratique: contribution à un nouveau contrat social* (pp. 47–71). Sion: IUKB/IDE.

Stoecklin, D. (2009b). Réflexivité, participation et capabilité. In J. Zermatten & D. Stoecklin (Eds.), *Le droit des enfants de participer. Norme juridique et réalité pratique: contribution à un nouveau contrat social* (pp. 75–109). Sion: IUKB/IDE.

Stoecklin, D. (2013, November). Theories of action in the field of child participation. In search of explicit frameworks. *Childhood*. Issue 4, pp. 443–457.

Stonge, J. (2000). The education of homeless children and youth in the United States: A progress report. In R. Mickelson (Ed.), *Children on the Streets of the Americas* (pp. 66–76). New York: Routledge.

Swart, J. (1990). *Malunde: The street children of Hillbrow*. Witwatersrand: Johannesburg.

Taçon, P. (1981). *MyChild minus two*. Unpublished UNICEF report.

Taçon, P. (1985). *A UNICEF response to the needs of abandoned and street children*. Geneva: UNICEF.

Tanon, F., & Sow, A. (2010). *Unaccompanied migrant minors from Africa: The case of Mauritania*. Paper presented at: Seminar on youth migration and transitions to adulthood in developing countries, Rio de Janeiro, Brazil.

Thapa, K., Ghatane, S., & Rimal, S. P. (2009). Health problems among the street children of Dharan municipality. *Kathmandu University Medical Journal, 7*(3): Issue 27, 272–279.

Tronchet-Pradhan, C. (2011). *Participation in the child and youth clubs of Nepal and experience of non-discrimination and equality rights. A field testing with the kaleidoscope of experience*. Thesis for the Master of advanced studies in children's rights. Sion: IUKB.

US Department of State (US-DOS). (2005). *Human Rights Report 2004, Bangladesh*. Washington, DC: US-DOS.

Uvin, P. (1998). *Aiding violence: The development enterprise in Rwanda*. Boulder: Kumarian Press.

Veale, A. (1996). *An empirical and conceptual analysis of street children in Sudan and Ethiopia*. PhD dissertation, University College Cork, Cork.

Veale, A., Aderfrsew, A., & Lalor, K. (1993). *A study of street children in four regional towns in Ethiopia*. Report for UNICEF in conjunction with the Ministry for Labor and Social Affairs, Ethiopia. Cork: University College Cork.

Veale, A., & Dona, G. (2003). Street children and political violence: A socio-demographic analysis of street children in Rwanda. *Child Abuse & Neglect, 27*, 253–269.

Whitbeck, L., & Hoyt, D. (1999). Nowhere to grow: Homeless and runaway adolescents and their families. *Youth & Society, 22*(1), 109–125.

Williams, N., Lindsey, E., Kurtz, P., & Jarvis, S. (2001). From trauma to resilience: Lessons from former runaway and homeless youth. *Journal of Youth Studies, 4*(2), 233–253.

World Vision. (1998). *Child-headed households in Rwanda: A qualitative needs assessment*. Technical report. Kigali/London: World Vision Rwanda and World Vision UK.

Wright, J., Kaminsky, D., & Wittig, M. (1993). Health and social conditions of street children in Honduras. *American Journal of Disabled Children, 147*, 279–283.

Young, L., & Barrett, H. (2001). Issues of access and identity: Adapting research methods with Kampala street children. *Childhood, 8*(3), 383–395.

Zhang, Q., & Yang, H. (2002). The situations and relief countermeasures towards street children in China. *Social Welfare, 9*, 18–22.

Chapter 5
Programs: Typical and Exemplary

Comparison of Programs for Homeless Youth and Street Children

Before we can begin to introduce models of intervention and present some current practices and programs, we will contrast programs for homeless youth and street children. Then, we offer a system of classifying different programs.

In contrast to the developing world, the wealth in the developed world is so substantial that for the most part we have to consider programs for homeless youth and street children separately. In a program for homeless youth the typical benefits include housing (usually a foster home), food, and medical care including mental health care, schooling, transportation, clothing, and support for extracurricular activities. In the developing world, the State rarely even responds to a child leaving home. If the child is resourceful, he or she can find a drop-in center run by an NGO where services usually consist of a bowel of porridge and sometimes a night's shelter.

So when we talk about programs for homeless youth, the bar is at the high end to begin with. But this doesn't mean that what is offered is successful. One problem is that most homeless youth in the developed world leave home out of desperation to avoid (further) abuse. Bao et al. (2000) report from the US Network of Runaway Youth Services that 70% of adolescents in shelters have been abused either physically and/or sexually by family members. More than a third of the young women said they were forced to have sex with an adult caretaker.[1] Programs usually address their homelessness through physical infrastructure and support (shelter, food) that is given without question, but do not address the abuse they endured.

There is some evidence that the programs which address both homelessness and abuse are effective, particularly for girls (Paradise and Cauce 2002). But even for girls the cycle of victimization slowed or stopped only for some. The authors were not able to discern why it was valuable for some and not others.

[1] Sexual orientation that is unacceptable to parents is another issue for fleeing.

L. Aptekar and D. Stoecklin, *Street Children and Homeless Youth: A Cross-Cultural Perspective*, DOI 10.1007/978-94-007-7356-1_5,

In a cross-cultural study of programs serving homeless youth from the USA, Canada, and S. Korea, Alteena et al. (2010) noted that the programs that focused on substance abuse were not attentive to overall quality of life, which might be why this study could not show much empirical evidence for effectiveness. When the programs provided help for the quality of life of the homeless youth (and drug abuse), they had more success. One form of psychotherapy, cognitive behavioral techniques, appeared to offer help with substance abuse and depression compared to the control group, but it did not help with the overall quality of life.

They noted that some programs included independent living designed to teach homeless youth the skills to support themselves. After two years of services these skills did increase, and there was some psychological help for the research group, but in both cases there might not have been, according to the authors, enough to justify the expense of the program. Brief motivational interventions, essentially consisting of inspiring interviews with a lot of positive talking and brief feedback showed no difference between the control and experimental groups, nor did peer-based intervention show differences after the program. Programs that helped homeless youth with money, assuming with cash they would feel better about their situation, showed that the experimental group had a slightly more favorable life satisfaction and enjoyed their family contacts more than the control group, but the differences were not significant.

After the evaluations were complete they concluded that it was difficult to know which part of any program was responsible for what success it had. They could not draw conclusions from the title of the program and its stated aims regarding the reasons for success. Likewise, it was not known which homeless youth gained from which program. Overall, they felt there were just too many programs for drug and alcohol abuse and not enough on critical living skills, including healthy interpersonal relationships (Alteena et al. 2010).

It just might be as Paradise and Cauce (2002) found in their examination of the history of homeless youth, that they are not easy to care for; they show a lot of difficulty sustaining attention and controlling their impulses and they make parenting even more difficult. In the latter case, the authors suggested that the children might have an innate temperament which leads parents and children to fall into a sliding cycle - irritable children brings irritable parenting, or vice versa leading to the mental disorders in the children and the dysfunction of the family. Empirical evidence from another source indicates the direction is the other way (Garder et al. 2006). Because three-quarters of the mothers of homeless youth have substance abuse problems and problems with the law, the fact begs the question of which comes first, the difficult to manage children or the substance abuse among parents?

Not making things easier for homeless youth is that the fact that in the US welfare assistance, as in some other countries in the developed world, has gone from abundance to scarcity; recipients are now expected to help themselves a lot more. Epstein (2000) argues that the State is only willing to address the needs of homeless children if pushed to do so, and the controlling political interests make this unlikely. So, more and more homeless youth must find their own means to overcome their living conditions and solve their personal problems.

Even when a supportive government provided housing for homeless youth so they had a secure place to live and adequate supportive services, there were plenty of problems. Three-quarters of these shelters have a fixed a time limit on staying, and very little attention is given to children in homeless centers - only about half of the shelters offer specific assessments of children's needs. This however, can only be seen in a comparative framework. What is left after what has been taken away is still a multiple of what is offered to street children.

When it comes to the education of homeless youth in the USA, the primary problem is not a lack of resources, but what is usually called government red tape. For example, while the McKinney-Vento Act of 1987 was helpful in enrolling homeless students who lack the required documentation, particularly the residency requirement, common problems still exist that prevent homeless youth from going to school. These include not having access to records from prior schools they attended, most importantly their medical and immunization records, or not having complete and up-to-date papers for their guardianship. Either one of these could be used by a school to bar homeless youth from attending. Nor does it help that teacher training does not focus directly on the unique needs of these children (Epstein 2000).

Kidd et al. (2007) studied 15 successful homeless youth workers in Toronto, Canada and found that they felt hemmed in by programs, because they said they were not flexible, or because they were forced to follow a pre-packaged curriculum or because the programs demanded religious affiliation. The youth workers who were successful were able to develop a plan based on two assumptions: that homeless youth could succeed and that success required a meaningful relationship with a single runaway youth. The fact that this is not a cost-effective effort has some bearing on programs for street children.

The skills the youth workers developed were not the result of the programs they were working in, only through time on the job did they learn how to work with homeless youth. What they learned among other things was how to work around the rules and develop their own counseling model, which (in addition to the two parts mentioned above) empathized with the situation of the youth including their reasons for leaving home. The successful youth workers allowed the youth to make mistakes without being lectured to and showed that failure did not hurt his or her relationship to their youth worker. This helped homeless youth to learn by modeling legitimate power and benign authority. When they did this, they were able to accept authority without becoming self destructive.

Peer relationships are an essential element of life for homeless youth as they are for street children. They are the main strategy for survival that allows homeless youth to come into adulthood (Paradise and Cauce 2002). Through a system of sharing they learn to improve their self-esteem and separate themselves from the problems of their families of origin (Schaffner 1999). Yet, the social service system moves homeless youth around without taking into account or respecting this aspect of their needs (Bao et al. 2000).

Similar to peer support is the importance of siblings. Given the trouble of family life, siblings either support each other by acting as buffers to their parents, or they turn against each other, as a way of taking out their anger. In one study sibling relationships among homeless youth went from love to hate, from being uninvolved to very protective, but more often than not in the long run they supported each other (Schaffner 1999). Older siblings felt guilty when they ran away because it meant abandoning their younger siblings at home in such bad situations.

Children in street situations have many coping mechanisms including peer support, help from siblings, an ability to make quick decisions, flexibility in dealing with problems, and an unusually developed sensitivity to adults. These unique strengths must be taken into account in educating and serving them.

Davies (2008), working in Western Kenya, found that street children in groups were in effect in an apprenticeship for the economic circumstances of urban poverty, which is entirely small scale and entrepreneurial, and where, if need be, the line between legal and illegal can be shifted a bit. Specifically, he mentioned informal jobs, and making contact with business people who can service them as middle men. Among his group of street children, he found little begging or stealing, which was frowned upon by their peers. Nor was there much scavenging, finding food that was only partially eaten. In this way, they were different than other children on the streets. Importantly, he notes that if street children were to list what they wanted from programs, and that might include better food and shelter and school, it would not include dropping their peers.

Krabanow (2003) suggests that in order for programs for homeless youth to be successful a well-rounded effort is necessary. First, he suggests providing food, shelter, and clothes. The next step is advocating for the children in the community and providing alternatives to street life. He points out the advantages of starting with the basic necessities. Toronto's Covenant House provides immediate help for basic necessities. Casa Alianza in Guatemala works in a very similar fashion. These programs allow children in street situations to see themselves as human beings worthy of the basic necessities and to know there are caring adults who will help them eat and provide for their medical needs. After time, this approach allows children to feel that they have a reliable benefactor and as word gets out and many homeless youth gather to access the services, a sense of community develops. Dans la Rue (in the street), provides essential services, but they do not have much in the way of structural costs, as they operate out of a mobile unit, carrying food, some medical supplies and hygienic materials.

Teaching skills can lead to employment, imagination and some business acumen. Street Kids International in Toronto for example, built up an educational system that was able to place some youth as couriers riding bicycles carrying documents or notes from one place to another (Fig. 5.1). A Child's Place is a nonprofit community-based program in Charlotte, North Carolina that provides many services to homeless children and their families (Yon and Mickelson 2000). It serves children from preschool to six years of age by locating and bringing them into the program, providing education and helping their families by setting up a variety of social service programs. While the results of this program are clear, since 1989 when it started, hundreds of children's lives have been improved; they have not been able to make a dent in changing the conditions that underlie homelessness in the USA or in the developed world, let alone in the developing world. Like almost all programs, A Child's Place does not directly address the underlying issues of abuse, an approach that could raise the tide sufficiently to allow all boats to float.

Fig. 5.1 Teaching skills

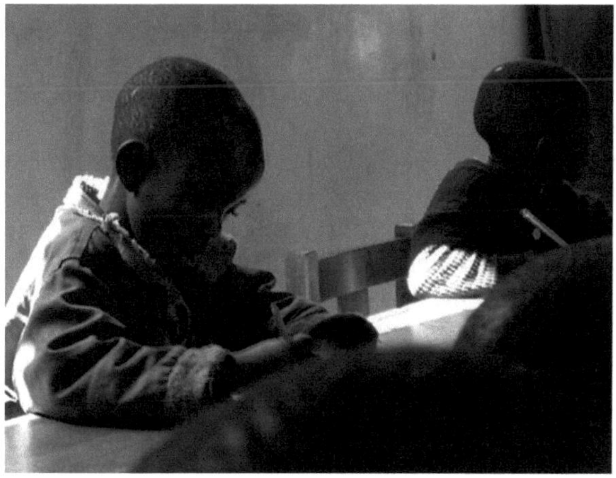

Epstein (1996), analyses how state and non-governmental organizations respond to homelessness of youth and children in Brazil and the USA (the developing and developed worlds). This cross-cultural comparison is used to understand the relationship between homeless youth and street children and the global neo-liberal economy. He takes as a starting point the conflict between homelessness and the State's stated aim of social and political inclusiveness; or otherwise stated the conflict between the morality and the reality of taking care of the basic needs of its citizens.

Epstein (1996) argues that street children and homeless youth are so different than what the State assumes is a proper way for children to live that when the State tries to educate these children it is clear that the value of the State toward these children is pejorative. The next step of the argument moves toward a critique of whether or not the State can reform its existing programs to include the special needs of street children and homeless youth.

One of the values of this article is to reflect on what characteristics are unique to homeless youth and street children. First, the author says is the fact that living in full public view means that the children's poverty is no longer private and their status as victims is always available to the public's eye. Secondly, because of the immediate necessity of life on the streets, planning for the future is limited, if not non-existent. Thirdly there is a reduction of personal space so the parts of life that were private become public (staying clean, eating, talking to others, etc.). Finally there is not only a reduction in personal belongings, there is not even a sense of being able to protect what few possessions they have left. The same can be said of one's social connections, they too change dramatically. What this means is that the lives of homeless youth and street children challenge the ability of the State to take care of its duty to a socially and economically diverse citizenry. But it is more than this. Together these features raise important issues concerning the workings of the State and its ability to protect those who benefit from social inequality. They can only do this by masking the coercive policies toward children in street situations.

When the children in street situations go to school, they often fail academically, and among the reasons they feel are the cause of their failure are being abandoned or poor, or socially unacceptable, or being homeless. They are embarrassed and made to feel embarrassed by their peers, even by those who try to help them, if for no other reason than accepting help is to accept the low status that necessitates the help in the first place.

The State has its challenges as well. While its representatives try to help, what they can do is limited because political and economic factors always keep them from making the deep changes that would deal with the causes. The author argues that as long as some people are impoverished others can benefit from their cheap labor and the need to purchase at least the basics of human life, if not of dignity.

Epstein points out that real solutions, such as affordable housing, reducing unemployment, raising the minimum wage, etc. cannot occur because they would cost too much and cause negative responses to the current beneficiaries of the market economy, because wages would go up and then housing costs and taxes would increase.

Epstein (1996) criticizes the McKinney Act of 1987, which gives some benefits to homeless youth in America, such as transportation costs that allow children to go to school but does nothing to reduce the systemic problems that led to being homeless in the first place. Nor do excessive degrees of fear about safety and order in shelters that lead to such a harsh climate of authority in the shelters for children.

Finally, he argues that programs for homeless youth do not consider the skills they have learned from being homeless which include valuing the current, understanding the self interests of authority and the values of living without many physical extras. Instead of using these skills the educational program demands the children adjust to their existing curriculum. There is also an accepted school philosophy that rewards individual success through competition based on accepted standardized criteria. There is little value given to the self-reliance skills than many homeless youth must learn to survive. He makes it clear that there are exceptions.

Epstein (1996) then turns his attention to comparing street children in the developing world with homeless youth in the developed world. The literature on homeless youth in the developed world, he says, has little to say about their resilience, while there is a body of research on street children that points to their resilience. The State in the developing world, (his example is Brazil) is not able to provide street children access to what the State's mandates say they should have; political and economic promise for all. This is why NGOs have evolved, and why most of the programs for street children have come from the non-governmental sector including churches (again using Brazil as an example). The State's educational approach in developing countries has been to teach vocational skills and practical academics.

There has been more flexibility in the non-governmental sector, even in some cases accepting how street life has changed the children and how these changes have contributed to having new skills. The flexibility, according to him is because programming has not been taken over by the government. He points out that NGO type organizations in the developed world have worked with and taken on the existing bureaucratic points of view.

As he talks about Brazil, he begins with its dismal history of having a very wide inequality of income distribution based on an extremely unprotected market place. Thus when street children threatened some small scale businesses by begging in front of their stores or begging from tourists, the children received an exaggerated violent response. While this violence was not directly from the State, it was clear that the State did not have the desire or power to oppose what the mercantile class wanted. As the violence escalated, the authority of the State was threatened.

Rather than continue with repressive measures, the State after some gruesome and well publicized violence against street children involving assassinations, established under the new civilian government, a permissive agenda to enforce children's rights.

Epstein (1996) shows that the Brazilian case is illustrative, and raises several important points about how the State and NGOs in developing countries can work together to meet the needs of street children. He points out two particular problems, the need to encourage and protect the grass roots approach and the threat of being taken over the more powerful State institutions. He believes that the most important goal of NGOs in developing countries is not just to increase the economic power of the poor, but to lead them into having more democratic power.

He has shown that in the developed world, homeless youth threaten the sacrosanct notion of equal access to public institutions. This is why, he claims, educational programs for them do not readily admit their skills or adjust their programs to them. Instead of receiving special programming, they become part of the larger and multi-dimensional group of "children at risk" that only stigmatizes them.

For him street children who are educated in the developing world have another type of problem, which is that they remain among the marginalized no matter what education they receive. Even if the curriculum is aimed at working with the skills that street children have developed as a result of street life, it is dismissed by authorities as less academic and valuable. What he wants to see happen in the developing world is not just educational reform but justice for the violence and other human rights abuses street children face.

In the end, the lesson to be learned from programs for homeless youth and street children is how the State and its citizenry can and might work toward social justice for all marginalized groups. He believes these are the lessons that can be learned in the developed and developing world.

Plummer and Wambui (2009) interviewed professional social service workers from different tribes in Kenya to ascertain the risk and protective factors related to sexual abuse of children. While there were many similarities there were also different opinions among tribal cultures. The endorsement of FGM (Female Genital Mutilation, or Female Genital Cutting) was seen as a risk factor among several tribes, but it was considered valuable and was still practiced as a rite of passage in some others.

The authors warn against accepting programs based on Western culture without taking into account cultural differences within Kenyan society and by inference other African communities. In fact, they want the term "community" to be more clearly defined within a cultural context. In contrast to the West, where community might mean something like neighborhood (a place where people live in close proximity, where their children go to school, and has common places for recreational and social events), community in the African context has more to do with kinship and tribal affiliation. There are also considerable differences among collectivistic and individual cultures, the level of acculturation to Western culture, and the degree of patriarchy, types of child rearing, etc. among tribes. While there were some similarities among the different communities, this study showed many disagreements about the causes of sexual abuse. Some of the professional workers lauded traditional culture as a preventive factor, while others blames traditional culture, citing it is a risk factor for sexual abuse.

Analysis of Programs from the Micro to the Macro Level

Programs are inevitably embedded in multilevel interdependencies, that we may situate at micro, meso and macro levels. The way a problem is publicly defined is here of major importance. We can be inspired by the way Knoepfel et al. (2007) make a distinction between target groups (those who cause the problem) and final beneficiaries (those who experience the negative effects of the problem). Public policies, including programs that the State subsidizes to the private sector, are very much framed by how this distinction is made. In other words, when a social problem becomes a public problem, it is because some powerful actors have the means to frame or define the problem in a particular way. Children in street situations are mostly excluded from this definition: they are framed, not framing. And, most of the time, those who frame the problem make a confusion between target groups and final beneficiaries. When this confusion is made, programs "target" street children and consider them as the beneficiaries of their interventions. And they are consequently trapped into a needs-based intervention. Because treating children as objects to be changed before they would have a place in the program, and hence in "society", is typical of this confusion between target groups and final beneficiaries. Being at the same time target and beneficiary, the child is in a double-bind relationship: the child is asked to change before the situation can change. This is why needs-based programs are bound to fail: they offer help only if those who are helped accept the dominant definition of the problem, which is impossible for them as this acceptance would negate their own perspectives and recognition of their competences. The double-bind lies in the contradictory expectations: submission and (before) liberation. It is as if the child would be told "you can become what I want you to become" or "you are free to choose my wishes".

The authors we will refer to in this section make different classifications of programs, according to their appraisal of their aims and qualities. We think that these classifications make sense only once the overarching question of "who defines the problem" has been addressed. For instance, de Benitez (2011) has developed a system of classification of programs for children in street situations into three categories: 1.) the correctional, reactive or repression-oriented model, whereby children in

Table 5.1 Classification of levels of interventions

Policy approach	Conceptualization of street children	Abstraction	Target levels
Repression	Deviants	Public order	Children in street situations (micro level)
Protection	Victims	Authentic child	Dysfunctional Families and communities (meso level)
Rights-based	Citizens	Child rights	State, historical and economic factors (macro level)

street situations are seen as deviants; 2.) the rehabilitative or protection-oriented model, seeing children in street situations as victims; and 3.) the human rights-based approach which considers children in street situations as citizens whose rights have been violated.

This approach however always depends on whether one defines children in street situations as deviants, victims or citizens. In the first case, they are seen as threats or potential threats to the public order. Defining them as victims is done by emphasizing the deficient conditions of street life. And the rights-based approach sees them as citizens who are discriminated against and whose access to rights as children is denied or unsecured by society. Measured against an ideal child, the programs try to cure the adverse factors: the public order threatened by children; the authentic and powerless child, threatened by street life; and the rights of the child, threatened by social discrimination. In other words, the target groups, those who are the groups that cause the problem, are different in each approach. For the repressive approach, those causing the problem are the children themselves. For protective approach, the target groups are all those who cause the departure to the street such as poverty, the dysfunctional family, abusive adults, gangs, drug dealers, exploiters, etc. For the rights-based approach, the target group is the State, which has ratified the UNCRC and therefore bears the responsibility to see to it that all rights are made accessible to all children. This approach ties the mirco, meso and macro levels together.

Programs can be aimed at working with all or some of the three levels, namely the target groups that cause the problem (families, neighbourhoods, gangs, etc.), the recipients who experience the negative effects of the problem (children in street situations), and the political-administrative authorities who develop and implement a given policy (the State). The following table based on de Benitez (2011) is helpful in seeing what we mean by working with children in street situations at all three levels (Table 5.1).

At the macro level the State, as a result of public policies and historical factors, is responsible for children in street situations. The policy questions at the macro level become: How is access to rights distributed in the population? What are the obstacles faced by children in street situations with regard to the accessibility of rights? These are questions that are challenging the State and their answers will have much more influence than protective and repressive programmes that live or die on the numbers of children rescued or kept away from street life. Addressing the causal factors raises questions around the unequal distribution of wealth. In this approach, then, the best practices are the ones linked to efforts directed towards the questions of social justice and equality. Some rights-based programs go as far as to advocate redistributing economical resources for the optimal well-being of all.[2]

Needs-Based Personal Aid Model

Under the needs-based aid model, projects for children in street situations "rescue" them from the streets. They are based on the perception that children need to be saved. Typically, in this model, street children are met by street educators: young adults, men and woman, sometimes former street children, who go to the streets to make a deal with the street kids, suggesting that if they join they will get some pretty handsome benefits (Fig. 5.2). If the street children take the bait, they begin their participation in a step-by-step model that often involves giving up street life for increasing programmatic rewards, which starts with going into the drop-in center, sometimes called a storefront where they might receive some food, cold showers, and minor medical care, and which could lead if they stick to their part of the bargain to shelter and vocational and educational opportunities. Note that in programs for homeless youth, these rewards are usually given without the child having to do anything.

Most children enter these programs without a heartfelt desire to change their ways; they see their commitment to the program as just another way of earning a living. While the program offers some of what the children need, it takes away from their work time and if it does not provide shelter, it leaves children, at the end of the day, to fend for themselves.

Conticini (2008) examined Needs-Based Programs for street children in Bangladesh and Ethiopia Subsequently, Conticini and Hulme (2007) asked why children left home. They argued that without knowing this, it would be difficult to establish a needs-based program to help them. They knew that in Bangladesh, as in many developing countries around the world, there was a tendency for policy makers and professionals to believe that street children left home because there was no money at home. Their choice was based on economic factors. Yet, they point out that there were a great number of empirical studies which suggest that it is not poverty per se, but the relationship between the family and the child that was most salient. In particular, they believed that violence was what caused children to leave home and go to the streets. Their work was devised to examine this question. For policy makers to be successful at reducing the numbers of street children, they would have to prioritize policy that was directed at reducing the excessive control and consequent emotional, physical and sexual violence that was occurring at home. While they acknowledged

[2] Schumacher (2011) deplores that it was not possible to find any published best practices or similar reports about programmes concerning children in street situations in South Africa.

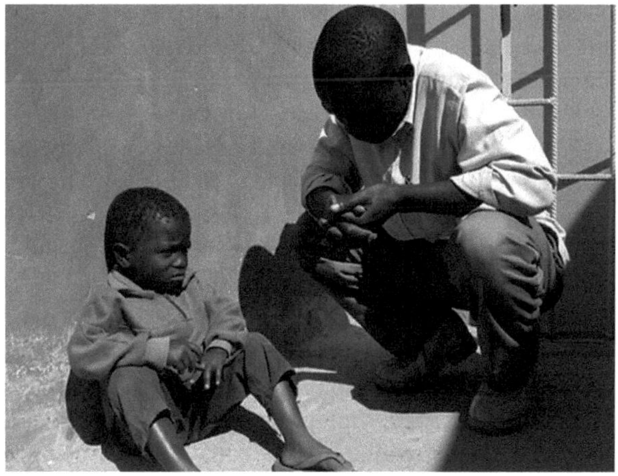

Fig. 5.2 Needs-based at a personal level

that economic growth and the reduction of poverty would be helpful, they argue that it would not be sufficient. They refer to a 16 year old boy in their study who said it was not poverty that led him to leave home. He left because his parents were violent and continually telling him that he was not a good person. Yet, he told potential benefactors he left because of poverty so they would give him money.

There are about a half million children living on the streets in Bangladesh, but nearly a billion who suffer from poverty. What the authors set out to prove was that these children are not just on the streets because they are poor. They argued that in Bangladesh children move to the street not simply because of economic factors as is commonly assumed. Rather, they say it is because their human rights are abused. At home there is violence and in the streets there is camaraderie.

While UNICEF (2000) argues for poverty reduction, Conticini and Hulme (2007) argue that improved economic conditions will only supply a limited amount of help. They point to several studies which suggest it is non-economic factors that explain why street children leave home. They also point out that being on the streets is not just about having come from abusive homes, it is also about the empowerment they get from having left and the support they find once on the streets. As they say, making the choice to leave is a tribute to their personal agency and if examined closely can illustrate how they cope with their circumstances.

Their study began with field research in Dhaka from August 2002 to July 2003. They followed 93 children in street situations of which 62 were boys and 31 were girls. They estimated that the ages ranged from 4 to 18 years old. They found that most of their subjects were not involved with programs run by NGOs, although two-thirds of them had been previously.

In addition to participant observation, their methodology included techniques in which the children acted out certain roles and scripts, followed by group discussions. In some cases followed by in-depth interviews. They also had 8 boys and 8 girls from their sample who served as advisors to them about how their research was going. They administered, at the end of their data collection, semi-structured questionnaires to triangulate the qualitative data. The authors define a child in a street situation as a child who provided his or her own daily basic needs without the support of their parents or guardians. They also included in the definition that a street child was actively involved in finding his or her own caregivers.

They started out with several assumptions, which they mention and therefore help the reader accept their results in spite of what might have been a bias. They argue that if family income or poverty were the motivating forces for migrating to the street, than they would have expected many more millions of children to be street children. They highlight that out of the total number of children living on the streets, only a small proportion of children were living below the poverty line in Bangladesh. Secondly, they note that not all street children in their study were from destitute households. In the study, the poverty line was defined as the daily expenditure needed for a consumption of 2,100 calories per person per day. They defined the severe poverty line as the daily expenditure needed for a consumption of 1,950 calories per person per day. Vulnerable households were defined as those with a per-capita expenditure that was above the poverty line by no more than 30%.

The authors commented on the fact that many of the programs the children participated in gave them food. And, rather than returning to their families after eating their needed calories, they went back to the street. They found that once their basic survival was secured, many of these children chose to live on the street rather than return home. Finally the authors found that even though the children might report that economic reasons were why they left home; the truth seemed to be that as long as they were earning enough money while they were on the streets, they could in effect buy their independence from an abusive home.

Conticini and Hulme (2007) point out that there is an inherent economic bias in many studies, particularly those that used instruments that are not normed such as questionnaires and surveys. These instruments over-report economic causes as the main factor for leaving home. Many street children in these studies told the authors that they responded this way because they thought that was what the researcher wanted. They reported that many of their responses were chosen to make a positive impression on the people administering the protocols. In fact, it was a lot easier than actually having to answer more honestly. Even with a close relationship between street children and the test giver, the bias is not easily eliminated. It might be argued that the closer the relationship, the more likely the street children know what the test giver wants and the more likely they are to provide those answers.

It is to the authors' credit to contextualize their data by pointing out that corporal punishment and violence against children are widespread in Bangladesh and are rarely considered wrong by parents, children or society. Thus, when the child leaves home because of violence they should not expect support from adult society. In fact, the more the child uses this as the reason for leaving home, the more likely they are to be lectured to by adults who are likely to say that submission is the proper behavior. Even professional social workers or police working with children are likely to see this child as a child who needs another beating.

Some street children complained to the authors in a very telling narrative that their mothers and fathers and the other adults who were involved in their child rearing all told them that they should stay home in spite of being beaten because at home they have something to eat, a place to sleep and their school fees paid for. Incredibly, the street children asked the researchers why they didn't also ask about love from parents. In contrast to the adults, a child living in the streets had very little social capital. Adults could rely on their neighbors, especially in a crisis, and they could rely on the fact that they were not breaking the laws, nor violating community mores. When the children left home, they went directly into a group to hang out where they found empathy with their problems associated with physical abuse. Their peers were saying we support your right to live another way. Only when the community mores change will the violence at home change.

When the authors talked to the children about how they viewed the violence they were receiving at home, and if it warranted their leaving home, the children carefully distinguished violence that they thought was illegitimate and punishment based on their idea of justice. They said that fair punishment was when they were misbehaving, but unfair punishment was violence when an adult abused them for reasons having nothing to do with behavior. This was why only some children who were being physically beaten were leaving home. The ones who stayed thought the punishment they were getting was just. But if the children thought there was no reason for the abuse, they began to distrust the punisher. They viewed them less and less as worthy of taking care of them. At some point the child had had enough and left to join his or her peers. The authors said that as hard as it was to receive physical punishment, even sexual abuse from their parents, if the children felt it was part of what they saw as justice for their misbehavior they could endure it. What they could not endure was what they considered unjust punishment and the more they were punished the more their relationships to their parents or guardians broke down.

What often followed after a child left home because of unjust violence, was a lowering of the threshold for any violence. The result was that family ties were severed to an even greater degree. Just as this is a process of growth, so too was leaving home. In this case, most children said it was not a particular heinous event, but a process that finally reached its climax.

Yet the children knew that the streets were not free of violence. So how they did decide to leave one place of violence for another? It was not the intensity or the frequency of the violence that was the issue, it was the identity of perpetrator and the respect or lack of it the child had for the perpetrator. On the streets the child is not likely to know the perpetrator and thus the violence is less charged; there is no trust that is broken. At home it is not the physical pain but the feelings that hurt. By the time the children had gained some street experience, there was almost no trust of their parents remaining.

Seventy-eight out of the 80 kids in their sample were either physically abused or sexually abused, or both, the year they left home for the streets. They were abused by parents, step-parents, relatives and neighbors. What was even worse, many adults who should have protected them did not.

The authors say that the idea that reducing poverty will help children from going to the streets is unlikely to be successful. Instead they want policies to focus on reducing abuse and violence. They note that in the case of Bangladesh (and in our opinion in many other countries) this will be difficult because society will have to accept a very different form of child rearing.

In an analysis of programs in Mexico, Magazine (2003) found that programs which began with the philosophy of helping street children become functional members of society often backfired because they treated them as objects to be changed. This was particularly manifest in programs that did not realize the importance of peers in the street children's lives. He found that most street children were in programs that did not have respect for their peer networks and their minds never changed about the disadvantage of home and the advantages of peers and the street. The needs-based aid model made the children give up what being on the streets offered them, which often meant their peer relationships, which are so germane to the children's well-being and enjoyment of life. The result is that many of the children who come to the needs-based programs are dubious from the onset. As time goes on, even the children who entered into what they thought was a good deal begin to challenge the "this for that" thinking, creating a feeling that the program and the child are working against each other.

In the needs-based model, the counselor's role is of a substitute adult family member. In demanding that children in street situations give up something before they can begin, they give the message that the children are pathogenic, which from the children's point of view is another rejection (often felt like a family rejection). By withholding shelter until the children perform to a certain level, the dynamics become highly charged reminders of their actual family life. It is difficult for street children to relive a similar untenable situation, comparable to the one they had left. There are similar feelings among homeless youth.

Ordonez (1994) describes a good example of a particularly well appointed needs-based program in Lima, Peru. The program provided shelter, nutritious food, new clothing, medical and psychological attention, education, but only if the children give up what they have used to cope in the streets, including peer support. (The street children found themselves getting peer pressure which made fun of the fact they were willing to give up so much.)

In this program, children lived in well provided quarters with a small number of street children and an adult supervisor. The rules of the house included what the program refers to as a democratic child-centered government that would include the children making decisions weekly on each house's problems and tasks. However well meaning, the rules do not really give the children a true voice in what is important to them, they can only vote on things that are either trivial (how many times each child has to take out the garbage) or already in place (attending the daily activities), which is already set and beyond the children's voice in changing. The notion that children need to be changed, without their participation in the how and why of the change is also characteristic of the needs-based aid model in the developed world.

Behaviors in many needs-based programs are regulated by a behavioral management plan (without input from the children) that uses a token system for access to privileges and usually also has sanctions. The behavioral plan operates on the premise that the children's character has to change, which would be best accomplished by eliminating through reinforcement and punishment the rewards of street life. The problem is that for many children in street situations, street life is their only way to strengthen their self-esteem and sense of achievement. The behavioral schemes also give little thought to the children's connections to family, community, culture, and other aspects of their environment that are meaningful to them.

The needs-based approach also raises serious questions about its long term viability. While it can offer remedial support to a minority of those in need, it does nothing to stop the flow of children becoming homeless. The needs-based aid model also favors the values of the State, and the State in return grants them money, which to some degree imbues them with the power of the State. Because the media portrays children in street situations as delinquent menaces, the State also can use the media to convince the populace that the needs-based option is more efficacious than other programs, particularly measures in which children have a real voice.

Scivoletto et al. (2011), working in the Department of Psychiatry at the University of Sao Paulo, Brazil found that among street children there were high levels of domestic violence, mental illness, and alienation from authorities. At that time, for street children to get services they had to have an appointment to go the hospital clinic, which was located far from the areas of Sao Paulo where they lived. The authors wanted to change this.

To assess how to proceed, psychiatrists interviewed some 60 street children. They found that many of the children knew what they needed. They wanted medical care, help with substance abuse, and help with their psychological problems. The children also said they did not want to leave the streets, go back to school, be placed in foster care, or perhaps most importantly be separated from their friends.

To address these problems, the authors developed The Equilibrium Project (Programa Equilíbrio, TEP). The basic doctrine of the project was to involve the street children in all aspects of their care. They went from a traditional professional clinic to a community-based center, sponsored by many psychosocial caregivers, medical service providers, and law enforcement agencies who offered a variety of services. The development of their current program was the result of continued input from street children and their families. The center has become the key place which professionals use as a conduit between the children and their families.

During each phase of the building of the program, street children were consulted and were allowed to provide input about which services to offer and how to offer them. In addition to this, the authors say that other essential features of TEP are the offering of bundled services in the community. To make the program more client-friendly they inserted recreational activities and included learning in basic communication skills by starting a child-led newspaper and radio program. One of the important (and interesting) components of the program is that they communicate directly with the children. They do not work through other NGOs, not even through child advocacy programs.

When they assessed the program they found that many of the adverse symptoms of mental health receded once the children were able to get into a safe place with a comprehensive program. The authors suggest that this proves that the children's hostility and mistrust were components of their coping strategies. Thus they suggest that before completing diagnostic reports they should give the children plenty of time to adjust to their new environment. They also suggest that it is better not to focus on their substance abuse problems without getting a global assessment of their family situations. Finally and importantly they found that the children who left the program did so because they did not want to be patients in a health center. By changing this perception, the center kept more long term clients.

In a cross-cultural study of a needs-based reinsertion program, (Harris et al. 2011) found in Peru and Brazil about half of street children were able to return to their homes. Their success rate was related to several demographic variables, including why and how the children were referred, how long the children stayed in the program, and the amount of education a child had before entering the program.

Finally, in a crosscultural comprehensive bibliographic study of non-formal education (NFE) methods for working with street children in developing countries, Shephard (2011) found that of the millions of street children, the vast majority were either not successful at school or not even in school. Schooling provides opportunities for street children to become empowered. Feeling empowered contributes to breaking the cycle where the sons and daughters of street children become street children themselves.

Shephard (2011) made an electronic search of 34 data bases. He ended up identifying 9,258 relevant titles. This review highlights the need to conduct rigorous effectiveness studies of NFE for street children and street youth in order to ensure that they are indeed effective.

His operational definition of NFE was any organized, structured, systematic learning that was outside of formal schooling. It also had to be cost and time effective. The curriculum had to be centered on the learner's needs. The NFE for street children provided basic skills up to the point of literacy and basic arithmetic. It has to include life-skills. It could be arranged so students could transfer into regular schooling.

He believes his study provides the most exhaustive information of NFE for street children in developing countries. Before presenting his results, he laments the lack of high quality research. The problems include, but are not limited to, the ethical and political challenges of creating a control group of disadvantaged street children who do not receive educational assistance. Therefore, while it appears that NFE is good for street children, say as opposed to providing funding for street children to attend regular school, it is not empirically proved. The people who are teaching street children or providing them with NFE should be very careful to monitor their work and have high standards for evaluations for both the good and the not so good of NFE.

Needs-Based Institutional Model

Another type of needs-based program takes children in street situations out of the city and places them into institutional care, where they sleep, eat, and are educated without being able to return to the streets (Fig. 5.3). They live in large dormitories with rules imposed upon them for almost every type of behavior (when to go to bed,

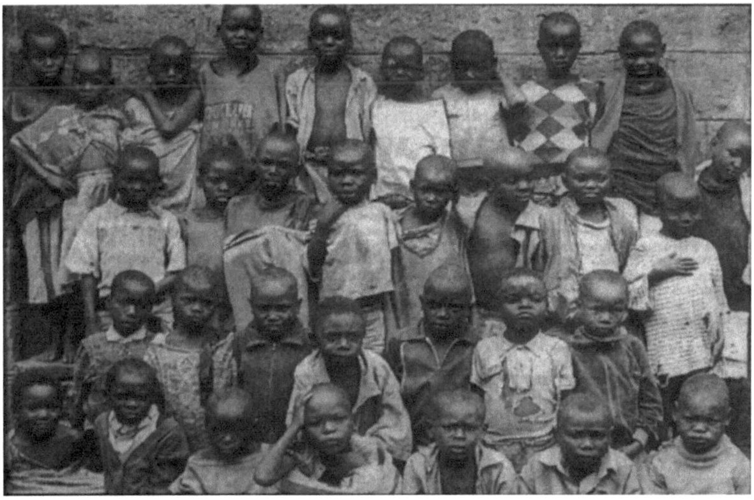

Fig. 5.3 Institutional model

how and when to clean their belongings, what they can say and not say, etc.). These programs like the other needs-based programs above have the final goal of making street children "productive members of society", but they don't. Mtonga (2011) noted that the one of the major reasons why street children in Zambia do not stay in the institutional programs that are designed to help them is that these programs infantilize them. On the streets they are earning money and spending it as they want, while in institutional programs they are forced into complete dependence. As Mtonga points out institutional programs take away their social agency, thus making the streets a socially healthier place for them, than the institutions. This is why Huang and Huang (2008) found that the success rate for institutional care programs for street children in La Paz, Bolivia were between 1% and 3%.

It is not surprising that the institutional model is disliked by children in street situations. Cheng (2006, 2008) conducted an ethnographic study of children near the Shanghai railway station and showed how badly the children perceived the government-run Protection and Education Centre for Street Children (the State's detention centre). Even though the centre provides food and lodging, the children prefer to keep away from it. Like anyone else they do not like to feel or be incarcerated. Nor do they like being under a bureaucracy that is so foreign to their street lives. They are also aware that the assumption behind institutional care is pejorative because it assumes they are deviant, or criminal, and thus in need of "rehabilitation". Fundamentally, because they are not on the streets, and are forced to give up their social networks, children in the centre are constantly thinking about escaping.

Institutions also undermine family and community care. Often people do not look at finiteness of giving, namely what giving does to other forms of care. For example, in institutions, the children might receive drug therapy, and individual or small group counselling, as is common for child delinquents in developed countries or for children in situations considered likely to be traumatic, such as armed conflict. While the expense and limited potential for expansion of this very professional-intensive approach is obvious, the obstacles it places in the path of developing more accessible, effective, efficient and culturally appropriate approaches is not. Two examples come to mind, the history of the community fostering of children and female-headed families linking together to help each other.

Other, but higher scale total immersion (institutional) programs are run by well funded international agencies, such as SOS Children's Villages, which is the world's largest charity dedicated to orphaned and abandoned children. In the SOS program in Swaziland, for example, the children were living in very well constructed small houses with 6 to 8 others and two adults mimicking a nuclear family situation. They were well fed, and clothed, and their medical attention was beyond what almost all Swazi children had. Their schooling is based on a European curriculum and they were taught by trained teachers in small classes. In some ways nothing bad should be said about this, but if nothing else, providing so much to so few does little to help with the problems facing street children in the aggregate.

Human Rights Model

The contemporary era of aid of the rights-based approach of assistance begins with the adoption of the UNCRC. Since the UNCRC was adopted, street children (and supposedly homeless youth) have been given a different role. They are no longer seen as pathological objects but as social actors who could and must have significant roles in their own aid-based programs. For example, the Child-to-Child program has a philosophy which includes an approach to learning and a set of activities promoting the active and responsible role of children in the improvement of their own health and well-being (and to their younger siblings and peers, and their family and community.) Since 1979, Child-to-Child programs run by Providing Education and Empowering Youth (PEEY) have worked in 80 countries, both in the developing and developed world.

The first step in the Child-to-Child program is for the children to understand what the organization is trying to do; they are told that they will be involved in activities that include reading, writing, discussions, and role playing about the lives of children in street situations like themselves. They will have members from the community who will listen to them tell their stories, and be told that they can ask them questions and initiate discussions with them.

The second step for the children is entering the local community to gather information about other children in street situations: such as who they are, why they are on the streets, how is their psychosocial health, etc. They do this by conducting a survey, observing, and having discussions with other children in street situations and with key community members. Then they carry out a needs analysis by identifying the key problems of children in street situations in the community.

At the third step, children bring the information they have gathered back to the Child-to-Child program where they discuss the issues as they affect them, their families and their community. The adult facilitator working with the children helps them look at the information they have gathered with respect, but not without asking critical questions. They discuss ways in which they might be able to address these problems. When they are finished the facilitator helps the children design solutions that are manageable, and helps them communicate their plans clearly and accurately to others.

At the fourth step, children take action at school and in their families and communities. They may be communicating information to others, demonstrating skills to others, working with other children or leading by example. Step five is about helping the children evaluate the effects of their work on others and on themselves and identifying if there are ways they can improve their ideas. Step six is the revision, which gives them a chance to make messages clearer, to reach other people more effectively and generally to improve upon what has gone before so that desirable changes made as a result of the project become permanent. It is also the step at which new ideas for new issues to explore further become apparent.

Another example of the Human Rights Model is Street Kids International (SKI), which is based in Canada, and offers a wide range of services for homeless youth and street children. Since there is only a small group of adults at the head office, the work depends on its success in using children in street situations in all aspects of their work, including research and dissemination (Sauve 2003).

By rejecting the needs-based paradigm of adults telling the youth what to do, SKI affirms that children are not objects to be changed, but social actors with active minds, dreams, desires, and particular visions and possible initiatives. According to SKI, while the children may not have the same scientific knowledge base as the adults, the children's unique intellectual skills are valuable and worthy of a true partnership.

By politically empowering children in street situations, SKI promotes their legal rights, including the right to earn a livelihood, because without access to their own money, they cannot get proper health care, food and shelter. They encourage the use of micro-credit, even though this is in contrast to many in the international culture of the NGOs who do not see children in street situations as fiscally responsible.

Yunus (1999), a pioneer of micro-credit, gives loans of small amounts of money for up to a year's time to the poorest 20% of the population, a group which includes children in street situations. Repayment begins one week after the loan originates, and the interest rate is 20%. Borrowers are in groups of five, if one defaults they all do, thus they can help each other from defaulting. This model fits the peer groups of children in street situations, who have a strong connection to one another. Yunus gives very little training and does not like training programs, because he believes that the poorest of the poor do not need to be trained, they are already entrepreneurs. They do not lack skills, they need capital. This is similar to many children in street situations.

Having said all that is good about micro-credit schemes, there are also criticisms that need to be addressed. Most micro-loans go to single parent female headed households, which won't include children in street situations. In the typical example, a woman takes a loan to produce and sell some item, but what happens is that the children do the selling, which in fact prohibits them from going to school according to Nieuwenhuys (1994, 2001) in Addis Ababa, and Wydick (1999) in Guatemala.

Ferguson (2007) runs a program for homeless youth in the Los Angeles area. Her model is called Social Enterprise Intervention. She feels that the needs-based approach provides the basic needs of homeless youth (and street children) but it does not do much to address their mental health needs. Likewise she had rejected the micro-credit approach, because it does not help low income women escape poverty.

From these criticisms she built Social Enterprise Intervention which she sees as a preventive program that offers homeless youth vocational training and small business skills which include building human capital from a clinical mentor trained by them. The mentor, in addition to providing direct mental health care, also helps the youth find other services which would not, given their low status, be available to them without the help of a middle class professional mentor. Covenant House and Casa Alianza are working with her to incorporate the model.

In addition to her work in Los Angeles with Social Enterprise Intervention she had done a comparative study of three faith-based programs: for homeless youth in Los Angeles in which they say there is separation of State and religion; for street children in Nairobi where the authors feel there is an integrated faith-based State; and a program in Mumbai where the State, according to the author is secular (Ferguson et al. 2013). The authors note the differences. In Los Angeles for example, homeless youth were not able to be financially independent and became icons for parental and societal failure. While in Mumbai children on the streets were earning a living and living with families. They are not viewed as failures but are seen as productive family members. In Nairobi, because of the AIDS epidemic many street children are orphaned, and in some cases heads of households.

What is interesting is that when the faith-based programs were evaluated, all three had positive outcomes. All three reported they were able to help out with basic necessities, simple health care, and some education and vocational training. While the authors do not believe there is a single model that is cross-culturally effective (in fact, quite the opposite), they do see that goals and in some sense outcomes are similar.

In addition to using micro-credit for financial independence, Street Kids International (SKI) in Canada promotes children's civil rights and works toward reducing the numbers of future children in street situations. SKI understands that the advancement of rights for children in street situations will not come in a vacuum, so they began working with local agencies of government, the police, and other community leaders to train them on understanding how traditional values toward children in street situations and the consequent programs they have had, work to keep the children down. They encourage seeing children in street situations in a more positive way, which would help both the children and the community.

The pedagogy of SKI is that of storytelling with children in street situations as the protagonists, the makers of the fictional narrative and the tellers (and actors) of the story. When they are acted out or shown in videos, it helps both the children and their potential benefactors talk more easily about the lives of the protagonists. By discussing the story or video, as one would in a literature class, the stories can be seen in all the human dimensions that go into a character's life and behaviors. One goal of this method is to teach the public about street children, according to how the children want to represent themselves.

In addition to working on the public's attitude toward children in street situations, SKI's goal is to build the children's abilities to make up their own minds and become fully functioning citizens. This, as we saw, is similar to the goals of the needs-based aid model. But SKI goes about it much differently, particularly in regard to the youth's participation. By following the SKI program, children in street situations can become members of the civil politic able to think critically, understand different possibilities, and be flexible in getting their goals met.

Positions on the role of the child in the Human Rights Model can be divided into four categories; Paternalism, Welfare, Emancipation and Liberation (Hanson 2012). Paternalism regards children not in their own right, but with regards to what they will become as adults.[3] The child is "incompetent" and protection is the main need of children. There is a clear divide between children and adults. Paternalism advocates for children as a category of people deserving special protection. The paternalistic essence is that programs adopt the idea that the child has almost no agency in absolute terms, regardless of the context, of age, and of culture, etc. Thus childhood exists as a category with specific and naturally shaped competencies that all children share (Esser 2004; Stoecklin 2009a, b).

On the other side of the spectrum are the Liberationists who consider children as beings with a presumption of competence and therefore with equal rights to those of adults. Liberationists emphasize the right of children to self-determination (Hunt 1994). Thus they consider children to be independent citizens (beings) who are competent to make rational decisions (Hanson 2012). Liberationists advocate for equal rights, like the right of children to work (Liebel 1997), the political rights of children (Franklin 1986), claiming against the paternalists that special rights on the basis of children's vulnerability or other ideologically constructed notions of incompetence, leads to a *de facto* discrimination against children.

In their perspective, the participation rights accorded by the UNCRC means shifting the burden of proof to adults who would have to systematically demonstrate that the child is not competent to justify their decision of not considering the child's view. For the Liberationists, participation rights supersede protection rights (Archard 2004).

In the middle of the spectrum is the Welfare approach. This position carries a more nuanced position than Paternalists and Liberationists. It tries to set the balance between the two extremes, with a preference for protection rights but combined to include participation rights. For example, they consider that treating children

[3] As Verhellen (2000) says in this perspective children are considered as "*not yet being*".

equally as adults does not recognize children's special needs. This approach is largely dominating today's sector of child welfare, at national and international levels, including leading organizations such as UNICEF (Hanson 2012). The balance between special and equal rights goes more in the direction of guaranteeing adequate response to children's special needs. The child is considered incompetent, unless one proves the contrary.

Emancipation is a perspective which uses similar nuances as the Welfare approach, but this time the balance is more directed towards autonomy, participation rights and equal rights. The child is considered competent, and the burden of proof otherwise lies with the adult who is obliged to listen to the child and to take his or her opinion seriously unless it can be shown that the child does not have sufficient maturity in the matter at hand. In this perspective, children are seen as being competent in certain matters and becoming competent in others in a progressive way. Programs in this perspective start with the importance of participation rights that help to best implement protection rights (Verhellen 2000; de Langen 1992). They consider children not as passive objects of intervention but as bearers of rights.

The legacies of the different models have diversely impacted today's debate on the implementation of the UNCRC and programs for children in street situations. The majority of researchers and programs lie between the two middle approaches of Welfare and Emancipation, leaving the two extremes as minorities (Paternalism and Liberation).[4]

Problems with the Human Rights-Based Approach

While Child-to-Child and SKI provide positive approaches to working with the human rights model proposed by the UNCRC, Nieuwenhuys (1994, 2001) who studied street girls in Addis Ababa, showed that there are some dilemmas that the UNCRC poses for girls and their families. While it is good that the UNCRC and the NGOs working under its auspices have reduced or dropped charitable needs-based approaches to helping street children and replaced them with programs focusing on children learning their human rights, it might not be so easy for children in street situations to go from charity to self-support.

She argues that the human rights approach of the UNCRC as it is being played out in an Ethiopian program she studied, and by inference in other programs, in essence forces street girls into accepting self-exploitation. This is because, she argues, that at the same time the UNCRC is bringing human rights advances, the new

[4]As in any debate, the differences began with a strong opposition towards traditional views, as it was in the *children's liberation movement*, also called *kiddie libbers*, which in the 1970's attacked the long-standing and dominant paternalistic approach to children (which led toward needs-based humanitarian programs). Another example is the strict interpretation of the caveats of children's right to participate (Gross and Gross 1977).

liberalization in the world economy is withdrawing basic social services, so whatever small resources from the State these children had are no longer available, forcing them into the market to earn the small amounts of money they were previously getting for lunch.

She describes one of the program's goals, which was to ask street girls to pay a modest amount for a lunch so they wouldn't become dependent. The hope was that once they learned to do this they would promote the same thing among their peers. In the past, lunch was free. So when they started the new program, the girls said their parents had no money for them, and this new policy was forcing them into the street. They said they preferred to go hungry than to beg for the money to pay for lunch. Imagine this on a broader scale by substituting lunch with a host of free services provided to homeless youth and you have a comparable situation in the developed world.

As can be seen in the above example, there are cultural problems that have to be considered when working through a rights-based approach. For example, one problem is the difficulty of how international law plays out in different cultures. In the Ethiopian case, the program's policy was to help only one person per family, and that recipient had to go to school. While there were good intentions on the part of the people responsible for the program, the rules came from far away and the organizers were not aware of how their rules would affect these girls who went to school and ate special lunches. The girls felt isolated and guilty at home, because they were the only family member to have an assured meal, while other family members had to fend for themselves in a very difficult open market. The author tells the story of one young girl who was being supported to attend high school, but her grandmother had to beg for food. The girl had to leave home because she couldn't stand seeing her grandmother beg while she was eating free food; in fact she preferred contributing to her family, even if it meant prostituting herself. Furthermore, it was local custom that parents disciplined their children by withholding food. This meant that while girls were in the program, the parents could no longer parent according to tradition. Also, in some cases, the largess that the girls received from the program gave them a step up on their families and they refused to be disciplined at home. Some eventually preferred going to the streets to enjoy their new-found freedom.

So it turned out that this program was rights-based on paper but not in reality, because the best interest of the child article of the UNCRC states that children must be a major consideration but not necessarily the major consideration. The interests of other people defined by the local culture (here the parents and grandmother) must also be taken into account. Actually, many programs claim that they are rights-based while they do not take into account this more subtle point of the UNCRC.

Some programs see handouts as problematic because they makes street life bearable. And because handouts are not sustainable they creates dependency. Should there be a free lunch? In Ethiopia it didn't work because of poverty and culture. Some people say there is no need to worry about creating dependence, while others in favour of the lunch program just want children to get enough nutrition to participate in life.

We should add that while it might be easy to enforce laws related to children who are physically abused, sexually exploited, made to be soldiers, etc. it is harder to enforce more subtle yet important rights like what the UNCRC calls "participation rights". These are the right to be heard (article 12), the right to freedom of expression (article 13), the right to freedom of thought, conscience and religion (article 14), the right to freedom of association and peaceful assembly (article 15), the right to privacy (article 16), the right to have access to information (article 17), and the right to participate freely in cultural life and the arts (article 31). They are difficult to enforce in part because they can work only when children's agency is acknowledged (Freeman 2007).

There are troubling yet culturally acceptable child rearing practices. For example, how do we apply the law to the case of child prostitutes in Thailand (Montgomery 2000)? According to article 4 of the UNCRC, it is the responsibility of the State to take all available measures to make sure their children's rights are respected, protected and fulfilled, and this includes funding of their social, legal, health and educational systems. But it still is a long way to make these normative claims integrated in people's code of conduct in situations where people don't have the necessary means to survive.

From our perspective (Montgomery 2000), these Thai children are not street children. They are neither abandoned nor abandoning. They are in touch and have good relationships with their mothers. Neither the children nor their parents feel they are doing something wrong, even though the children are being asking by their parents to engage in what the West believes is prostitution. As part of the Buddhist tradition, the children are told they are making "merit" for their parents, which both the parents and the children believe will lead toward negating the immorality of prostitution in the next life. Also, and importantly for our discussion, the children are giving their family what they need to keep them all together. Their parents don't see that allowing their children to be prostitutes is bad for their children; they see it as the only way to make enough money for the family to survive. Obviously, according to the UNCRC these parents do not have the right to have their children live this way. And we in the West are unlikely to change our attitudes.What is the role of well-to-do Westerners in enforcing laws or children's codes of conduct in situations where they and their families do not have the necessary means to survive?

Another problem for the UNCRC, as for any international treaty with a large scope based on principles, is its inability to adapt policies to quickly changing political realities. Take for example Haiti, where we showed how street children became pawns in a political struggle. At first, programs for them were orphanages and run by Christian clergy. One of these, Lafanmi Selavi (Family is Life), operated in accordance with former President Aristide's religious affiliation, which followed the theories of liberation theology, such as dignity in poverty, democracy and reconciliation. Lafanmi Selavi was teaching street children (at one point more than 190 boys and 160 girls) to find their political voice along the liberationists viewpoint.

When Aristide's government lost power the new government brought a violent end to the Lafanmi Selavi program. Then Aristide came back into power and Lafanmi Selavi reopened. It became even stronger, the children began a children's radio station which gave them a voice that met a wide public audience.

But politics changed, and with time the program was no longer politically advantageous for Aristide to support. Lafanmi Selavi fell into disrepair. The children did not get enough food nor health resources, and there were accusations of rape, and physical abuse. On Kovats-Bernat's (2006) last visit to Lafanmi Selavi he found it heavily guarded, the radio program barely broadcasting, and a security dog (supplied by the USA) discouraging anyone trying to come in or leave the compound.

Haiti illustrates how the realities of children's rights can change rapidly. First there was freedom. But when the second Aristide government came to power, it broke the law regarding children's rights of free speech and assembly. The mechanisms of the UNCRC could not respond rapidly. And it is not only in Haiti where the Children's Rights Movement has been a challenge to the authorities. As pointed out (Hanson 2012), the same has happened in other situations where children's rights run into political and ideological problems with entrenched power.

Another problem is that the UNCRC fudges on its own laws. Take the right for a child to be heard, which is considered the centrepiece for child participation:

> States Parties shall assure to the child who is capable of forming his or her own views the right to express those views freely in all matters affecting the child, the views of the child being given due weight in accordance with the age and maturity of the child (UNCRC 1989, article 12.1).

The fudging is that this leaves open the question of how we assess "*in accordance with the age and maturity of the child*" because there is no specific criteria to evaluate maturity. The rather large spectrum left open in the interpretation of this article obviously poses difficult questions.

Because of the ambiguity in many situations such as the ones we have presented above, we are left with a lot to be decided by the assessment of the decision-makers, who of course have their own constituencies. For example, the right to expression is usually only recognized if it is expressed in such a way that it is acceptable to the broad consensus. It is clear that many adults are simply not ready to hear voices of children. In fact we are sure that there are many more parents who adhere to the statement "*children should be seen and not heard*" than there are for its converse.[5]

There are significant differences between child participation in the developing world and in the developed world. In the developed world, there is an individualistic conception of participation; children are encouraged to participate in activities that allow them to acquire useful skills for their future lives as adults. In the developing world there is a collectivist conception of participation; child participation is seen as a social obligation to share the duties that contribute to the immediate well-being of the group.[6]

---

[5] This is also why, we said, street children tend to express themselves in a way that is socially acceptable when they want to gain some advantage. The adaptation skills of street children are very high. The challenge is to really hear what they have to say and not just listen to what they are saying.

[6] Mason and Bolzan (2010) have suggested that the developing world favours the liberationist argument because it values participation communally, even in situations that are difficult, such as children's right to work in dignity.

Programs from the Micro to the Macro Level

While all three human rights programs mentioned are providing services to children, they work less with families and local communities, and almost not at all with the larger factors of poverty and abuse which also impinge on the lives of children in street situations.

To see what this means, we can go back to four schools of thought in children's rights: paternalism, protection, emancipation, and liberation (Hanson 2012). Most programs as we have seen fall into the two first schools of thought or what we call the micro level; that is programs which offer direct support and services in street situations. We also see that programs should be involved at the meso level which involves families and local communities and thirdly at the macro level which includes the economic and political realities of the cultures where services are being provided.

As an example, we take South African extended families which are similar to many families in the developing world, where parents and children, grandparents, uncles and aunts, relatives by marriage, cousins, and even persons that are not related by blood are considered family, and often live closely together. Therefore, children are not necessarily brought up solely (if at all) by their biological parents (Schumacher 2011). In fact, the African extended family has elements of an effective welfare system, it supplies child care for working parents, it cares for the elderly, it feeds the unemployed and shelters the homeless, the disabled and mentally ill. By redistributing human and financial resources between the haves and the have-nots, the extended African family holds together the poorest of the poor.

But family structure is affected by macro-level events and there are historical, economic and political factors at the macro level that have changed family structure in ways critical to children in street situations. Perhaps, it is the legacy of Southern African Apartheid that shows how macro-level historical events have put children into the streets, although the situation can be extended to other places. The laws of Apartheid violated basic human rights for the vast majority of children who were denied access to a decent life, including adequate nutrition, housing, health services and education (UNICEF 2000).

With the first fully democratic elections in 1994, a new Constitution was adopted. All residents of South Africa became rights holders, including children. However, they all still didn't have the same opportunities: Poverty, HIV/AIDS, child-headed households, child labour and street children mostly found in rural areas and urban townships, were unduly affected by Apartheid (Schumacher 2011). Recipients of programs dedicated to the alleviation of factors contributing to children in street situations therefore were affected by macro-level factors including the lack of access to health care, education, nutrition, housing and other forms of social assistance. It wasn't enough for a program for children in street situations to be concerned only with direct care at the micro level.

This political legacy has made the challenge huge. There are about 20 million children under the age of 18 some 41% of the total population of nearly 49 million,

(Hall and Meintjes 2010). In 2008, nearly two-thirds of these 20 million children lived in households below the poverty level (Hall 2010). Extreme poverty touched almost two-thirds of households with black children, but only 4% of households with white children (UNICEF 2000). The richest 20% of the population earned 73% of the total income, while the poorest 20% received less than 2% (UNICEF 2000).[7] Also, some 28% of children are not registered and therefore are not entitled to claim social and legal services (Schumacher 2011). School fees, uniforms and materials make school enrolment and attendance difficult for non-registered children all over the world. As in many other places in the world, the political legacy, in this case of Apartheid (a macro factor), also affected children in street situations at the meso level (family and local community). Unemployment in South Africa is high but proportionally highest among black Africans (Statssa Quarterly Labour Force Survey 2010). The available jobs take the workers away from home, to diamond or gold mines or domestic work, making further demands on the extended family and the local community.

The well-known downward cycle by which poverty causes disease, which in turn reinforces poverty, is similar around the world (Benn and Weinreich 2003). In fact there are many macro-level health problems that impact families (meso-level). For example, in South Africa there is a very high HIV prevalence; an estimated 5.7 million people are infected, and there are 3.7 million AIDS orphans who lost one or both parents (UNICEF 2000). The HIV/AIDS pandemic stressed the extended family to an unprecedented level. While fostering orphans is a common cultural practice in nearly all African societies, the rapid rise in the number of orphans overwhelmed the traditional fostering system, simply because the loss of heads of households earning a living was so great at the same time that the number of orphans was increasing. Households became too poor to take in additional orphans. Inequality of access to health care, job opportunities and education also leads to limited accessibility of basic human rights due to the political and economic segregation that affects primarily the children of non-white communities. The social consequences of these political and economic legacies were made worse when the AIDS pandemic overwhelmed the fostering capacity of the extended family model.

In short, macro and meso factors, and not just micro situations, concern children in street situations. The best practices regarding intervention programmes are therefore bound to include human rights and address macro level factors. What happens is that because of the macro economic and political factors, meso factors in extended families change, leading to micro factors causing children to go to the streets. While the street is the place where these marginalized children become visible, it is also the place where intervention takes place, usually through the provision of basic necessities (the old needs-based aid model). But this is far from sufficient to reduce

[7] In 2006, about 10 million South African children lived in rural areas (Berry and Hall 2006) of which 2.3 million lived in shacks or backyard dwellings lacking the infrastructure of formal dwellings, without adequate housing or sanitation (Schumacher 2011). According to UNICEF (2000), more than half of all African children still use inadequate toilet facilities leading to a disproportionate number of cases of childhood diseases.

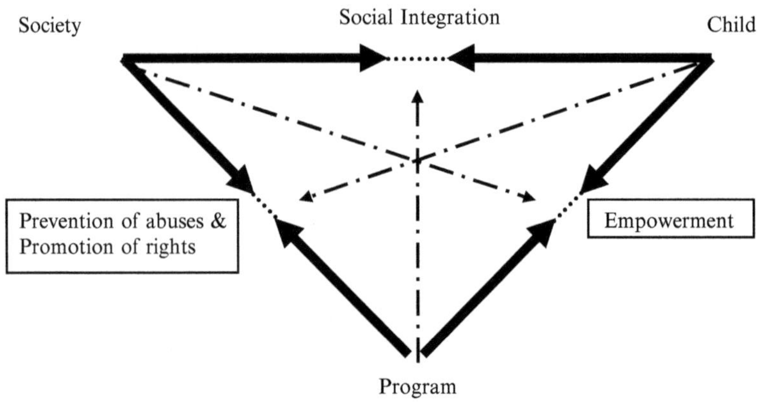

Fig. 5.4 Social integration in a rights-based approach

the problems of children in street situations. Providing for children in street situations at the micro level is only one step of intervention.

Historically, the needs-based approach was seen as the most relevant intervention as long as children were depicted only as victims. The same could be said for the approach that sees these children mainly as delinquents. The needs-based approach defines the symptom as the problem: the presence of children in street situations. On the other hand, a rights-based approach deals with situations depriving children access to their basic rights. The rights-based approach deals with street situations, with the relations among people, and not primarily with the specific characteristics of the children themselves. This is where the expression "children in street situations" gets its practical relevance and its huge consequences in the practices of intervention.

We can refine the human rights programmatic approach by referring to Sen's (1999) view that focuses on the lives people can choose, which he calls a person's "capability". A person's capability depends on numerous elements including personal characteristics (micro factors) and the socio-cultural situation (micro to macro factors). The diagram above is a reflection of this (Fig. 5.4).

This diagram follows Sen's capability approach whereby the child's empowerment depends both on the personal characteristics of the child and on social organisation. The large arrows in the diagram symbolize concrete interactions, while the dotted arrows symbolize the influence of one actor on interactions of the other two. For instance, we can see the direct interaction between the street child and the programme's street educators who help them and the indirect influence of the program (dotted arrow) which shapes the relationship between street educators and the street child.

The diagram shows the principles: Let the child participate in identifying his or her own needs and capacity-building activities. Let the child feel free to participate or not. Promote the children's active participation in carrying out the project's activities. Value children's capacities acquired on or off the street such as sharing, solidarity and critical thinking.

This is the framework that has been integrated into the Terre des Hommes' (TDH) policy regarding children in street situations (it is also related to the Child-to-Child program and the SKI program). Founded in 1960, TDH is a Swiss NGO. They help build a better future for children in street situations in 9 countries (Afghanistan, Brazil, Burundi, Egypt, Lebanon, Mozambique, Pakistan, Sri Lanka, Vietnam). The framework developed by Stoecklin (2007) and adopted by TDH (2012) addresses the dynamics linking together three major factors: the intervention programme, the child (including his or her family), and society (from the micro to the macro level).

This model of intervention uses the capacities of street children. For example, a child who is a leader on the street has an organisational competence which can be redirected towards advocacy campaigns. It also encourages children in street situations to voice their views. The children understand their own rights whenever a program starts from children's experiences, rather than a top-down teaching of abstract principles. The idea is to find a dialogue that empowers children in street situations to transform their individual conflicts into collective positive actions. The goal is an interactive adjustment of individuals and institutions.[8]

Friends International has worked in Southeast Asia with some success, especially in Cambodia. According to their web site (http://www.friends-international.org) they conduct outreach programs and have drop-in centers where they provide education and reintegrate the children back into formal schools. It may be that their success comes from their well rounded program. In addition to direct care, they provide indirect care by giving the children parents' vocational training. They work on prevention through education by emphasising safe migration and providing support during the migration as well as working toward preparing a safe return when they can re-integrate a child with his or her family.

Stoecklin (2000b) has worked on profile identification in Chittagong, Bangladesh. He identified six profiles of children in street situations (see chapter 2). Here we look at his corresponding recommendations. First, for the heroes, help them get better working conditions in the street. Allow them to deposit their savings in a bank to reduce snatching by police. Have an outreach team that leads talks and negotiations with community leaders, especially employers, in order to help heroes within non-exploitive street or shop work environments. Help them realize their wish for more respected positions; provide opportunities for the vocational training of their choice: (driver, vendor, businessman or policeman). Sensitize the community on child rights and give these heroes a key-role in the project's advocacy activities. These children can be examples to modify the public prejudices against children in street situations. Develop a drop-in center for them and arrange family visits to solve problems with parents and siblings.

---

[8] Sen (1999) sees poverty as a lack of freedom to lead a suitable life, a lack of "capabilities". The question is: how can we transform our human and material resources into better development for children in street situations? The way a society or community "transforms" material wealth into symbolic wealth (culture) helps us understand diversity in social integration and/or social exclusion. The competencies (instrumental and symbolic) of children in street situations can therefore be considered as a "reflection" of the social structure of their societies/communities.

The second group are the hard workers who can be encouraged to attend Street Schools, where among other things they can be engaged in discussions about returning to their families or pursuing vocational training. The emphasis is on reconstructing or reinforcing familial ties with special attention to assessing the hard-working child's role and importance for family income. It is also possible to see that hard-working children are connected to adult competitors to negotiate ways of cooperation in order to improve the children's working situations. Also, sensitize the community, by having these children (along with the "heroes") be involved in advocacy activities.

Third are the ambivalents, who should be invited to join a Street School to discuss their experiences and to help them form a clearer and more balanced picture of their street lives. Further recommendations would depend on the results of this counselling activity.

The fourth profile group are the survivors who, given the high degree of suffering experienced coupled with their low level of street skills, need shelters and drop-in centres. They should be given psycho-social counselling similar to what is used for traumatized children, and in groups they can be motivated to seek out alternatives to the street. At the same time, they need family counselling to help them with their parents or step-parents and to get support from their siblings.

The fifth group are the dependent abused whose relatives (mothers, step-mothers, step-fathers) can be approached with a proposal for their children to attend a Street School. Then, contacts and negotiations should be intensified with the children's families or guardians according to the appraisal of risks and envisaged solutions. Don't ask the children to disclose things in the presence of their guardians.

Finally, training should be provided for policemen on the UNCRC and juvenile justice principles. In all cases, consideration should be given to the children's competencies in order to use these abilities as resources, and redirect them in positive group activities. Consider local cultural ways where children function in symbolic roles and use them as ways of enhancing child/community relations.

Another classification of programs for children in street situations is provided by Rizzini and Lusk (1995) who divided them into four programmatic approaches based on assumptions about street children. The correctional approach assumes children in street situations are a delinquent menace to public safety and the result is to put them into institutions. The rehabilitation approach sees the problems with children in street situations as being part of the children's pathology. But rather than jail the children, this approach tries to rehabilitate them by protecting them from becoming more pathological by offering services to help them change. The third approach is educational. In this case the assumption is that the children are without pathology but the society which they come from is deficient in taking care of them, mostly because the society is too poor or too abusive to do so. In this approach, the programs try to empower the children to increase their abilities to change the civil politic. Finally there is prevention, which works to eradicate the reasons that cause children to become homeless. The prevention programs are community-based and offer activities that might reduce the possibility of going to the street, such as after school programs, organized sports, theatre arts, etc.

Problems with the Best Practices Model

We believe the best programs for children in street situations must work at all three levels (micro, meso, and macro). While immediate opportunities via special protection programmes at the micro level are vital for the children already facing the hardship of street life (Volpi 2002), children can gain from being more than passive beneficiaries of direct help. They gain by participating in developing programs at all three levels. For example, children in street situations can help us prevent violations of their rights that affect reintegrating them back into in society. They can do this by participating in data collection, doing the kind of street work that is done by street educators, and developing educational programmes for children in street situations. They can act as health educators, giving information to their peers. They can learn how to triage patients, care for minimal wounds and determine where to send others who might need more care, as prescribed in the book, *Where There is No Doctor* (Werner 1994). It is this kind of activity that would prevent children in street situations from getting sexually transmitted diseases because if they know how their bodies work, they will be more careful in their sexual experiences. They should also avoid pre-packaged educational programs, particularly ones that replace insight with fear in issues such as drug usage or HIV infection.

While we provided several examples to illustrate how children can participate in all three levels of programmatic support, below are some examples of very well run rights-based programs but which nevertheless have some problems associated with initiating or assessing the rights-based programmatic approach. The *Fundacion Junto con los Ninos* (JUCONI) targets young children, adolescents and their families. The programme is based in Puebla, Mexico, and began in 1989 with the goal to improve the lives of street children (de Benitez 2001). It has been further developed in order to help children find solutions through access to their rights. In 1994, UNESCO recognized the JUCONI model as the most innovative and promising program for street children (Volpi 2002).

The JUCONI model is comprehensive, including street work by street educators, an educational programme, shelter, family reunification, a community-based programme, an after-care programme as well as a prevention programme that advocates for the rights of the child using the UNCRC for its overarching goals. There are three steps that characterize the program, initial contact, intensive change and follow-up service. The initial contact stage has a different approach for each of the three categories it identifies: Street-living children; street-working children; and market-working children; children who work in the street markets but do not always live with their families.

Each child's capacities are strengthened with a focus on the skills the child needs most. Academic learning blocks are developed for each child. After this intensive phase of intervention, a follow-up is directed towards the child and his or her family. Prevention is also used, especially with the siblings of 'street children' considered as likely to end up in a street situation.

The definition of street children given by JUCONI, with the three subdivisions, focuses on the needs and takes into account different situations. By having data on children in each situation, they can measure each sub-group based on international standards, particularly by using the educational approach in which the children and working staff share the same language, tools and goals as other educational programs so they can work together.

The question of applicability of international standards to the local reality remains a problem in many settings and it would be surprising if this would not be the case in the Mexican reality. Typically, the top-down approach and "common language" reflect the social relationships that the planning process itself produces (Mosse 2001). This has been observed in many programmes for runaways and street children which are still mainly directed according to adult intervention agendas and children's views are not taken into consideration (Parazelli 2002; Rizzini et al. 2007; Stoecklin 2007).

There are some other weaknesses of the JUCONI programme. Despite Mexico being a party to the UNCRC, the JUCONI model is still not fully rights-based. Like other programs, JUCONI finds it difficult to use the UNCRC to plan abstract concepts, for instance the "best interest of the child", because they are so difficult to measure (de Benitez 2001). But in fact there is an acknowledgment that the best interest of the child is a general principle of the UNCRC and its implementation and evaluation should be done on a case-by-case basis (Zermatten 2005). Yet at the level of child's rights, the program runs into a typical dilemma. So many of the children's rights are violated that one organisation cannot address all of these violations simultaneously. This is the case in almost all settings and it would therefore not suffice as an excuse to refrain from implementing a rights-based approach. Another way to look at this would be to consider the holistic nature of the UNCRC, whereby the rights are all linked together so that an action in the direction of access to one right has consequences over some other rights, and possibly over all of the rights.

To its credit, JUCONI has identified some of the lessons learned. One of them was that there was no lasting effect from outreach services (de Benitez 2001). Another was that the streets seemed to be an unfavourable place for learning. Consequently, the programme changed so that the educational and therapeutic work takes place at a half-way house.

One problem is that while the UNCRC is often displayed as being the core principle, the JUCONI program (like many other rights-based programs) conducts evaluations based on the numbers of children leaving the streets and not based on access to specific child rights. For instance, the latest available numbers given by JUCONI show that 96.5% of children using their services are no longer working or living on the streets, and that 80% of JUCONI graduates break out of the cycles of chronic poverty and violence to achieve their permanent social integration. These are exemplary results, but an additional, and probably more difficult, assessment about how they have affected the children's human rights would be valuable.

As we go on to the next example, non-formal education (NFE), we can clarify the findings of JUCONI that the streets are an unfavourable place for learning. To do this, we look to Shephard (2011), who as we said previously provided the first systematic review of the effectiveness of non-formal education for children in street situations. The search was conducted in thirty-five structured databases and numerous online publication lists. Forty-two organizations and twenty-six experts were also contacted.

Non-formal education is operationally defined as any organized, structured and systematic learning service delivered outside the framework of the formal school system. It is tailored to a particular audience for a particular objective. It strives to be low-cost both in time and in resources. The method of delivery is determined by the learner's objectives and styles of learning (Thompson 2001).

It is appropriate for children in street situations for several reasons: it can provide basic skills such as literacy and numeracy, and by being time efficient and flexible it can help street children and homeless youth acquire catch-up knowledge and academic skills so they can transfer into the formal education system or vocational programs (Etling 1993; Thompson 2001).

Most NFE programs rely on a curriculum that has an intrinsic interest and value. With children in street situations, these programs can use materials about oppressed and marginalized people, which have a parallel in street life. NFE's flexibility and its sharing of decision-making also complement the independence of street life and street children's mistrust of formal adult society (Aptekar 1988; Bar-On 1998; Cheng 2008).

The ability of NFE to focus on basic academic skills, such as literacy in an accelerated, condensed curriculum, matches the needs of many illiterate children in street situations. Because they must generate their own income, NFE programs focus on vocational training and life-skills is suited to their needs. And, by improving their skills and providing pathways into formal education or vocational skills, NFE has the potential to give the children a more positive future orientation (Freire 2003; Huang and Huang 2008; Zimmerman et al. 1992).[9]

However, it should not be assumed that NFE is suitable for children in street situations merely because it claims to match their needs. Future research and program monitoring is needed (Zutshi 2000). Other potential weaknesses of NFE include (1) a lack of resources and suitable (safe and quiet) locations, (2) poor teacher training, (3) abuse resulting from a lack of accountability and training, (4) the inability of many NFE programs to grant any meaningful qualification after completion, and (5) the lack of vocational training that is sensitive to street youth aspirations and local economic circumstances (Rodriguez 2004).

Pavement schools are common in India, and both authors of this book are familiar with *Proyecto Alternativos* in Honduras which does not have a school room. They use market space that is temporarily available. When Aptekar visited the school in 2004, street children were learning among hung bananas, which

[9] The Axe project started in 1989 in Salvador, Brazil, and from the start it worked with the National Movement of street boys and girls in Brazil (MNMMR) (Almeida and de Carvalho 2000). Its goal was to restore street children's lives so they could become functional adult citizens. Its approach was to adopt Paulo Freire's methodology of education, what they termed, "the pedagogy of desire".

frankly was as nice as the four concrete walls that he was using in his teaching at a University in Tegucigalpa.

The extent to which NFE programs are designed around principles of critical pedagogy, empowerment, and participation varies greatly, which is too bad because there is merit in teaching without a pre-arranged curriculum, which can lead to passivity. The latter is more likely to promote engagement. It is better to develop a curriculum based on the students' interests. Few NFE programs actually transfer any decision-making power to the students and most use didactic teaching methods.

The Mkombozi program in Tanzania was granted the Impact Award in 2008 for excellence by the Stars Foundation. The organisation began in 1997 as a residential centre and a place of safety for children living on the streets and developed over the years with the aim of ending the abuse and neglect of children, ensuring that children's rights are recognised, and identifying opportunities for intervention before a child migrates to the street. They target over 1,000 families and children a year and offers protection services, research, advocacy, and education (Schumacher 2011).

Mkombozi emphasizes active child participation in decisions concerning the children's own lives. It has made great strides in doing this. Voluntary participation is fostered on the basis of the child's wish to join and change in order to become part of the programme. This means that participation can only follow the child's acceptance of a process that is already functioning, which therefore actually does not leave much room for negotiation.

Participation is not an either/or phenomenon. This type of participation would locate somewhere in the middle of Hart's (1992) eight step ladder of participation. The levels begin with participation by manipulation to participation by tokenism, such as having one street child on a city committee that is making decisions for street children. In the Mkombozi program, the children are operating beyond these levels. Their programming is between level four, where children are assigned to a program but are also informed about it, to a higher level (5 or 6) where they are being consulted about belonging. They fall below levels seven and eight where children are truly acting as fully fledged citizens and participants.

The Mkombozi project has an evaluation component, but the research is mostly needs-based and the program analyses its own results by referring to reports on best practices (Dybicz 2005; Volpi 2002). What the Mkombozi programme learned was that a needs-based response can have side-effects. For instance, they began handing out food based on responding to an immediate need of hunger, but rapidly noticed that there were unexpected negative outcomes of this good intention, such as finding that some children and youth became dependent on the programme rather than self-reliant, and that it caused some children to leave their homes because they could eat better in the program than at home (Mkombozi 2010).

While the program is extraordinary in what it accomplishes, it does raise questions about how such a program might increase its rights-based programming. In this case, the program does not have staff with specific expertise on legal questions. It is quite important to have legal expertise to help children who are stigmatised and sometimes even put in prison just because they are in the street. This issue is a major one, as was shown by Wernham (2004) who said that the majority of street children processed through justice systems were not in actual conflict with the law, but detained for activities like running away, vagrancy, begging, or for their own protection.

In St-Petersburg, Russia, a billboard recently appeared explaining that taking children off the streets is a matter of public security (UNICEF CEE/CIS 2010, p. 34). This reinforces the observation that the vast majority of street children have to face the stigma of perceived rather than actual conflict with the law (Wernham 2004). Cheng (2008) shows how China still applies a protective model associated with forceful measures to send the children back home, a policy which has not much changed in the last decade (Stoecklin 2000a).

Problems with Macro Level Human Rights Programs

It may well be that it is typical of programs that claim to be rights-based to revert to the micro level. They do this by starting with the premise that it is necessary to clearly define the population and adapt the intervention to be relevant and specific to the needs of that population. Sometimes such programs divide the population into sub-groups, which can be helpful because some children require only a very light and temporary support from one organisation, while others face multiple deprivations which require a well-coordinated interventions through a network. And, there are networks within a needs-based framework.

But most self-proclaimed "rights-based programs" are not yet functioning on the premise that intervention should be primarily directed at redressing violations of specific human rights. This is still seen as too abstract. Program managers and donors find it easier to assess the successes and failures in terms of the numbers of children "processed" through the different components of a project. In most cases, data about failure or success of the programme concentrate on numbers of children that have benefited from the programme and not on the progress of law implementation regarding specific rights enshrined in the UNCRC that the signatories to the Convention have agreed to implement.

There are other problems with human rights programs related to not evaluating child participation in planning, implementing and monitoring programmes. In part, this depends on the way child participation itself is conceived. If it is only tokenistic, whereby children have an influence over secondary or tertiary aspects in a daily routine, there is only a small chance that child participation will be of value. If child participation is part of a rights-based strategy that touches all three levels of intervention (micro, meso, and macro), and children and decision-makers meet and discuss the issues, there is a greater chance that child participation will be valuable. However, this is demanding on the staff because, among other things, it really requires a certain acceptance of younger people having a true voice in adult decisions.

Institutional and private donors need to consider the possibility of making a difference with a strategy targeting less immediately visible results and favouring long-term human rights development. If the State re-assumed its role in a child-rights approach, it could replace NGOs which are carrying out activities that the public sector has abandoned. In the present neo-liberal ideology, it is quite the reverse: a multiplicity of NGOs are striving to achieve a comprehensive or "holistic" approach (which is an opportunity to expand the market for their services). While there are networks conceived to achieve a comprehensive service-delivery model (if an NGO cannot respond to a specific need, the child will be referred to another NGO), this is only at the micro level of programming.

There is also a problem of scale: what is the financial volume that is necessary to make a difference regarding a child rights approach for children in street situations? A fully funded rights-based approach, monitoring all rights violations and intervention impacts, requires a lot of human resources that are beyond the capacity of many organizations. Because of their limited resources, they choose to concentrate on direct aid and services, which are the elements that can be made visible for donors and help to gain more funding.

As we have touched on the question of the scale of finances, it is quite interesting to see how a big financial institution sets its own programme for children in street situations. The Asian Development Bank (ADB) does not work directly with children; instead it funds NGOs and other organisations.[10]

It was established in 1966 with the mission to help developing countries to reduce poverty and improve the quality of life of their people. It has partners in the private sector, among development agencies, community-based organisations, and foundations. With reference to the UNCRC, the ADB adopted the core values of protection and participation as the two key principles for working with street children (ADB 2003).

From 2001, the ADB has been working to reduce poverty (macro level), which they see as the problem behind children in street situations. The impact of this big financial institution combining direct services at the micro level and macro level work is difficult to judge because, strangely, the ABD hasn't developed a monitoring system that helps follow up on the progress of children's rights.

Indicators of Child Participation

Indicators of child participation should include the quality of participation (Lansdown 2010). Thus, she suggests assessing if the participation is voluntary, respectful, relevant, child-friendly, safe, sensitive to risk, and accountable.[11] The children should be involved in the evaluation of child participation. This has been

[10] The Asian Development Bank sees handouts in the streets as problematic because, according to their policy, they make street life bearable, and because they are unsustainable and create dependency (ADB 2003).

[11] Information on the rights of children should be taught for all ages and abilities, and with increasing sensitisation and awareness among adults. There should also be systematic mechanisms for influencing public decisions at all levels, for both remedy and redress.

done within several member states of the Council of Europe including Finland, Slovakia, and Moldova (Stoecklin 2013).

The UNCRC proclaims that children have a right to be heard and therefore there is an obligation of State signatories to insure this (Zermatten 2005). Although, the degree to which the child's voice is to be taken into consideration depends upon the age and maturity of the child (Pufall and Unsworth 2004).

The Convention also implicitly recognizes the child as a social actor. The notion of social actor thus becomes central to understanding how State parties can guarantee child participation. Yet this notion remains largely undefined in spite of an increase in articles and books using the concept.[12]

Even though participation (including speaking one's mind) is a street child's right, most people would prefer that children express non-challenging points of view, even though these are often not reflective of the real experiences of children in street situations (Woodhead 2010; Percy-Smith and Thomas 2010). As difficult as it may be to hear what they have to say, their right to speak and be heard is instrumental in developing their capacity to make decisions (Woodhead 2010).

As the child acquires the competence and willingness to bear accountability, a transfer of responsibility from adults to children should be granted. This would have to be judged case by case, because the capacities of the child, the levels of risk involved, the degree of support available, the level of understanding of the nature of the risks involved, and the child's own views change in different circumstances (Lansdown 2010).

A Rights-Based Strategy for Children in Street Situations

A child-rights approach to children in street situations contributes to a child's social integration, but this is the case only if there is a process of mutual adjustment (Stoecklin 2007). Children have to be socialized to become members of society, while society has to adapt to the children's rights and abilities. The UNCRC offers the legal framework to empower the child as a "social actor", meaning the child is the owner of his or her human rights, and a participant in his or her social reality.

In spite of current conceptions of street children as social actors, they are still portrayed only as "outcomes" of poverty or abuse and viewed as strange, irrational and/or dangerous (Stoecklin 2007). Even the label "street child" leads itself to ready-made prejudices as well as dismissing the children's points of view about their own situations as superfluous. The way forward is to build a civil politic in which citizens will assume the responsibility for giving voice to children in street situations and where the parties will make the mutual adjustments necessary to social integration.

[12] See for instance the *Special Issue on Children as Social Actors; The International Journal of Children's Rights, Volume 15, No 1, 2007.*

Dyregrov et al. (2002) studied children who have been through a war, some of whom will become street children. While there was resilience and vulnerability in these children, the authors ask what, if any, psycho-social program can be used to reduce suffering. They ask important questions. Should psycho-social support come from Western style counseling or indigenous methods? Whatever the source of support, it is important before helping to respect the principle of allowing full child participation and human rights. The authors own longitudinal study and others cited in their paper suggest psycho-social help is justified.

They point out the value of addressing the issues using Western approaches, but advise being clear about the limitations. They acknowledge harmful possibilities while suggesting that the best method is to involve both traditional and western ideas in a thoughtful, integrated fashion. The evidence suggests that such an approach is valuable. The question of ethics always looms. There is not only the requirement to do no harm, but also the questions that arise when there are more needs than resources: Who gets help? How? How and when do interventions stop? These are still issues which have not been studied.

Elsewhere, Wessells (2006) said that psychosocial counseling should include the physical, psychological, social and spiritual aspects of life. It is different than therapy in that it is not exclusively treatment of mental disorders. There is a need to document which services are effective, and important to consider that the very services one is trying to provide can also be harmful. A lot of the Western styles of talk and art therapies have not really been justified empirically. Or they have been used at the wrong time or carried out by inexperienced people. On the other hand, many traditional approaches are reported only through anecdotes. There are no studies which look directly at the issue of doing no harm, which is vital to the children's human rights.

The issue of how to help in the cultural context is always problematic. The best approach is to respect and encourage indigenous forms of healing such as dancing singing, and rituals surrounding coming of age and dying. The more these ceremonies can be continued in spite of the absence of the surroundings that are usually associated with them, the better.

Empirical studies also need to be developed to contribute to a scientific framework on how to guide children's voices in the process of decision-making (Stoecklin 2007). These studies would be seen in a different light than empirical studies based at the micro level. Take for example the problem of the numbers of children in street situations we were speaking about earlier. He draws an important distinction regarding the use of numbers in a human rights-based approach (something we have touched upon earlier). He gives an example from Chittagong, Bangladesh, where he was conducting a study with Terre des hommes and Aparajeyo-Bangladesh (Stoecklin 2000b). The team of inquirers interviewed 246 children, out of a total number of street children that was first estimated at 5,000. The sample of 246 represented the desired 5% of the total target population. However, when talking with people in daily contact with these children (railway staff, policemen, judges, etc.), they estimated the total number of street children in Chittagong as being fewer than 1,000 children. This was not only fewer than the 5,000, but also far removed from the estimate of "100,000 street children in Chittagong" announced by the UNDP.

The important point Stoecklin makes is that in a child-rights approach, rights are not to be seen in relation to the numbers of cases involved, because every single child is entitled to the same rights. Therefore, even if estimates would be less alarmist, "small" numbers should not be viewed as unimportant.

As is always the case with those on the margins of society, children not only adapt to the situation; they actively try to surmount their difficulties by joining and creating their own world. Economic competition is compressing wages and economic policy is dismantling the public sector, which increasingly condemns large sectors of the population to social exclusion. The weight of this economic model of development over people's lives is only "seen" when we eventually encounter children looking for opportunities in the street in order to survive. We see more children surviving in the street environment, more children exploited by growing mafias, including grown-up former "street kids", (even without forgetting the numerous cases of children physically eliminated by vigilante groups).

The difficulty of fully implementing a rights-based approach can be illustrated with numerous international NGOs. Take Terre des hommes as an illustration.

Terre des Hommes is an international organization that develops and implements projects designed to improve the living conditions of disadvantaged children. TDH set up its first project aimed at protecting children in street situations in 1986 in the northeast of Brazil. Since then, TDH has been increasingly concerned about the enormous vulnerability of children in street situations and has expanded its involvement to other urban areas all over the world particularly affected by this problem either by supporting local partners or by carrying out actions of its own.

In these 25 years, TDH has acquired considerable experience working at the micro and meso levels. It offers support or strengthens already existing programs that empower children and families and communities. It also does advocacy work for children's rights, and works at the international level in analysis of programs related to children's rights and collaborates with other large institutions such as UNICEF, UNESCO and the International Labour Organization (ILO) through discussions and networking of efforts. TDH also contributes to reports for the UN Committee on the Rights of the Child. It often reports on how rights are applied or violated. Thus, TDH helps build local and national capacities to ensure a system of complete protection, acts as a catalyst in network advocacy, and encourages participation in organisations that defend and promote rights and draw up and present public policies. What makes operational organisations like TDH special is that they are in a position to promote and facilitate the UNCRC's implementation plans through the flow of information from the micro and meso levels of their programs to the groups in the international arena such as the Committee on the Rights of the Child, and other United Nations bodies. But do these organizations systematically address the rights enshrined in the Convention on the Rights of the Child? Or do they rather pick up some examples of what they and somehow relate them to the UNCRC as a general framework that guides their intervention? To some extent, the latter is what many States do when submitting their periodic reports to the UN Committee on the Rights of the Child. But a real rights-based approach would require more systematic implementation and follow-up of every right enshrined in the UNCRC.

Almost every country is a party to the UNCRC.[13] The rights enshrined in the UNCRC assure that all children have the same rights independent of their backgrounds and current situations of their lives. However, being declared a "subject of rights" by internationally recognized law does not necessarily mean that the child's rights will be attended to. This is problematic because children in street situations are not specifically mentioned in the UNCRC.

Of course there are important general principles that apply to street children and homeless youth. These include among many others the right to non-discrimination (Article 2), the principle of the best interests of the child (Article 3), the right to life, survival and development (Article 6), and the right to be heard (Article 12).

While the principle of the best interests of the child (Article 3) for example says that in all actions concerning children, the best interests of child should be given primary consideration. This seems straight forward, but one of the most difficult rights to guarantee, because by law the best interests of the child have to be assessed case by case (Freeman 2007). Case by case is particularly difficult for refugee children and street children who are refugees. As they suddenly flood into a new environment, there simply are not enough people to serve them.

To help with this type of situation, the UNHCR (The Office of the United Nations High Commissioner for Refugees, May, 2008) developed a set of criteria that guides the assessment of unaccompanied minors. The UNHCR guidelines includes a step by step procedure. In this way they can determine the best interests of the child in a formal process with procedural safeguards, proper documentation, and in front of a trained decision maker who is required to weigh all of the factors of the case before coming to a lawful conclusion. One is asked to look at the long term best interests of each child, even while making temporary care decisions. In this way hands are not tied to offering short term help. Without going into all of the details here, we recommend that professionals who are working with children in street situations pay careful attention to the UNHCR guidelines.

People working with children in street situations should also pay attention to Article 9 of the UNCRC which concerns the circumstances under which children can be taken away from their parents. The child cannot be taken away against his

---

[13] The UNCRC (United Nations Convention on the Rights of the Child), was adopted by the UN General Assembly (1989) and entered into force in 1990, is the most widely ratified human rights treaty in history. The treaty has been very quickly ratified in all countries, except three, namely Somalia, South Sudan and the USA. Somalia is currently unable to proceed to ratification because it has no recognized government. The United States of America has signed but not yet ratified the treaty. Many countries have also ratified the Optional Protocols to the UNCRC, namely the Optional Protocol to the Convention on the Rights of the Child on the sale of children, child prostitution and child pornography (adopted in 2000 and entered into force in 2002) and the Optional Protocol to the Convention on the Rights of the Child on the involvement of children in armed conflict (adopted in 2000 and entered into force in 2002). A third Optional Protocol which allows children to bring complaints to the UN Committee on the Rights of the Child regarding the violation of their rights, has been adopted in December 2011. It has been signed by 37 countries and ratified by 6, but the numbers are growing. This Optional Protocol allows children in street situations, in the States which are parties to this OP, to directly bring complaints before the UN Committee.

or her will without a full judicial process based on appropriate laws and procedures. This might be necessary in cases of abuse or neglect, which of course can be common in children in street situations. If the child must be separated from the parents, the law demands that the child see his or her parents regularly (if they are not dangerous to the child).

Those who are working with children in street situations must deal with several other articles of UNCRC that indirectly deal with street and homeless children. These include most notably Article 27 (poverty, standard of living and lack of shelter) and Article 37 (children deprived of liberty). We have noted that in some countries, the ethnic, racial and religious identification of street and homeless children plays a significant role in how they will be treated, which is discriminatory in nature.

Poverty, poor standards of living and the lack of shelter (Article 27) are conducive to multiple issues of deprivaton. Children in street situations who, in addition to having problems of health, might also be HIV positive or have AIDS (many African children with AIDS end up in the streets). Homeless youth in Canada are 6 to 12 times more likely to get HIV than any other group of youth (Rotheram-Borus 1993).

Article 23 refers to disabled children. Similar to children suffering from HIV/AIDS, many disabled children are forced to take refuge in the streets; in certain countries, children are abducted, disabled and then forced to beg in the streets.

Articles 28 and 29 refer to education. Street and homeless children are generally denied equal access to education. Although a number of innovative models have been developed to ensure their proper education, few have been properly evaluated.

Article 32 refers to economic exploitation including child labor. In many countries, street children are engaged in hazardous labor at extremely low wages, and all children in street situations are vulnerable to inappropriate work. Articles 33 (substance abuse), 34, (sexual exploitation and sexual abuse) and 35 (abduction of, sale of or traffic in children) and 36 (all other forms of exploitation) are of particular importance for children in street situations. Street and homeless children are victims of these abuses.

Articles 37 refers to cruel, inhuman and degrading behavior towards children. This includes victimization by law enforcement authorities, and organized crime. Articles 38 and 39 refer to children being recruited into armed conflict. Children in street situations, particularly in the developing world, are often forced or lured into joining one side or the other in situations of armed conflict. And of course many children in street situations are dealt with as children in conflict with the law, and are most of the time denied the provisions of Article 40 (the right of children alleged as, accused of, or recognized as having infringed the penal law to be treated in a manner consistent with the promotion of the child's sense of dignity and worth).

NGOs working at all levels of programs (micro, meso, and macro) can strengthen the implementation of the UNCRC articles, as the micro and meso levels are of crucial importance for the work to be done on the macro level. They can bring in all that is diverse among the cultural variations of children's lives. They can contribute to defining what is universal about children's rights, and therefore help link the rights of children in street situations to the reality of all children's rights, including those outside of Western cultural contexts.

This is not without problems. For example, how does the Convention deal with differences in ages? The classical child development approach to legal law used age as a general measure of the level of individual cognitive development.

A newer paradigm should look at children's age and maturity in more detail. There are two extremes to avoid. The first is to consider children as proto-adults (Matthews 2004). The second is to consider children's agency as attached to children themselves. Whereas the older approach emphasised age and cognition, the newer approach should emphasize age and social constraints. Some extreme interpretations of the new paradigm have given rise to a rejection of any criteria that would place a divide between children and adults. This may lead to treat the constraints children are facing as similar to adult problems. But one cannot just ignore the huge differences that are at play in the structural forces that shape the phases (school/work/pension) of a life cycle. These are fields with distinctive stakes and challenges. To treat school – or any institution that is age-specific – as leading to exclusion of children from the adult or "real" world, or as overprotecting them, paradoxically runs the risk of naturalizing the neo-liberal philosophy of the "free market", where competition should rule everywhere, and where, consequently, individual responsibility is the norm by which people are entitled to have a say. A slogan-like discourse on agency is likely to fall into the trap it wanted to avoid: naturalizing the dominant force (competition) that tends to run through every sphere of human activity. The discourse on the "competent" child is full of traps (beginning with the word competence which has the same root as competition). The most important trap to avoid is linking agency with individuals, rather than seeing agency in the relationships between individuals. And one should consider that the UNCRC is precisely dealing with these relationships: it says how the relations with and among children should look like. The extensions and limitations of children's agency are therefore clearly bound to the scope of their rights and interpretations of the latter. Children in street situations are a clear illustration of this: although they are to be considered as holders of the rights enshrined in the UNCRC, they experience important limitations in the exercise of these rights, and these limitations are both socially and individually shaped.

The position considering children as generally competent agents regardless of their age and specific situations shows its limitations when it comes to interventions with real children. Dealing with a child or a teenager with such general stances about autonomy is not of much help. To work with children in street situations, we recommend creating linkages between individual competencies and social opportunities to work with children in street situations. We take the stance that a child is a subject of rights from birth onward and at the same time a social actor with evolving capabilities. This perspective, trying to reconcile what has been somewhat artificially separated (being and becoming), seems a more promising way to consider how different children in diverse contexts exercise their rights in their daily life.

To demonstrate this, we examine the distinction between assigned and acquired status. A newborn possesses an assigned status conferred by others, according to their normative socio-cultural framework. The inclusion of children's rights into this framework doesn't change the fact that an assigned status (in this case the legal status) is always conferred by others. The newborn is unable to recognize or practise social roles. It is through the process of socialization that the child progressively internalizes social norms and cultural values that are commonly used to give meaning to interactions. The UNCRC also considers the evolving capacities of children's ages. Ignoring and not documenting the range of sophistication of children's agency overlooks important differences. The systemic theory called "the actor's system" (Stoecklin 2009a) and its corresponding tool, the "kaleidoscope of experience" (2009b) help uncover these differences, as their are concretely expressed by actors in terms of activities, relations, values, images of self and motivations therefore also help having children in street situations included in project programming through respect of their levels of agency.

Article 12 is concerned with how views are expressed (freely), and the range of matters on which these views are expressed (all matters affecting the child). We note that this article gives consideration to the child's views in accordance with the age and maturity of the child. There are two elements of this article that impose some restrictions according to the capacity of the child. The formulation, "*the child who is capable of forming his or her own views,*" leaves open the question of how we assess this capacity. The consideration given to these views, "*in accordance with the age and maturity of the child*" also does not specify the criteria to evaluate maturity.

While the UNCRC sets no age limit on participation rights, we clearly see that implicit restrictions are left to the assessment of the decision-makers. One challenge is therefore to make the criteria as transparent as possible, even if they are left to the decision-makers' discretion. How "free" is the building of one's views at different ages and in different settings? Expression and recognition are interdependent: a discourse can be recognized only if it is expressed in such a way that it can be socially shared. Here, the distinction we make between the subject of rights and the social actor clearly shows.

The formation of "one's own views" expressed in a socially recognizable way is a culturally acquired competence. The social actor is acting in a pragmatic way which derives from experience, allowing for the adjustment of thoughts, expressions, and lines of conduct, through interactions with others. The evaluation of one's maturity is therefore bound to these adjustments: being able to recognize the points of views of others and being open to information. The child's competence of building views that would be socially considered as mature is in fact matured through interactions. It is hard to think of an opinion that would be absolutely free of influences conveyed by the opinions of others. Participation is itself the process whereby children acquire the capacity to build their "own views".

How to take into account what children express is of crucial importance. This is particularly difficult and important when it comes to children suffering from a stereotyped definition of their situation, such as that conveyed by the category "street children and homeless youth". These labels are a limitation to the free expression of opinions by children who are not listened to just because they are surviving on the streets. What this shows is that there are social and individual limitations to the exercise of children's rights which reinforce each other circularly and cumulatively. To break this cycle, we have changed the labels (street child and homeless children) into more neutral wording (children in street situations). We believe that this obliges one to listen to these children in order to identify the breaches of rights that have led to their particular situations. Words count. They determine how we act. When associated with approaches documenting and strengthening the cumulative and recursive nature of action, like Stoecklin's "actor's system" (see Chapter 4), the cycle of negative limitations can be replaced by or inverted into a cycle of positive reinforcement of children's agency through respect of their rights.

Prevention

Preventive programs (like most macro level programs) are difficult to assess, because they focus on large goals without easily identifiable conclusions, such as reducing poverty, changing public opinion, and empowering the community. Prevention programs which address "root" causes; for example poverty in the case of street children, are facing a task beyond any but the largest organizations.[14] The most difficult and perhaps most important work is to address the public's, (particularly people with community influence), negative feelings about children in street situations, and to get the public to lobby for community support for poor children, or other children at high risk. The problem is that for many preventive (and macro level) programs, the financial needs are so great. Thus whenever humanitarian aid focuses on particular groups, others in the community or family are left out. The pie is only so big and the needs are always greater than the resources (Aptekar 2010). Focusing on children in street situations takes money away from programs that deal with the much larger issues such as generic poverty (Ennew 2003). For children in street situations, the biggest problem is living in poverty, which is a far greater risk to health than living without adult authority (Panter-Brick 2004).

There are 1.3 billion people in the world, a quarter of whom live in absolute poverty, meaning among other things, that they survive on less than one dollar a day. If you increase the poverty line to two dollars a day, more than half (56%) of the people in the developing world live in poverty (Bassuk and Donelan 2003). There are 472 million children who, because of malnutrition, live with a compromised immune system, anemia, and impaired cognitive development.

Does living on the streets represent a mental health emergency worse than this? Is it right to assume that psycho-social intervention for children in street situations prevents the development of serious and long lasting health problems? It may well be that living on the streets has more mental health benefits that living in an abusive home, or a home so poor that it cannot feed all of its children. Thus needs-based programs which make the children's vulnerability the focus of funding, can miss the real problem of the cycle of poverty.

[14] However, on a smaller preventive scale things can be done: food can be given to high risk families, either directly or to working children who are not making their quota.

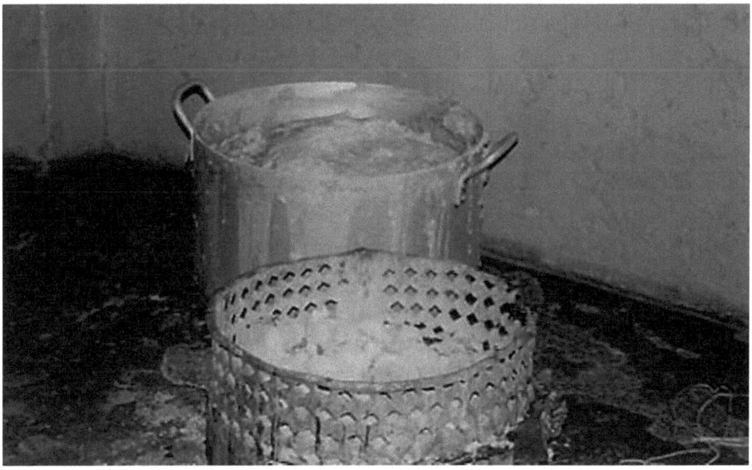

Fig. 5.5 They feed them like dogs

Are the Right Services Being Provided?

In Nairobi, Kenya there were many programs that serve street children (Aptekar and Ciano 1999), but there were disconnects between the programs' written philosophies and the actual experiences of the children, making it difficult to easily determine which programs would be helpful and how. In some cases, the official philosophy was benevolent, but the children were treated poorly by the adults they interacted with. In other situations, the children appeared to be treated very well, even though the stated philosophy seemed quite rigid or even out of compliance with UNCRC. The results from programs for children in street situations might have less to do with the programs' written goals, the funders and the parameters of the funding, than they do with the people the children interact with.

Numbers can hide important differences. Take the case of feeding programs. Many micro level programs give food to street children. It is usually cooked in institutional size pots and pans, and consists of the local gruel plus some greens. The food is ladled out while the children sit in lines against a wall waiting for their turn (Fig. 5.5). As a rule the food is adequate, supplies calories and has some nutritional value. It is not interesting or a balanced diet.

Why aren't food programs serving family type meals in a civilized fashion? That so many people see children fed this way without thinking it could be different speaks for itself. In Maputo, Mozambique, one program teaches the children how to appraise an animal on the hoof by estimating its weight, and then how to make an intelligent bid. If they have the winning bid, they take the live animal home where other children who have learned how to butcher take over and prepare the animal to be cooked. Still others set up tables that serve six or eight children. The tables are laid with cloth table covers and cloth napkins. When the children sit down to eat, they feel that they are participating in a family meal for which they have offered their expertise in preparation. And the cost is less than the institutional fare.

Why haven't other programs adopted this method? Is it that in the more traditional meal for street children, the feeding is set up to be efficient, not humane, and represents a diminished view of them, that they are more like animals or convicts than children? The current feeding system cannot help but to communicate a message to those who eat the food that they are not worth much.[15]

It is also difficult to tell which programs are effective because there is so much competition among programs, and among personnel working in different programs. All over the world, it is not uncommon to have people working for one program discount the work of a neighboring program, as if they could only cheer for one. There is also a lot of gossip about who is doing what, or who isn't doing what. Innuendo and scandal are always in the wings. None of this favors street children or homeless youth.

This begs the main question: are there too many programs for street children? For every project for working children living at home there are multiple projects for street children, in spite of the fact that working children outnumber street children many times over (Ennew 1994).

Even if there is a plethora of programs, do the children know of them? Nieuwenhuizen (2006) reports in her study in Bangalore, India that the street boys she worked with were unaware of the programs available to them, or were aware of the programs, but didn't think they could actually help them with their problems. On the other hand, Aptekar and Ciano (1999) found that the street children in Nairobi, Kenya were very aware of the different feeding programs, including what kind of food was being offered each day. They went where they could get the best fare.

Another question is: are there too many programs providing the same services? And not enough providing some needed services? We have suggested already that there are too many micro level needs-based programs and not enough human rights programs that include work at the macro level. In Nairobi, at the micro level, there was over-programming for food. As a rule, street children are not more in need of food relative to other impoverished children.[16] It was not uncommon for street children to talk about what programs were serving what, and where to go or what to avoid. As we have said, because the larger the number of children served means a greater likelihood of getting funding, there is a significant inflation in numbers. Hecht (1998) says of Brazil, only slightly tongue in cheek, that there were more people working for the programs than there were street children.

At the micro level, programs can have too much success. By offering too much they become too attractive, so instead of serving only street children, they

[15] Marquez (1999) notes that once the Mexican street boys are incarcerated they are considered as the lowest marginalized group. They are given food only to reduce hunger and avoid starvation. The kitchen areas are dirty, with many pests. This is not so different than most NGO feeding programs for children who have never committed a crime.

[16] There is evidence that they weigh more than their domiciled counterparts (Wright et al. 1993). The hungriest children are those cases where the mother has had to go out to work and the oldest female child stays at home to help with child care.

end up serving working children who might become more involved in street life once they have access to the services the programs offers. Programs for street children can actually bring domiciled children from their homes into the streets. It is easier eating for free than it is working for food and taking the money home, particularly if the home is not a comfortable place to be. It is also possible that a successful micro program blocks indigenous forms of helping, such as fostering needy children or establishing child-headed families that might be an available alternative.

As we have said, the programs that are most needed are at the macro level, those designed to change the public's attitudes towards children in street situations, to help reduce the repression and anger of the police and other members of society. In some places, organizations have given street children identity cards that allow children to be on the streets without being harassed by police. Of course, the police have to accept the identity card as a free pass, and allow organizations to work in that manner. Another approach is to agree with the police and the courts to designate a certain portion of urban physical space "out of bounds" to the police, in essence offering the children, as long as the children can obey the project's rules, temporary sanctuary.

The UNCRC remains the main strategic lever to advocate for the respect and protection of children and therefore to encourage the development of a society of social integration providing basic services for all. But there are problems. Street life is highly invested in political interests either to shine on it or to cover it up. The media too often creates and maintains the labelling of outcasts. The general suspicion among the public that such labelling produces limits the skills and competencies of children in street situations. There is another consequence; the initial labelling of children in street situations diminishes the capacity of ordinary citizens to see these children in ways that would contradict their pejorative prejudices. There is a double-victimization of children in street situations: not only are they denied access to fundamental rights, they also have to face the barriers implicit in peoples' hostile stares. It is reasonable to think that we first have to remove the obstacles that diminish human rights and to allow children in street situations to live within an accepting society.

We should consider that when it comes to helping children in street situations, we might be misplacing our efforts. Summerfield (1999) believes that psychology has replaced religion as a way to heal spiritual wounds, even difficult ones that come from war trauma or rape. We have, according to him, obscured the boundary between normal reactions to difficult situations and mental disorders. While he is talking primarily about people traumatized by war, there are some analogies that might help us think about children in street situations.

As he says, most people in war-torn areas (he mentions Rwanda and Cambodia) worry more about health care, food, and shelter than they do about the disturbing and intrusive memories suggestive of post traumatic stress disorder (PTSD). Is this similar to children in street situations? If so, the programs which focus on psychological "rehabilitation" will not be as helpful as those that focus on food, health care and shelter, nor would they be as helpful as changing the public's attitudes.

By looking at what Summerfield calls seven false assumptions about PTSD, we can see that while there is misery it does not in the vast majority of cases lead to mental disorders. What are these assumptions and how do they play out in our context? The first is that the stresses of the street are so extreme that they produce trauma. While the streets can be inhospitable, even deadly in some cases, for the "average" street child or homeless youth, being on the street does not and has not led to a mental disorder.[17] There is no universal response to highly stressful events. Even in the worst of circumstances, the question is not what victims feel, but whether or not their reactions stop them from adapting to a future life.

This means that people who work with children in street situations should look less for signs of mental disorders, and concentrate more on how children in street situations cope with life. Summerfield (1999) found that people affected by war tended to look outward on how to deal with life's problems, rather than dwell on their inward mental processes. Thus most people traumatized by war do not need professional psychological help, they, like children in street situations, need to focus on economic problems, food, shelter, health care and safety.

As we have pointed, out most humanitarian assistance in response to war works on the needs-based model rather than focusing on human rights and justice. In this case, maybe they are right. But we suggest that what is needed is a plan to eliminate or at least drastically reduce the waging of war. Thus the needs for macro level interventions cannot be ignored.[18]

What specifically can you do to help street children? Here are what we consider to be the ten most important directions for working with children in street situations:

1. Examine your culturally bound beliefs about the families of children in street situations and about the psychological functioning of the children.
2. Embrace alternative family structures as legitimate.
3. Don't confuse poverty with psychopathology.
4. Accept young people in adult roles.
5. Understand that one barrier to success is not using the children as resources for programs.
6. Work with children in street situations without forcing them to accept your moral point of view.
7. Refrain from quick judgements against others who work with children in street situations from different cultural points of view.
8. Give psychotherapy only to those who need it. Give the rest of the children practical help.
9. Do your best to increase income generation and self-efficacy.
10. Educate the public, the most difficult, and potentially the most rewarding of tasks you can do.

[17] Summerfield believes that PTSD is what can be called a category fallacy. The same symptoms can be found in different cultures, but they have different meanings in the different cultures.

[18] See Brown et al. (2002) for how kinship care and foster care are related in the case of African-American runaway youth.

These directions are convergent with the ones given in numerous guidebooks and packages for intervention. They, however, do not cover all of the different areas where advice can be given. Actually, a synthesis of all the lessons learned and consequent advice is hardly possible as the selection of best practices is always bound to a certain philosophy and vision of intervention. The directions we have selected and considered as the ten most important ones are following a rights-based approach, considering children in street situations as social actors who have some agency to change the environment surrounding them. This confirms that programmes are always bound to a certain vision of childhood and a corresponding theory of action. There is no intervention with children that does not reflect a certain theory about childhood. Therefore, an overarching recommendation we can make, both as academics and consultants engaged in intervention, is to make the theoretical frameworks explicit (Stoecklin 2013).

Conclusion

This chapter compares programs for homeless youth and street children; noting that the different economic levels not only are materially different, but can focus on different interventions. We showed how difficult it is to ascertain the effectiveness of programs serving homeless youth. Even though some youth show some improvement, it is difficult to know why. Cognitive behavioral therapy seemed to be effective. Drug and alcohol treatment programs without additional services do not appear to be helpful. In some cases one could argue that the results did not justify the money spent. Education for homeless youth has been criticized for its excess of regulations, which makes it difficult for homeless youth to receive a public education. People working in programs for homeless youth also felt hemmed in by paper work.

We created a categorical method of analysing programs which depended on where the services were provided, from individual (micro) to communal (meso) to societal (macro).

We also divided programs by philosophy; some were based on the needs of the individual child, and some on the rights of children as defined by the UNCRC. The latter can be difficult to use because of cultural difference, and because to follow the law the children must be involved in all aspects of the program, from planning to implementation.

We showed several best practice programs and other programmatic philosophies. These included *Fundacion Junto con los Ninos* (JUCONI) in Mexico, which has a comprehensive needs-based model with significant meso level programs. The Mkombozi program in Tanzania ensures that children's rights are recognised; identifies opportunities for preventive intervention before a child migrates to the street and works to advocate for them. The Asian Development Bank (ADB) does not work directly with children. Instead it funds NGOs and other organisations. Terre des Hommes (TDH) offers support for existing programs that empower children and families and communities. It advocates for child rights, collaborates with large institutions such UNICEF in discussions and network implementation, and contributes to reports for the UN Committee on the Rights of the Child.

In the area of preventive approaches, the most difficult and perhaps the most important work is to address the public's, (particularly people with community influence), negative feelings about children in street situations, and to get the public to lobby for community support for poor children, or other children at high risk. We also wanted to be sure that some programs work preventively, including dealing with the large scale social problems (such as child abuse and the lack of basic financial opportunity) that result in children going to the streets.

References

Almeida, F., & de Carvalho, M. (2000). Projeto Axe: Educating excluded children in Salvador. In R. Mickelson (Ed.), *Children on the streets of the Americas* (pp. 172–183). New York: Routledge.

Alteena, A., Brilleslijper-Kater, S., & Wolff, J. (2010). Effective interventions for homeless youth: A systematic review. *American Journal of Preventive Medicine, 38*(6), 637–645.

Aptekar, L. (1988). *Street children of Cali*. Durham: Duke University Press.

Aptekar, L. (2010). *In the lions mouth: Hope and heartbreak in humanitarian assistance*. Bloomington: Xlibris.

Aptekar, L., & Ciano, L. (1999). Street children in Nairobi, Kenya: Gender differences and mental health. In M. Raffaelli & R. Larson (Eds.), *Homeless and working youth around the world: Exploring developmental issues: New directions for child and adolescent development*, Number 85 (pp. 35–46). San Francisco: Jossey Bass.

Archard, D. (2004). *Children, rights and childhood* (2nd ed.). London: Routledge.

ADB (Asian Development Bank). (2003). *Working with street children; Exploring ways for ADB*. Assistance: http://www.adb.org/Documents/Books/Street_Children/working_with_streetkids.pdf

Bao, W., Whitbeck, L., & Hoyt, D. (2000, December). Abuse, support, and depression among homeless and runaway adolescents. *Journal of Health and Social Behavior, 41*, 408–420.

Bar-On, A. (1998). So what's so wrong with being a street child? *Child & Youth Care Forum, 27*(3), 201–222.

Bassuk, E., & Donelan, B. (2003). Social deprivation. In B. Green, J. de Jong, M. Friedman, A. Marsella, et al. (Eds.), *Trauma interventions in war and peace: Prevention, practice, and policy* (pp. 33–55). New York: Kluwer.

Benn, C., & Weinreich, S. (2003). *AIDS – Eine Krankheit verändert die Welt*. Otto Lembeck: Frankfurt am Main.

Berry, L., & Hall, K. (2006). Children's access to education. In J. Monson, K. Hall, C. Smith, & M. Shung-King (Eds.), *South African child gauge 2006* (pp. 80–82). Cape Town: Children's Institute, University of Cape Town.

Brown, S., Cohon, D., & Wheeler, R. (2002). African-American extended families and kinship care: How relevant is the foster care model for kinship care? *Children and Youth Services Review, 24*(1), 53–77.

Cheng, F. C. (2006). The street children's street life and the victimizations against them: An ethnographic study. *Youth Studies, 9*, 1–9 (in Chinese).

Cheng, F. C. (2008). *Negotiating exclusion: An ethnographic study of the street children in Shanghai, China*. Unpublished doctoral dissertation. Hong-Kong: University of Hong-Kong.

Conticini, A. (2008). Surfing in the air: A grounded theory of the dynamics of street life and its policy implications. *Journal of International Development, 20*, 413–436.

Conticini, A., & Hulme, D. (2007). Escaping violence; seeking freedom: Why children in Bangladesh migrate to the street. *Development and Change, 38*(2), 201–227.

Davies, M. (2008). A childish culture? Shared understandings, agency and intervention: An anthropological study of street children in northeast Kenya. *Childhood, 15*(3), 309–330.

de Benitez, S. (2001). *What works in street children programming: The JUCONI model*. Baltimore: International Youth Foundation.

de Benitez, S. (2011). *State of the world's children: Research* (Street children series 2). London: Consortium of Street Children.

de Langen, M. (1992). The meaning of human rights for children. In M. Freeman & P. Veerman (Eds.), *The ideologies of children's rights* (pp. 255–264). Den Haag: Martinus Nijhoff Publishers.

Dybicz, P. (2005). Interventions for street children: An analysis of current best practices. *International Social Work, 48*(6), 1–9.

Dyregrov, A., Gjestad, R., & Raundalen, M. (2002). Children exposed to warfare: A longitudinal study. *Journal of Traumatic Stress, 15*(1), 59–68.

Ennew, J. (1994). *Street and working children – A guide to planning* (Developmental manual #4). London: Save the Children.

Ennew, J. (2003). Difficult circumstances: Some reflections on street children in Africa. *Children, Youth and Environments, 13*(1), 120.

Epstein, I. (1996). Educating street children: Some cross-cultural comparisons. *Comparative Education, 32*(3), 289–302.

Epstein, I. (2000). Dependence served: Rhetorical assumptions governing the education of homeless children and youth in the US. In R. Mickelson (Ed.), *Children on the streets of the Americas* (pp. 99–107). New York: Routledge.

Esser, F. (2004). Agency and generational difference. Einige Implikationen der indheitsforschung für die Sozialpädagogik. In H. Homfeldt, W. Schroer, C. Schweppe (Dir.) *Vom Adressaten zum Akteur: Soziale Arbeit und Agency* (pp. 133–153). Leverkusen, Germany: Barbara Budrich Publishers.

Etling, A. (1993). What is nonformal education? *Journal of Agricultural Education, 72–76*.

Ferguson, K. (2007). Implementing a social enterprise intervention with homeless street-living youth in Los Angeles. *Social Work, 52*(2), 103–112.

Ferguson, K., Dortzbach, K., Dyrness, G., Dabir, N., & Spruijt-Metz, D. (2013). Faith-based programmes and outcomes for street-living youth in Los Angeles, Mumbai and Nairobi: a comparative study. *International Social Work, 51*(2), 159–177.

Franklin, B. (1986). Children's political rights. In B. Franklin (Ed.), *The rights of children* (pp. 24–53). Oxford: Basil Blackwell.

Freeman, M. (2007). *Article 3; the best interest of the child. A commentary on the united nations convention on the rights of the child*. Leiden: Martinus Nijhoff Publishers.

Freire, P. (2003). *Pedagogy of the oppressed* (Trans: M. B. Ramos, 30th anniversary edition ed.). New York: Continuum.

Garder, F., Burton, J., & Klimes, I. (2006). Randomized controlled trial of a parenting intervention in the voluntary sector for reducing child conduct problems: outcomes and mechanisms of change. *Journal of Child Psychology and Psychiatry, 47*(11), 1123–1132.

Gross, B., & Gross, R. (1977). *The children's rights movement: Overcoming the oppression of young people*. New York: Anchor Books.

Hall, K. (2010). Income poverty, unemployment and social grants. In M. Kibel, L. Lake, P. Pendlebury, & C. Smith (Eds.), *South African child gauge 2009/2010* (pp. 105–109). Cape Town: Children's Institute, University of Cape Town.

Hall, K., & Meintjes, H. (2010). Demography of South Africa's children. In M. Kibel, L. Lake, P. Pendlebury, & C. Smith (Eds.), *South African child gauge 2009/2010* (pp. 99–104). Cape Town: Children's Institute, University of Cape Town.

Hanson, K. (2012). Schools of thought in children's rights. In M. Liebel et al. (Eds.), *Children's Rights from Below. Cross-cultural Perspectives* (pp. 63–79). Basingstoke: Palgrave Macmillan.
Harris, M., Johnson, K., Young, L., & Edwards, J. (2011). Community reinsertion success of street children programs in Brazil and Peru. *Children and Youth Services Review, 33*(5), 723–731.
Hart, R. (1992). *Children's participation from tokenism to citizenship*. Florence: Innocenti Research Centre.
Hecht, T. (1998). *At home in the street: Street children of Northeast Brazil*. Cambridge: Cambridge University Press.
Huang, C., & Huang, K. (2008). Caring for abandoned street children in La Paz, Bolivia. *Archive of Disabled Children, 93*, 626–627.
Hunt, F. (1994). Rights flow downhill. *The International Journal of Children's Rights, 2*, 343–368.
James, A., & Prout, A. (1990). A new paradigm for the sociology of childhood? Provenance, promise and problems. In A. James & A. Prout (Eds.), *Constructing and reconstructing childhood. Contemporary issues on the sociological study of childhood* (pp. 7–34). London: The Falmer Press.
Kidd, S., Miner, D. W., & Davidson, L. (2007). Stories of working with homeless youth: on being "mind-boggling". *Children and Youth Services Review, 29*(1), 16–34.
Knoepfel, P., Larrue, C., & Hill, M. (2007). *Public policy analyses*. Bristol: The Policy Press.
Kovats-Bernat, J. (2006). *Sleeping rough in Port-au-Prince: An ethnography of street children and violence in Haiti*. Gainesville: University of Florida Press.
Krabanow, J. (2003). Creating a culture of hope: Lessons learned from street children agencies in Canada and Guatemala. *International Social Work I, 46*(3), 369–386.
Lansdown, G. (2010). The realisation of children's participation rights: critical reflections. In B. Percy-Smith & N. Thomas (Eds.), *A handbook of children and young people's participation. Perspectives from theory and practice* (pp. 11–23). London/New York: Routledge.
Liebel, M. (1997). Children want to work. *NATs: Working Children and Adolescents International Review, 3*(3–4), 79–81.
Magazine, R. (2003). Action, personhood and the gift economy among so-called street children in Mexico City. *Social Anthropology, 11*(3), 303–318.
Marquez, P. (1999). *The street is my home: Youth and violence in Caracas*. Stanford: Stanford University Press.
Mason, J., & Bolzan, N. (2010). Questioning understandings of children's participation. Applying a cross-cultural lens. In B. Percy-Smith & N. Thomas (Eds.), *A handbook of children and young people's participation. Perspectives from theory and practice* (pp. 125–132). London/New York: Routledge.
Matthews, G. B. (2004). Children as philosophers. In P. Pufall & R. Unsworth (Eds.), *Rethinking childhood* (pp. 38–53). London: Rutgers University Press.
Mkombozi. (2010). *Think piece: External analysis of Mkombozi's streetwork*. Mkombozi. http://www.mkombozi.org/publications/think_piece/2010_04_12_think_piece_externalanalysis.pdf. Accessed 7 May 2012.
Montgomery, H. (2000). Abandonment and child prostitution in a Thai slum community. In C. Panter-Brick & M. Smith (Eds.), *Abandoned children* (pp. 182–189). Cambridge: Cambridge University Press.
Mosse, D. (2001). People's knowledge, participation and patronage: Operations and representations in rural development. In B. Cooke & U. Kothari (Eds.), *Participation: The new tyranny?* London: Zed Books.
Mtonga, J. (2011). On and off the streets: Reasons why street children escape institutional care and their survival on the streets. Unpublished Master's Degree. Trondheim: Norwegian Centre for Child research (NOSEB).
Nieuwenhuizen, P. (2006). *Street children in Bangalore, India: Their dreams and future*. Antwerp: Het Spinhuis Publishers.
Nieuwenhuys, O. (1994). *Children's life worlds: Gender, welfare and labor in the developing world*. London/New York: Routledge.

Nieuwenhuys, O. (2001). By the sweat of their brow? 'Street children', NGOS and children's rights in Addis Ababa. *Africa, 71*(4), 539–557.
Ordonez, D. (1994). *Metodologia: De Pirana a Delfin*. Lima: CEDRO.
Panter-Brick, C. (2004). Homelessness, poverty, and risks to health: Beyond at risk categorizations of street children. *Children's Geographies, 2*(1), 83–94.
Paradise, M., & Cauce, A. (2002). Home street home: The interpersonal dimensions of adolescent homelessness. *The Society for the Psychological Study of Social Issues, 2*(1), 223–238.
Parazelli, M. (2002). *La rue attractive. Parcours et pratiques identitaires des jeunes de la rue*. Sainte-Foy: Presses de l'Université du Québec.
Percy-Smith, B., & Thomas, N. (2010). *A handbook of children and young people's participation. Perspectives from theory and practice*. London/New York: Routledge.
Plummer, C., & Wambui, W. (2009). Cultural protective and risk factors: Professional perspectives about child sexual abuse in Kenya. *Child Abuse & Neglect, 33*, 524–532.
Pufall, P., & Unsworth, R. (2004). *Rethinking childhood*. London: Rutgers University Press.
Rizzini, I., & Lusk, M. (1995). Children in the streets: Latin America's lost generation. *Children and Youth Services Review, 17*(3), 391–400.
Rizzini, I., Mandel-Butler, U., & Stoecklin, D. (2007). *Life on the streets. Children and adolescents on the streets: Inevitable trajectories?* Sion: Institut International des Droits de l'enfant.
Rodriguez, D. C. (2004). *Empowering urban street children: Freirean and feminist perspectives on non-formal education in Mexico*. Ph.D. Los Angeles: University of Southern California. Retrieved from, http://proquest.umi.com/pqdweb?did=795927031&Fmt=7&clientId=15810&RQT=309&VName=PQD
Rotheram-Borus, M. J. (1993). Suicidal behavior and risk factors among runaway youth. *American Journal of Psychiatry, 150*(1), 103–107.
Sauve, S. (2003). Changing paradigms for working with street youth: The experience of street kids international. *Children, Youth, and Environments*, 13(1). Retrieved August 25, http://cye.colorado.edu
Schaffner, L. (1999). *Teenage runaways: Broken hearts and "bad attitudes"*. New York: Haworth Press.
Schumacher, S. (2011). *Children in street situations in South Africa*. Master of Advanced Studies in Children's Rights. Sion: IUKB.
Scivoletto, S., Fernando da Silva, T., & Rosenheck, R. (2011). Child psychiatry takes to the streets: A developmental partnership between a university institute and children and adolescents from the streets of Sao Paulo, Brazil. *Child Abuse and Neglect, 35*, 89–95.
Sen, A. (1999). *L'économie est une science morale*. Paris: La Découverte.
Shephard, D. (2011). *Non-formal education for improving educational outcomes in street children and street youth in developing countries: A systematic review*. M.Sc. Thesis. Oxford: University of Oxford.
Special Issue on Children as Social Actors. (2007). *The International Journal of Children's Rights, 15*(1).
Statssa (Statistics South Africa). (2010). *Quarterly, Labour Force Survey, 2010*. http://www.statssa.gov.za/publications/P0211/P02111stQuarter2010.pdf. Accessed 7 May 2012.
Stoecklin, D. (2000a). *Enfants des rues en Chine* (Street Children in China), Paris: Karthala.
Stoecklin, D. (2000b). *A baseline survey of the street children of Chittagong city in Bangladesh*. Dhaka: Aparajeyo-Bangladesh/Terre des hommes.
Stoecklin, D. (2007). Children in street situations: A rights-based approach. In I. Rizzini, U. Mandel Butler, & D. Stoecklin (Eds.), *Life on the streets. Children and adolescents on the streets: Inevitable trajectories?* (pp. 77–97). Sion: Institut International des Droits de l'enfant.
Stoecklin, D. (2009a). L'enfant acteur et l'approche participative. In J. Zermatten & D. Stoecklin (Eds.), *Le droit des enfants de participer. Norme juridique et réalité pratique: contribution à un nouveau contrat social* (pp. 47–71). Sion: IUKB/IDE.
Stoecklin, D. (2009b). Réflexivité, participation et capabilité. In: J. Zermatten & D. Stoecklin (Eds.), *Le droit des enfants de participer. Norme juridique et réalité pratique: contribution à un nouveau contrat social* (pp. 75–109). Sion: IUKB/IDE.

Stoecklin, D. (2013, November). Theories of action in the field of child participation. In search of explicit frameworks. *Childhood.* Issue 4, pp. 443–457.

Summerfield, D. (1999). A critique of seven assumptions behind psychological trauma programs in war-affected area. *Social Science and Medicine, 48*, 1449–1462.

TDH (Terre des hommes). (2012). *Children in street situations – Thematic policy*. Lausanne: Terre des hommes.

Thompson, E. (2001). *Non-formal education in Urban Kenya: Findings of a study in Kisumu, Mombasa and Nairobi* (p. 71). London: Commonwealth Secretariat.

UNHCR. (2008, May). *UNHCR guidelines on determining the best interests of the child.* UN High Commissioner for Refugees. Available at: http://www.refworld.org/docid/48480c342.html. Accessed 28 Apr 2013.

UNICEF. (2000). *Poverty reduction begins with children.* New York: UNICEF.

UNICEF CEE/CIS. (2010). *Blame and banishment. The underground HIV epidemic affecting children in Eastern Europe and Central Asia.* Geneva: UNICEF CEE/CIS.

UN General Assembly. (1989). *United Nations Convention on the Rights of the Child.* New York: United Nations.

Verhellen, E. (2000). *Convention on the rights of the child. Background, motivation, strategies, main themes.* Antwerpen: Garant Publishers.

Volpi, E. (2002). *Street children: Promising practices and approaches.* Washington, DC: World Bank Institute.

Werner, D. (1994). *Where there is no doctor: A health care handbook* (2nd ed.). London: Hersperian Health Guides.

Wernham, M. (2004). *An outside chance: Street children and juvenile justice – An international perspective.* London: Consortium for Street Children.

Wessells, M. (2006). *Child soldiers: From violence to protection.* Cambridge: Harvard University Press.

Woodhead, M. (2010). Forward. In B. Percy-Smith & N. Thomas (Eds.), *A handbook of children and young people's participation. Perspectives from theory and practice* (pp. xix–xxii). London/New York: Routledge.

Wright, J., Kaminsky, D., & Wittig, M. (1993). Health and social conditions of street children in Honduras. *American Journal of Disabled Children, 147*, 279–283.

Wydick, B. (1999). The effect of microenterprise lending on child schooling in Guatemala. *Economic Development and Cultural Change, 80*(2), 853–896.

Yon, M., & Mickelson, R. (2000). From church basement to mainstream classroom: The evolution of a child's place in Charlotte, North Carolina. In R. Mickelson (Ed.), *Children on the streets of the Americas* (pp. 160–171). New York: Routledge.

Yunus, M. (1999). *Banker to the poor: Micro-lending and the battle against world poverty.* New York: Public Affairs.

Zermatten, J. (2005). *Les enfants ont des droits: une révolution?* Sion: Institut Universitaire Kurt Bösch/Institut international des Droits de l'Enfant.

Zimmerman, B., Bandura, A., & Martinez-Pons, M. (1992). Self-motivation for academic attainment: The role of self-efficacy, beliefs and personal goal setting. *American Educational Research Journal, 29*, 663. doi:10.3102/00028312029003663.

Zutshi, B. (2000). *Impact, community response and acceptance of non-formal education under the National Child Labour Project: A case study of the carpet-weaving belt of Mirzapur-Bhadhoi and Glassbangle region of Ferozabad.* New Delhi: National Human Rights Commission of India.

Chapter 6
Summary, Conclusions and Recommendations

The Cross-Cultural Approach to Children in Street Situations

We made an effort to be precise about our terminology. We used the term **children in street situations** to refer to homeless youth in the developed world **and** street children in the developing world. Children in street situations, both homeless youth and street children, across cultures often shared some antecedents which were rooted in poverty, family violence and individual psychology. But not all children in street situations have these characteristics, nor are their origins the same. In order to understand these differences, we continued our definitions.

We defined homeless youth as coming from the developed world and going to the streets to escape abuse. We showed that their origins were from all social classes. Almost always, they left home in their teenage years. The gender ratio was about even; their mental health problematic.

We defined street children as coming from the developing world. We showed that poverty was a necessary but not sufficient condition to explain their reasons for going to the streets. Sometimes there was abuse and neglect, but some boys chose to leave simply because their lives were much the same as other poor boys growing up in urban situations. In the developing world, 90% of street children are boys. The picture of their mental health was not clear, probably because it varies quite a bit, but boys generally fared much better than female street children.

At one end of the spectrum of mental health were the children whose vulnerabilities put them at the mercy of exploitation by unsavoury people. On the other end were children in street situations who coped and did better than their abused or impoverished domiciled counterparts. Successful coping was more likely among street boys, who showed diverse coping strategies, and strong peer relations. Many of them had resilient personal characteristics. To be sure, we also found less successful children, but we found they were fewer in number than what we were led to believe. How well children in street situations coped was dependent on what culture they lived in, and how much they functioned as "social actors" facing difficult

L. Aptekar and D. Stoecklin, *Street Children and Homeless Youth: A Cross-Cultural Perspective*, DOI 10.1007/978-94-007-7356-1_6,

situations for better or worse. We discussed the subcultures of street children and homeless youth which included a very strong peer culture of respect, dependence, and family. More than any other factor, their friendships with each other provided a floor upon which they could stand.

The contents of the book were slightly skewed in favor of street children for two reasons. One was that the sheer numbers of street children far outnumbered the numbers of homeless youth, and secondly the amount of resources in programs, research and writing for homeless youth far outweighed those for street children. While the research we present on homeless youth is not exhaustive, it will meet the needs of the reader whose focus is on how homeless youth in the developed world fit into the cross-cultural picture of children in street situations.

When we talked about homeless youth, we showed that their mental health was troubled; in part because they were the victims of abuse and neglect, but also because there were no cultural role models to follow. They were forced to be dependent on the State, which provided them with housing, food and medical care, but not with the freedom of the streets. Most were troubled. Altruism, even among themselves was rare. We showed that the State gave them very little room to be on their own, and they often languished in poorly run programs.

In contrast, we explained that in many ways street children were like poor adults; they had jobs, places to live, things they enjoyed, etc. And like adults living in poverty, with whom they shared the same general appearance of place and possessions, some were hateful, disloyal and self-serving, while others cared for the weak, respected their subculture, and aspired to belong to a better world.

Because of our cross-cultural emphasis, we showed that the terms "street child" or "homeless youth" did not exist in a vacuum: they are social constructions with a specific point of view that is predominant. We gave examples showing comunity members analysing children in street situations, using their own values, positions and interests; for some, these children were bandits, for others victims.

Programs that served children in street situations and the State that struggled to care for them, exaggerated their numbers and emphasized their problems. When these figure were presented to the public, as they often were, they increased feelings of insecurity among the middle and upper social classes, which, in turn, justified the State in "cleaning-up" the streets. Yet, we showed that in some places, their numbers were underestimated, their difficulties were over-simplified, and even talk about them was censured.

Children in street situations shared in being repeatedly marginalised by social and cultural forces. They experienced some form of conflict with the main institutions of socialisation and protection; school, family, and the State. In spite of international law, they were given little opportunity to contribute to decisions concerning themselves.

We follow with a series of questions, which are difficult to answer for people working with children in street situations and an opportunity for study for researchers.

Our historical information showed that children in street situations come from nearly every country, have existed for centuries, and endure to the present day. The cultural and historical comparisons we offered have enabled us to pose important questions: Why are there fewer than expected children in street situations in certain cultures and more than expected in others? Why do some children leave home, but their siblings do not, and what combinations of parenting practices contributed to or mitigated children leaving home? Why does poverty force some children to the streets, but not their siblings or peers? Does the subjective meaning of being a child in a street situation differ in different cultures?

We were able to answer some but not all of these questions, because even though we presented the pertinent information, there are considerable differences by place and from different researchers. The reader will know where and how to begin research, and what types of programs are justified by empirical data and what practices need to be avoided and how to change them.

What we did show with confidence is that some children in street situations were not abandoned, but were abandoning. We found that the reasons for this vary. In some cases children do the abandoning because they prefer the streets and the company of peers, over living with abusive parental discipline.[1] While in most countries children in street situations have the legal right to leave home under the United Nations Convention on the Rights of the Child (UNCRC), it is not likely they will be allowed to do so.

Children's Rights, the UNCRC and Cultural Differences

In this section we ask another round of questions, each of which present a moral dilemma for people working with children in street situations and a challenge for researchers.

We traced the history of children's rights from the first half of the 20th century, showing that the focus remained on the physical welfare rights of children. An important first step was the UN Declaration on the Rights of the Child (UNDRC 1959). It was not until the drafting of the UNCRC (1989) that human rights were seen in the broader context of defining what roles children should play in society. We gave examples, showing that carrying out this new focus has run into many problems, not the least of which were based on cultural differences. For example, while the UNCRC gives children the right of free speech and the right to make choices about where they live, etc., these rights are often in direct contrast with adult views of acceptable childhood and parenting. This allowed us to examine a variety of cultural differences among parenting and child development practices. While these differences appeared to be academic, we showed how in many cases they led to the persecution of children in street situations. Parents from the developed world would be unlikely to support for example, a child of 12 or 13 who decides to leave home, live with other children, and drop out of school. We from the West make the case that children of that age are not capable of making good decisions (although

[1] We also looked at conflicting interests between those of the parents and those of the child; particularly as they related to child participation in the UNCRC.

some of these same parents aren't capable at any age). But in the developing world, particularly among the poor, there is another point of view, which may be largely a result of the difficult circumstances that they face.

We showed that there are many problems that come from reliance of the UNCRC on the Westerners' version of childhood, that it should be a period of play, school, and freedom from major economic and social responsibilities. This is far from being the case among all cultures; and almost by definition not the case for street children, and unlikely to be the case for homeless youth.

Thus, increasingly the UNCRC is being interpreted to mean that prolonged dependence on the family and attending formal schools is the only context for rearing, protecting and socializing children. We did find empirical evidence to confirm this. In fact, children in poor countries flourish. They work and study, share economic and social responsibilities with adults, and have broad community access to the information and activities available to adults. On the other side, we attracted attention on the possible traps of the "competent" child discourse, whereby a romanticized view of children's agency and responsibilities might be used as a neo-liberal apology with the effects of undermining economic and social rights.

We showed that the UNCRC can be interpreted along diverging schools of thought (from paternalism to liberation) and consequently these different interpretations may collide in various ways with culturally accepted traditions. While there might be some parenting practices that can be universally accepted, the question is where among parental actions should we draw the line between cultural relativism and universalism?

For example, in the developed world, we showed that among homeless youth there are considerable numbers of children from nuclear families who have been abused. Is it better to force them to stay at home or better to allow them to leave? Who decides and how?

Among developing countries, perhaps the most cited question is how can we approve of female circumcision even if it is presented as having cultural meaning, or does any cultural argument ever justify mutilation? What about female children whose parents have their limbs amputated, or their faces burned by acid? What should Westerner's do if local authorities don't react to these human rights violations perpetrated within their jurisdictions? Do these abuses of human rights call for other nations to intervene? While the UN Committee on the Rights of the Child can put pressure on State parties who have ratified but do not follow the UNCRC, they have little authority to intervene. Should they have more? At this time under article 4 of the UNCRC it is specified that if a country is unable to reach the standards included in the law, it should resort to international aid. The legal means to "intervene" are not military, but linked to development and aid policies. What happens if there is not sufficient aid to do this?

We can be encouraged by the success of advocacy campaigns to improve implementation of children's human rights. For example, advocacy helped reduce the problems of child marriage in Nepal (Tronchet-Pradhan 2011), and protective associations of child workers in Latin America helped reduce abhorrent child labor practices (Liebel 1997).

How does this liberationist view of the UNCRC apply in the case of children in street situations? We showed that as the numbers of children in street situations grew, the more likely it was that the children were seen as a "problem" or a "menace" by international organizations. As the problem appeared bigger and more insoluble, it provoked a growing hostility on the part of the local populace toward the children in street situations.[2]

A cycle began; as society became more aggressive towards the children so the children became more aggressive in response, in turn provoking more violent reactions against them. At some point both sides were out of compliance with the law.

We showed that children in street situations should have the power to do more than just being allowed by adult authorities to talk and participate regarding only mundane or indisputable matters. They should be allowed to confront adult authority and learn by reasoning how to exercise their human rights. We think this can be done without escalating violence by having, as we said above, the power of an advocacy group to support them.

We believe there are many children in street situations who show us a new way for children to grow up in dysfunctional families and societies. We say this while knowing that many of the people we referenced in our book found that children in street situations live very negatively, so we must acknowledge that any comments to the contrary carry a heavy burden of proof. There is always the danger of minimizing their vulnerability and the future consequences that living on the street will have for them. We do know there are different reactions to street life, because some do better than others. What we don't know (and what would make for a good research project) is for all those who have survived and appeared in research studies as resilient, how many have not survived?

Likewise, when we looked across cultures, we saw so many abused and poor children that the pertinent question is not why there are so many children in street situations, but why so few? To address this, and indeed many of the questions we ask, we need longitudinal data. Without longitudinal data, we don't know if, as some writers suggest, living on the street is a passing phase and the children will successfully reintegrate themselves into society (Ennew 1994; Swart 1989, 1990), or whether it is a reality that reinforces their marginalization and social exclusion.

We have demonstrated that there are many problems with research including getting a random sample so that inferential statistics can be used. We showed some different ways that a random sample might be drawn. We emphasize the need to be clear about the characteristics of the sample group. We recommend the use of projective type instruments in lieu of those such as questionnaires and other paper and pencil tests that make it easier for children to adapt their responses to perceived expectations.

When we talked about defining street children clearly, we asked several questions including what amount of time spent in the street is required to be considered

[2] A good case study of this can be seen in Angola, where within five years the country went from no street children to many. At first there was a willingness on the part of the public to assist them as they were seen as victims of the war, but as the numbers grew they became from the public's point of view "thieves" or "delinquents" and full of "vices".

a "street child" or a "homeless youth". We suggested some ways that a career path from domiciled to homelessness could be demarcated stage by stage and offered some information from researchers, but more work on the long term psychological consequences and more longitudinal data are needed. At this point, there is a dearth of age-sensitive information, knowledge of the cumulative stressors these children have, and a careful plotting of a child's developmental path.

We stressed that development studies must take into account gender differences and to stop referring to studies on street children and homeless youth and to begin studies on street boys and street girls and homeless boys and homeless girls.

We also lamented the lack of comparisons between children in street situations and matched peers (either other poor children living at home, or siblings or relatives living at home) because we believe that this could help prevent children living a life that would be damaging. And, it is the only way we can bring clarity to the results of living a street versus a domiciled life.

There are few empirical studies that inform or lead policy makers (and researchers) toward evidence-based programs. This means, among other things, that there is no way of knowing if current funding is working or even effective. They warn, as we have also warned, against evaluative studies based on unacceptable methodology and often involved in conflicts of interest and producing biased data because the results are more about competing for funding than producing solid empirical evidence.

Without empirical evidence and longitudinal data, it becomes too easy to violate the basic ethical principle of doing no harm. Too often the aid community quotes articles that have used questionable research methods or assumed that the children were truly free to participate in research, even though the children may well have believed that if they dropped out they would have lost something valuable, and if they stayed in the study they would surely say whatever they thought would be most profitable to themselves. We do not believe that research that is focused on emphasizing children's problems will do justice to their resilience and it might make normal reactions to extreme stress seem like mental health problems.

We said we wanted to avoid using predefined questions and categories without taking into account the children's input into the research process. And we wanted to be sure that professionals from developing countries routinely are involved in supplying their expertise. We thought context in studies is often undervalued, and that there is little attempt to develop local scholarship. Similar comments might pertain to the use of children, which can promote better scholarship while not incorporating them might possibly be against the rights of children to participate in what affects them.

Working Children

We examined the majority of street in children situations, but we covered their work less completely. We did talk about begging; here we want to address the fact that these children are also child workers, and child labor is also subject to international conventions (OHCHR 2012). Working on the streets entails exposure to weather, environmental pollutants, and crime. For example, children working in the kilns in Pakistan (Awan 2008) carry heavy bricks to and from the machines, and it is not unusual for accidents to occur involving their hands and fingers. The dust can be unbearable and many suffer from respiratory diseases. Some children start working when they are 5 or 6 years old. Other children in street situations make their way by being porters, carrying heavy loads repeatedly. In the developed world, it is not unusual to see small children working long hours in agricultural fields, also exposed to the weather and environmental pollutants.

Abuse is also common among child workers. One study in India reported that two-thirds of the children were abused (Mathur et al. 2009). In Nepal, child porters were carrying loads that were more than their weight and also experienced abuse (Celik and Baybuga 2009). Garbage workers in Latin America were particularly exposed to environmental waste, and being ill with TB and Typhoid (Pinzon-Rondon 2010).

How Much Is Fair?

At some point we will have to find programs and policies which deal with the sheer magnitude of children outside of family care, some of whom are children in street situations. Boothby et al. (2012) quote the latest statistics: nearly18 million children are parentless. In the developing world, there are approximately 200 million children under 5 years of age who are slow to meet developmental milestones, due to poverty and its concomitant lack of nutrition.

About 1.8 million children have been sexually trafficked and 150 million girls and 73 million boys have experienced forced sexual intercourse or other forms of sexual violence. More than a million have been forced into labor, but about 115 million children are engaged in hazardous work.

The authors tell us that in spite of these staggering figures there is very little funding for programs or research for children whose lives are like these. Not all of these children are children in street situations. Some critics have argued that children in street situations are getting too much attention (and too much NGO money).[3] We said that street children make up only a very small percentage of poor children. And, that homeless youth are a small part of children who are abused. A case could be made that children in street situations have, in effect, diverted social services from the much larger group of poor and abused children who while living at home are in need of various kinds of essential help.[4]

The stark truth is that even if we fund programs for the grossest inequities of child labor, such as the child camel riders or the children who work in carpet factories, or

[3] Categorizations, "children at risk", "children in especially difficult circumstances", or "children in or of the streets", endure in spite of being stigmatizing, because the tags help the humanitarian aid community fight for funds. Funding them does little to alleviate the larger problems of children in street situations, which are poverty and abuse.

[4] Panter-Brick (2002) believes that help is focused on street children because they lived in public view and in the absence of parental attention.

the most traumatized children, such as child soldiers with their own or others' blood on their hands, and the children traumatized by disaster who lost, in seconds, whole families in front of their eyes; we will fall short of helping the children who grow up poor in the shanty towns of the developing world where they can't go to school, because what few scraps they can gather during the school hours are needed to feed the family. For these children, there are no inoculations to be had or food to be eaten. Because of poor nutrition, they have compromised immune systems, and because they live among free-flowing untreated sewage, (for which no projects are funded), and without clean water, they do not live as long as children with material resources. And during their lives they may never be really fully functioning.

The majority of poor children earn what money they can to help their families, yet because they are not living as premature adults in the central cities occupying valuable public terrain in full public view, they receive nothing from the State and not much from the international volunteer community. The research studies and the money go to the children in street situations, not because they are the neediest for humanitarian reasons, but for political reasons; they threaten the established order.

In the developed world, when we talk about runaway and homeless youth, we have a similar situation. To be sure, the slums in the developed world are less toxic in comparison to the shanty towns of the developing world, but the income differentiation between the poor and the middle class in the developed world has widened. And, while there are very few homeless youth who sleep rough in the developed world, because the State is too strong to allow them to do so, and the resources are sufficient to have options, the fact remains that political rather than humanitarian concerns govern who gets what, with the over-representation of homeless youth who might threaten the status quo and not enough resources for the poor who could benefit from the money that might bring about structural changes for preventing abuse. Nor is there access to equal funding for schooling, medical care, and economic opportunity.

There is, however, another side to this argument about children in street situations getting too much of the pie. As we have shown, in the few comparative studies many street children are coping as well as or better than their stay-at-home siblings, so teaching them to read and helping them to become leaders can be considered a more satisfactory way to provide aid than it would be to provide such support for their lower functioning stay-at-home siblings. Yet, the funding often goes in the other direction.

Almost any kind of help is good, but there is surely not enough to go around. We are still left with the question; who is to make these decisions, and how? And what, if any, should be the role of the UNCRC in this debate?

A Public Mental Health Model for Children in Street Situations

In Chapter 5 we discussed programs and policies for children in street situations on the basis of individual merit and in the relation to the three levels of help (micro, meso, and macro). We found a paucity of programs that deal with the macro level or working at all three levels. Here we propose a policy for helping children in street situations which uses a public mental health model. This is a major suggestion of on our part, because it establishes a blue print upon which one can see what services are being provided and what needs to be done.

We break it down into three forms of care, primary, secondary, and tertiary, each of which has two ways to offer help, direct or indirect.

Primary care provides help to homeless youth or street children usually at the micro level. It can be direct primary care which helps the children in street situations directly. For example, we could give financial vouchers to the children in street situations so they can attend school and get sufficient food. A program in Kenya which is run by International Childcare Trust, established a safe haven shelter for street children who were in crisis. The expectation was that the children would return to their families when the crisis abated.[5] Timing is a factor in direct primary care. For example, by focusing on the time when children are in high risk situations, we can get the most for our investment. When children first enter street life, it is an opportune moment for direct primary mental health care services.

Indirect primary care provides services to those who help the target group, such as making the homes of homeless youth less abusive which in turn helps homeless youth. In Brazil, for example, Rizzini (1992) found that street children reported higher incidents of corporal punishment at home, (63%) compared to (23%) of working street children. In Ethiopia, homeless children reported significantly higher levels of abuse at home in the form of violence, shouting among family members and beatings, than was reported by family-based street children (Veale 1996). In both cases, we can help the children (target group) by helping those who take care of them (indirect method).

Timing is also valuable in indirect primary care. For example, support is needed for parents of children in street situations when a household member dies, or is away for work or when there is war; because at these times the strains of being a single parent caregiver are at the highest. Such programs might focus on particular families with children in street situations who, if given help at the right time, would meet the supportive goals of indirect primary care.

The target group of secondary mental health services are those children who are already in street situations but are not coping or who have an additional problem, such as the need for medical care. Secondary care helps to reduce or eliminate their problem. In essence, secondary care is for those who are not coping well and who, hopefully, by virtue of receiving care will not get worse. It can be direct secondary care aimed directly at the target groups, such as providing appropriate mental health care, including medical treatment, to those children with these problems. Even those at the highest risk (low self-esteem, poor communication skills, drug abusing, abused, etc.) can, at certain moments, learn how to take advantage of what is being offered and learning how to identify new opportunities to take advantage of.

[5] This particular program was in a rural area. That is important to note because most programs for street children are found in the major urban areas. But as war becomes a more important causal factor, there are more rural children who become displaced, or orphaned.

Timing is also important in direct secondary care. There might be opportune moments to provide direct secondary care, such as when street children or homeless youth have already had their first contact with the police or the justice system. As they are being adjudicated for the first time, they are in crisis which is often the opportune time to listen and learn. It is better to strike before the problem is exacerbated.

Homeless youth and street children have developmental milestones that are predictable and difficult. Direct secondary care could provide support for those who are having a particularly hard time during the period of physical maturation into adolescence or the transition from street child to adult citizen.

Indirect secondary care supports those who are helping street children or homeless youth when the children are already showing signs of not coping well. This includes supporting drug abuse counselors, and the myriad of programs provided by the NGOs. Help might also be directed at community mental health programs that work with children in street situations who have mental disorders. It could also mean adopting an educational approach that would take into account the unusual skills children in street situations have as a result of street life.

Tertiary care focuses on the larger issues of prevention and education. There are two formats that have driven educational policy for homeless youth and street children. The first has a technical model which was developed from professional educators who adopted a curriculum designed to meet the problems of "at risk students". It can be used as a tertiary indirect method of mental health, if it educates teachers on how to prevent children going into street situations. It champions such things as a change in curriculum or a change in the delivery of the curriculum by building new curriculum (with the children's participation) or to have a new method of delivery with children in street situations teaching the prevention materials or by acting them out.

As we have said, children living in street situations, by assuming the right to live as they choose, have taken on many of the qualities associated with adulthood, (either attending or not attending school, entering public restaurants for something to drink or eat, by becoming intoxicated when and where they desire, and by working to support themselves). They have done this in full public view. As a result they have received sanctions, in many cases of immense proportion. We can help prevent this by educating the public about young children assuming adulthood earlier than certain cultural expectations allow. If we can do this, we might be able to negotiate a truce in the troubled space where children assume adult roles, and where the public views and responds to them with such fear and anger.

The second format of preventive education has a political model; this approach is usually community-based. In this case the education is not for correction or control but for teaching the community or nation how to support the human rights of children in street situations granted to them by the UNCRC, or how to teach police to provide the special protections for children in street situations that are guaranteed them in the UNCRC. This might be done in formal teaching or by providing community education, say through street signs (like those used in the USA to prevent smoking).

Direct tertiary care strengthens communities and institutions that can support children at risk, and helps grow a civic politic that is involved with children's welfare. At the local level a direct tertiary care program could identify high risk neighborhoods or groups, say where there is a demographic of a lot of child abuse, and plan a community wide education program of parenting to prevent family discord that might lead to abuse.

In a large community, indirect tertiary care could take the form of helping justice agencies refocus their efforts from adjudicating the petty crimes of children in street situations to the larger crimes perpetrated on street children and homeless youth. Indirect tertiary care could include teaching stakeholders that structural adjustment policies adversely affect vulnerable children.

Tertiary care can have a political agenda by supporting education to large social movements that give power to the excluded who then can force the government into making changes for the disenfranchised (Klees et al. 2000).

In 1986, as a result of prior political organization, the National Movement of Street Boys and Girls had their first public meeting in Brasilia. About 500 street children impressed the audience (with scores of media present) with their tales of violence perpetrated on them.

This movement joined forces with other political groups working on similar child related issues. Using the framework of the UNCRC, they were able to include a great part of their agenda into the newly forming constitution being written as the country went from military to civilian rule. The UN law guaranteeing the Rights of the Child was passed. The next political step was to lobby for implementation. This can be supported by ongoing tertiary care that promotes political pressure, rather than technical arguments.

Using a tertiary indirect model to change public opinion could follow up on the fact that almost all the research that has been done with street children has led to the conclusion that as difficult as life is for street children, the worst problem the children face is from the public. Nor is this problem only associated with street children; it is also a problem for homeless youth. In the case of street girls, this often takes the form of sexual abuse, in the case of street boys it often takes the form of violent hostility. In many places in the world, street children have been assassinated for no more than petty crimes and haughty behaviour. In fact, the number of street children killed in Brazil supersedes the total casualties in the civil war in Lebanon.

Simon, a child of 15 years of age, was murdered by a police reservist (Aptekar and Ciano 1999). So many poor unkempt children had already been mistreated that his demise would not have aroused much concern except that he was shot five times at point blank range, kicked into the gutter, and then spat upon. Evidently, Simon had stolen a signal lens from a parked car. There were no other complaints about Simon. No one said that he was belligerent or that he assaulted anyone. How was it that Simon's relatively minor crime aroused such anger in the police officer? Was he seen in the context of a grand menace? Was he used as a warning to the larger group of street children? If these answers could be found, we might be able to offer a preventive education to the public to help reduce this hostility.

We believe that children in street situations, in nearly all cultures in the world, have become symbols of moral judgement because they violate the norms that most cultures maintain regarding children. They do this by not being under the same roof as their parents, by working instead of going to school, and by assuming the right to enjoy the fruits of their work as they choose (such as consuming drugs). What makes the climate so volatile is that the phenomena of children taking on the roles of adults is peaking at a time when many societies are moving from traditional to modern codes of conduct; from codes related to birthrights and long accepted roles of authority to codes based on rational values, democratic choices, and a world-wide culture based on the western entertainment media.

Like the alleged murderer of Simon, who seemingly quickly (and falsely) made a connection between large-scale societal problems and the petty problems of minor delinquency caused by some street children, other murderers of street children justify their actions in self-righteous moral terms, seeing themselves as heroes in cultures rapidly approaching moral decay.

The study of street children and runaway youth brings to the table important issues and raises important questions. Is it the case that the children are at risk, or is it that the children are the risk? In the case of Simon, the case shows that a good boy who was a street kid was killed by police and that all over the world street children and runaway youth fear the police most. The public, thinking the kids are a menace, employs its public servants to eradicate the menace. But could not the case be made that the public is the menace? Are these children to be pitied because of a lost childhood, or admired for surviving against such odds, or feared for their gangs and delinquency? Do we assume the premise of *The Lord of the Flies*, that children-led groups lead to the powerful taking over the weak, or do we assume the inherent goodness of children?

These varied perceptions contribute to the confusing image of who the street children are and lead to several myths about the children. Each perception gives as much information about the perceivers as it does about the perceived. Aptekar (1988) places street children in the complex, if not ambivalent, feelings toward children's "place" as part of the everyday commerce between social classes.

Street children are in the grey area between sympathy and disgust, and are both a threat and a disgrace. In a good part of the developing world there are vast extremes of wealth and an ever-present possibility of a violent change in power. Defining the boundaries of the appropriate amount of submission to authority is a serious concern that affects everyone in the society.

Street children have become cultural scapegoats portrayed as carriers of all the large-scale social problems, including inequality of income, changing family values with concomitant alterations in the roles of men and women, and the reduction in personal security in the context of an overly romanticised past. Only when the vastness and complexities of this situation are confronted will the hostilities be reduced. There is an old African saying, "*if you want to get to the root of a murder, you have to look for the blacksmith who made the panga* (machete or cutlass)". This is to say that if you want to help street children, it is not the street children or their families, but the culture where they live that needs the help.

Our work has led us to believe that in spite of many fine programs at the primary and secondary levels, what we still need is a considerable effort in the area of tertiary care, particularly indirect tertiary care to resolve the issue of community violence. We also suggest combining primary, secondary and tertiary approaches.

We report below two examples of programs that are adhering to the public mental health approach we are suggesting. Using his work in Ethiopia and Bangladesh as case studies, Conticini (2008) broke down the process of leaving home and becoming a child in a street situation into stages beginning with the first days and weeks on the streets. His work is directed toward street children, we expand his ideas to include homeless youth. His model can be used as a guideline for understanding interventions based on psycho-social developmental periods.

At first children in street situations need street educators, (essentially former street children or homeless youth who can relate to street children). These should be the first interventions (indirect primary care), followed by assistance in temporary shelter and other basic needs which should be offered to new street children (direct primary care).[6]

The complete adaptation of the child or youth to the streets can take a year or two. During this phase the child begins learning how to deal with the informal market and how to generate income. By the end of this phase, the child has a peer network, is able to survive but likely does not have security. Because of their original trauma that caused them to leave home (if indeed this was the case) and the repeated interactions with adults who might want to abuse them, or arrest them, or otherwise take advantage of them, they are very wary of adults.

Instead of trying to encourage children in street situations to go back home, attention should be focused on having the family and community help the child without making a demand to return to what was an untenable situation (indirect primary care).

Once the child is accustomed to street life, he or she begins to help the newcomers learn the ropes. Counseling at this phase should be oriented to the future in which the child in a street situation, can look to the future by shedding past history, and thinking about starting his or her own family (direct primary care and in some cases direct secondary care).

Young adults must have a safe space, know where to move around to secure income, and have some positive relationships with adults. There are of course gender distinctions, girls having a harder time.

Because of the long history with police, drugs and sex, and possibly radical political groups, they can be encouraged to think what the future holds for them and they are making plans. Because they share a common history, group counseling is appropriate. Through group experience they might be ready to work on their

[6] He begins with a critique on current research practices, which he says are too descriptive without being analytical, do not look at how services can be provided, and focus on case studies without a theoretical framework. Above all, he is bothered by the fact that research talks more about the children's problems, than it does on their strategies for earning a living and becoming effective adults.

traumas (direct secondary care). The counselor can reinforce the positive skills the children have had because of their street experience, in particular economic skills that will take them out of the streets (indirect primary and secondary care).[7]

While there may be some success as the children and youth age into young adulthood, the route will not be continual. No doubt some will fall from time to time to less maturity. And some will never be able to cope well as adults. There are too many children in street situations who are working for drug lords or arms dealers, and too many are still prevented from moving forward by the police or societal attitudes.

They can certainly be helped with better living situations, (indirect secondary care). And they can benefit by having counselors who provide encouragement for what they have done and avoid criticism about earlier decisions (this is as an example of direct secondary care).

Any career and personal developmental model has the advantage of seeing how children in street situations cope over a time period. The direction seems to go from fear of securing basic needs with a low level of cognitive coping ability to a cognitively sophisticated strategy of forming a new life based on what they want and aspire to having.

Another public mental health approach was carried out in Ethiopia by Save the Children. They began by providing direct primary care to those children who were new to the streets by feeding and sheltering them (see Veale et al. 1993). After this first phase, they moved into a secondary indirect approach that dealt with reducing poverty for families whose children were failing. They began with having community members nominate those children and families who were at highest risk. Then they provided a micro-credit program for mothers to start income generating businesses.

They also targeted parents (indirect primary approach) in order to increase communication between them and their street children. They taught parents how to take care of their own personal needs without expressing anger toward the children. This was done through teaching self-discipline skills, and increasing self-esteem. The idea was that with better parenting children on the streets would be healthier mentally and physically.

They continued to work with parents, in this case those who were working all day, many of whom had a long uncomfortable commute. These parents were trying to support the household and usually had more than one child. When they got home they were often met by one or more of their children unwilling to accept their authority. These parents needed help to cope.

The program offered indirect tertiary care by providing public preventive education to the broader society about the dangers of street life. They worked in indirect tertiary care by training police to see street children as not necessarily being delinquent or a threat to the public order. They trained them about the UNCRC laws, telling them that these laws should guide their actions in dealing with street children. In doing this they were almost unique. Because there are tens of thousands

[7] Dybicz (2005) suggests micro-credit (indirect primary care), but only if the credit applies to earning an income in a better environment.

of people devoted to helping street children by working directly with them, but the important work of changing society's attitudes toward street children is almost completely neglected. Whether this is because direct care is easier to administer and evaluate than community development is not clear. But whatever the reason, ignoring the work of changing the public's perception is problematic.

Taking Care of Yourself

Finally we offer to those who work with children in street situations a message about the importance of taking care of yourself. You will need to deal with difficult ethical problems in a way that prevents burnout.

Since we believe that almost any effort to help children in street situations is better than none, the more you stay in the field, the more heroic your efforts. To do this, you might have to develop a different *modus operandi* than most program workers. For several years, Aptekar (2003) worked with an elderly priest who had been working with street children for nearly four decades. Each Monday night the priest conducted street work on the streets of a large city with several young men and women interested in learning how to work with street children. It was his pleasure to accompany him. One rainy evening they stopped to talk to a group of about a dozen boys who were living at the back of a dead-end alley. After talking with them about getting help, they bought each of them a bag of chips and then went off to the next group of children who received the same treatment. As was the custom, at the end of each evening they would sit down to discuss the evening's work over chicken and chips. Afterwards, as they were on their way home, they encountered a group of seven girls about 13–15 years old. They came into the street, stopped at their car, and pointed to one girl who stayed behind in the shadows. This girl clearly had a high fever and was delusional. She was either suffering from malaria, from an overdose of drugs, or even from syphilis. Whatever the reason for the girl's illness, they implored the priest to take their sick companion to the hospital. He refused and told them he would check on her in the morning. As we drove back to where Aptekar was staying, he asked the priest why he left the girl in such a crisis. The priest said it was past ten o'clock at night, and if he took her to the hospital he wouldn't get home until past one in the morning. He had mass to give at six and a full day of street work already planned to do afterward. "I have to draw the line somewhere", he said.

One fact of street work that needs to be learned is that there are always more troubled children than there are resources to help them. At some point everyone has to turn his (or her) back, if for no other reason than to move forward to the next day. The priest's refusal to administer to the sick child, a decision learned from decades of experience, was based on the greater good. Yet, when Aptekar saw him leave this sick young girl alone in the rainy night he felt betrayed. How could he let himself be mentored by such a person? The priest wasn't living up to the moral standards of his calling; Aptekar found himself evaluating 40 years of good work by a single late night decision.

Making moral judgments toward colleagues is rampant in this work. Aptekar, in this case made a judgement about what was appropriate and inappropriate for the priest. He did this in spite of the fact that each time he visited a program for street children, no matter what continent or hemisphere, people spoke disparagingly about another program across town. They also spoke badly about people helping in a different style than their own. He had seen the religious assail the secular, tough disciplinarians complain about the easy-going, those in favour of sheltering fight against those who favour fostering, etc.

Yet, there is little correlation between a program's official written policy and the ways that different children experience the program. There is plenty of room for nearly all philosophies and nearly every style of help. What keeps diversity, experimentation, and variety from flourishing in the work and what leads to burn out can often be traced to ethnocentric values and moral judgments made.

The work is fraught with ethical dilemmas (Aptekar 2003). The distance between those with wealth and children in street situations is so vast, that one has to ask himself why or how such a world as this can or should exist. Pragmatically, when is the time to give or to intervene and what is the amount to give, and worse when is the time to stop, and if you stop, how?

As we said in chapter 3, when we discussed Sister Mary, the Italian Comboni nun who specialized in working with "outcasts", the best way through the difficulty of keeping an ethical balance and to avoid burnout over time is to find your own way of working and your own illogical approach to it. Hers was filled with qualifications, omissions, and idiosyncratic rules. What we said in her case was that the idea was not to fulfill politically correct Western ethics, but to do what you can sometimes leaving your intelligence in a distant corner of the room, and bringing your heart to the forefront, and above all not worrying about covering your back or looking over your shoulder. Any help counts (Fig. 6.1).

Conclusion

In our final conclusion, we summarize some of the main points, beginning with defining children in street situations as including homeless youth; who come from the developed world, are equally divided by gender, likely to be abused and functioning poorly; and street children; who come from the developing world, are 90% male and who live much like the urban poor. We showed how the developmental paths are different for boys than those for girls.

The synopsis of research problems with children in street situations included unclear definitions, non-random samples, and poor choices of data collection. We gave examples to solve these problems, such as avoiding questionnaires, and using projective techniques. We explained the mental status exam and how it might be used to help get valid data.

There is a need for comparative research between children in street situations and their siblings at home or matched peers from the same circumstances. This would

Fig. 6.1 Any help counts

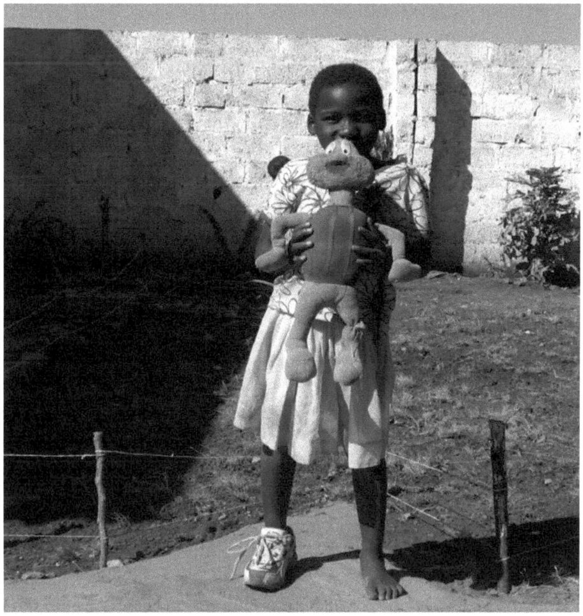

help us to understand why children go to the streets. We also spoke about the lack of longitudinal data, which could help us know the effects of street life on the eventual development of these children into adults. We mentioned research that outlined developmental phases, which was needed to understand children in street situations as they moved from home to being partially non-domiciled to full engagement in street life.

The adoption of the United Nations Convention on the Rights of the Child (UNCRC) meant that children's rights went beyond the physical well-being of children to the human rights granted adults. One problem with this is that the definition of children and their rights tends to use a Western model at the expense of different, but legitimate child rearing practices in other cultures. Thus, enforcing the UNCRC presented a lot of problems as cultural differences made for many ethical and practical questions. We gave some examples of this.

The children's rights movement has had some accomplishments in helping children in street situations access their legal rights. We compared the problems of children in street situations with the problems of other children at high risk to ask how the pie of assistance should be divided. We reviewed the arguments for more or less funding for children in street situations. We asked for programs to use empirical evaluative data and to avoid interventions that were not supported by research.

We presented a public mental health model of three types of services, primary, secondary, and tertiary care. Each of the three can be divided into direct and direct services. The former is helping the recipient directly while the latter is helping those who help them.

Primary care includes direct services to children in street situations, and indirect services to their families. Secondary care focuses on children who are already in street situations and who need help. Direct care would be providing mental or physical services for this group, while indirect care trains those who are providing the help. Tertiary care focuses on the larger issues of prevention and education. Direct tertiary care strengthens communities and institutions that support children in street situations; indirect tertiary care educates teachers and others on how to prevent children from going into street situations. We call for more funding for tertiary care. And, last but not least, we offer some examples to prevent burnout.

References

Aptekar, L. (1988). *Street children of Cali.* Durham: Duke University Press.

Aptekar, L. (2003). Cultural problems for Western counselors working with Ethiopian refugees. In F. Bemak, R. Chung, & P. Pedersen (Eds.), *Counseling refugees: A psychosocial approach to innovative multi-cultural innovations* (pp. 208–225). Westport: Greenwood Press.

Aptekar, L., & Ciano, L. (1999). Street children in Nairobi, Kenya: Gender differences and mental health. In M. Raffaelli & R. Larson (Eds.), *Homeless and working youth around the world: Exploring developmental issues: New directions for child and adolescent development*, Number 85 (pp. 35–46). San Francisco: Jossey Bass.

Awan, L. (2008). *Occupational safety and health hazards of brick kiln workers.* Lahore: Centre for the Improvement of Working Conditions & Environment.

Boothby, N., Balstera, R., Goldmanc, P., Wessells, M., Zeanahe, M., Huebnera, G., et al. (2012). Coordinated and evidence-based policy and practice for protecting children outside of family care. *Child Abuse and Neglect, 26*, 743–751.

Celik, S., & Baybuga, M. (2009). Verbal, physical and sexual among children working on the street. *Australian Journal of Advanced Nursing, 26*(4), 14–22.

Conticini, A. (2008). Surfing in the air: A grounded theory of the dynamics of street life and its policy implications. *Journal of International Development, 20*, 413–436.

Dybicz, P. (2005). Interventions for street children: An analysis of current best practices. *International Social Work, 48*(6), 1–9.

Ennew, J. (1994). *Street and working children – A guide to planning. Developmental Manual #4.* London: Save the Children.

Klees, S., Rizzini, I., & Dewees, A. (2000). A new paradigm for social change: Social movements and the transformation of policy for street and working children in Brazil. In R. Mickelson (Ed.), *Children on the streets of the Americas* (pp. 79–98). New York: Routledge.

Liebel, M. (1997). Children want to work. *NATs: Working Children and Adolescents International Review, 3*(3–4), 79–81.

Mathur, Me., Rathore, P., & Mathur, Mo. (2009). Incidence, type and intensity of abuse in street children in India". In: *Child Abuse and Neglect, 33*(12), 907–913.

OHCHR. (2012). *Report of the United Nations High Commissioner for Human Rights on the protection and promotion of the rights of children working and/or living on the street.* Human Rights Council, Nineteenth session, agenda items 2 and 3. http://daccess-ds-ny.un.org/doc/UNDOC/GEN/G12/100/74/PDF/G1210074.pdf?OpenElement. Accessed 7 May 2013.

Panter-Brick, C. (2002). Street children, human rights, and public health: a critique and future directions. *Annual Review of Anthropology, 31*, 147–171.

Pinzon-Rondon, A. M. (2010). Workplace abuse and economic exploitation of children working in the streets of Latin America. *International Journal of Occupational and Environmental Health, 16*, 162–169.

Rizzini, I. (1992). *Childhood and urban poverty in Brazil: Street and working children and their families* (Urban Child Series, No. 3). Florence: Innocenti Occasional Papers.
Swart, J. (1989). Community and self-perceptions of the black South African street child. In *Street children in the third world: A symposium on theory and practice* (pp. 49–57). Amsterdam: Caritas Neerlandica.
Swart, J. (1990). *Malunde: The street children of Hillbrow*. Witwatersrand: Johannesburg.
Tronchet-Pradhan, C. (2011). *Participation in the child and youth clubs of Nepal and experience of non-discrimination and equality rights. A field testing with the kaleidoscope of experience*. Thesis for the Master of Advanced Studies in Children's Rights. Sion: IUKB.
UNDRC. (1959). *UN Declaration on the Rights of the Child: Proclaimed by General Assembly Resolution 1386(XIV) 20 Nov 1959.*
Veale, A. (1996). *An empirical and conceptual analysis of street children in Sudan and Ethiopia*. Ph.D. dissertation, University College Cork.
Veale, A., Aderfrsew, A., & Lalor, K. (1993). *A study of street children in four regional towns in Ethiopia* (Report for UNICEF in conjunction with the Ministry for Labor and Social Affairs, Ethiopia). Cork: University College Cork.

Index

L. Aptekar and D. Stoecklin, *Street Children and Homeless Youth: A Cross-Cultural Perspective*, DOI 10.1007/978-94-007-7356-1,

MIX
Papier aus verantwortungsvollen Quellen
Paper from responsible sources
FSC® C105338

If you have any concerns about our products,
you can contact us on
ProductSafety@springernature.com

In case Publisher is established outside the EU,
the EU authorized representative is:
Springer Nature Customer Service Center GmbH
Europaplatz 3, 69115 Heidelberg, Germany

Printed by Libri Plureos GmbH
in Hamburg, Germany